# PEDIATRIC PHYSICAL DIAGNOSIS

**Balu H.Athreya M.D.**
Emeritus Professor of Pediatrics
Thomas Jefferson University – Jefferson Medical College
And
University of Pennsylvania, School of Medicine,
Philadelphia, PA, USA
And
Teaching Consultant
A I Dupont Hospital for Children
Wilmington, DE, USA.


With a Section on the Newborn
By
**Stephen A. Pearlman, MD**
Fellowship Director, Division of Neonatology,
Thomas Jefferson University – Jefferson Medical College
Philadelphia, PA, USA
And
Associate Director, Division of Neonatology,
Christiana Care, Wilmington, DE, USA

Anshan

**PEDIATRIC PHYSICAL DIAGNOSIS 2E**

By Balu H Athreya MD
Stephen A Pearlman MD
Foreword by Basil J Zitelli MD

Published in the UK by:-
Anshan Ltd
11a Little Mount Sion
Tunbridge Wells
Kent. TN1 1YS

Tel: +44 (0) 1892 557767
Fax: +44 (0) 1892 530358

e-mail: info@anshan.co.uk
web site: www.anshan.co.uk

© 2010 Anshan Ltd

ISBN: 978 1 848290 14 3

British Library Cataloguing in Publication Data
A catalogue record for this book is available from the British Library.

Copy Editor: Andrew White
Cover Design: Terry Griffiths
Cover Image: Science Photo Library
Typeset by: Graham Rich
Printed and bound in India by Replika Press Pvt. Ltd.

**Dedicated**

To all children, all over the world

To their innocence, curiosity, humor, and trust.

and

To the mother of three children I know best,

RAMAA

# CONTENTS

# PREFACE

Welcome to this new edition. There are two unique features to this book.

The first is a novel approach to recognition and description of physical findings. There are two parts to it. The first is definition of normality for each organ system and its components. The second is the logical definition of abnormal physical findings based on the components of normality. This is different from the traditional description of physical findings on the basis of inspection, palpation, percussion, and auscultation.

The second unique feature is the inclusion of evidence-based data for physical findings wherever such information is available. I have included data on the precision and accuracy of some of the physical findings under the heading "Evidence Based Data." These should be interpreted with caution since these come from clinical examinations of hospitalized adults performed by specialists and not strictly applicable to children of various ages and developmental stages.

The book is intended to encourage newcomers (medical students and house officers) and to refresh veterans in the skills of pediatric physical diagnosis. This revised new edition incorporates ideas received from the readers and reviewers of the earlier editions.

Good clinicians have always been aware of the need for careful observation, definitions of abnormalities and a logical approach in interpretation. In to-day's high-tech atmosphere and assembly-line approach to office visits, they are difficult to practice. For example, we all know that a precise description of a swelling, when we see one, will help in formulating an initial hypothesis. But we do not use this logical approach consistently. This book emphasizes the almost - forgotten fundamentals of physical diagnosis.

I was fortunate to observe and learn from great clinicians such as Drs. S. T. Achar, S. M. Merchant, K.V.Thiruvengadam, D. Buchanan, F. H. Wright, D. Cassels, and S. Tucker. Dr. Lewis. L. Coriell taught me how to think critically. My brother, Professor N. H. Athreya, taught me how to think creatively and sowed the seed for this book. He showed me the difference between mere competence and sheer excellence. Dr. H. S. Cecil showed me how to care for human beings.

I have always enjoyed my time with students and trainees. They asked some of the toughest questions and stimulated me with their enthusiasm. They charged my "battery" all the time.

Nothing gets done by one individual. Several people have been involved with this book since its inception in the 1970's. I owe them immense gratitude. Let me start with thanking Doctor Benjamin Silverman who helped me with the previous edition. I have left several of his editorial marks untouched.

A special note of thanks is due to Stephen Pearlman M.D. for re-writing the section on the examination of the newborn. In this era of high-technology care of the newborns and premature babies, he has taken a sound clinical focus. An additional note of thanks is due to Dr. S. Tucker for his review of the chapter on the central nervous system.

Several of my colleagues helped me with editing and checking for accuracy of specific chapters.

Dr. Rhonda Walter (A I Dupont Hospital for Children) helped review the Chapter on Behavioral and Developmental Assessment. Dr. Cindy Christian of the Children's Hospital of Philadelphia reviewed the section on Child Abuse.

Several readers from all over the world have written to me with comments and suggestions. I thank them all. I give special thanks particularly to two pediatricians who pointed out some errors and added some good ideas. They are Doctor Johnny Vincent and Doctor Sohrab Tomaraei.

Obtaining good clinical photographs with proper permission was a challenging task. Dr.Maureen Leffler offered her son Max as the subject for normal findings. Both the child and mother were gracious enough to spend an afternoon in our Photography department. Our award-winning photographer Ms. Cindy Broadway made sure the time spent was worth it.

Dr. Sharon Lehman of the A I Dupont Hospital for Children provided clinical photographs of eye diseases. Dr. Lawrence Eichenfield of the Children's Hospital of San Diego provided clinical photographs of the skin diseases. Dr. Suken Shah of the A I Dupont Hospital for Children provided clinical photographs of the child with scoliosis. I thank all of them for their time and generosity.

Kim Eissman is known for her quiet efficiency. Her help in getting the manuscript on time is greatly appreciated. Karen Ott is a fine medical illustrator and an artist. She has redrawn many of the line diagrams.

I am honored that Prof. Basil Zitelli was kind enough to write a Foreword for this book. It is amazing how the busiest people are the ones who get things done on time. I thank Prof. Zitelli for completing this task ahead of time and also for his helpful comments and suggestions.

Finally, I thank Mr. Andrew White for his interest and patience during the preparation of this manuscript.

I hope you find this book useful. Suggestions from the readers were extremely helpful in my revisions. I hope you will continue to share this book with your students and share your ideas for improvement with me.

Balu H. Athreya, M.D.

# FOREWORD

History and physical examination remain the foundation of the clinical evaluation of our patients. Study after study document the importance of these diagnostic skills. Yet, increasingly the skills of a careful history and detailed physical examination are being lost as physicians rely more heavily on technology to attempt to make a diagnosis. This book by Dr. Balu Athreya, a consummate clinician, refocuses the evaluation of the patient back to the basics. Dr. Athreya, through his years of careful listening to patients and families and his meticulous examination techniques, creates a new method for approaching the patient.

Dr. Athreya emphasizes that history taking is an art. The physician should not only focus on content of the history, but also the process itself, using the exercise to develop a relationship with patient and family, gathering information not only from verbal communication but also from subtle nonverbal clues. Careful listening is not passive. It requires patience and practice. The new method of physical examination uses an objective method for observation based on anatomical and physiological components of normality for each organ system. The examiner starts from normality, and if the organ system is not normal, then Dr. Athreya asks the physician to describe components that anatomically and pathophysiologically deviate from normal. The physician must know, define and be able to describe normality. When confronted with abnormality, students and physicians should ask, "What is it?" to define the problem; "What is it not?" to exclude disorders; and "How do you know?" to confirm the diagnosis. In the scientific method, the observer gathers data, develops a hypothesis, then tests the hypothesis through appropriate testing.

Abundant use of tables, figures and mnemonics guides the clinician through elements of the history and physical examination. In addition to the three general precepts to define, exclude and confirm, each chapter devoted to an organ system also includes evaluation utilizing William Osler's four dictums of examination, i.e., inspection, palpation, percussion and auscultation. Descriptions of normal and abnormal findings are noted, often with proper examination techniques, explanations and important questions to ask.

This book revitalizes the importance of the history and physical examination as the foundation of clinical evaluation. It provides invaluable hints, aids and guidelines for effective physical diagnosis. Clinicians who value these basic skills should not be without it.

Basil J. Zitelli, M.D.
Edmund R. McCluskey Professor of Pediatric Medical Education
University of Pittsburgh School of Medicine
Chief, The Paul C. Gaffney Diagnostic Referral Service
Children's Hospital of Pittsburgh of UPMC
3705 Fifth Avenue, 4B 480 DeSoto Wing, Pittsburgh, PA 15213-2583
Tel: 412/692-5135 Fax: 412/692-7038

# SECTION I

# CONCEPT OF NORMALITY

# Chapter 1

# DESCRIBING NORMALITY

Diagnosing a disease requires an ability to recognize abnormalities in the structure and/or function of various organ systems of the body. To recognize an abnormality one needs to know normality. How is one to recognize normality during physical examination?

A good history and a thorough physical examination help recognize abnormalities in the organ systems. Time spent on these fundamentals helps develop a relationship with patients and facilitates future communication. A thorough physical examination, in addition, is an essential part of reassurance therapy, particularly for patients with functional ailments.

Books on physical diagnosis generally follow the tradition of objective descriptions of physical findings based on the subjective faculties of the examiner, namely inspection, palpation, percussion, and auscultation. I take a different approach in this book, and suggest an objective method for observing, based on the logical anatomical and physiological components of normality for each organ system.

The traditional approach of descriptions of physical findings under inspection, palpation, percussion, and auscultation is subjective and is based on the faculties of the examiner (sight and hearing). For this reason, one student's inspection is likely to be more or less complete and revealing than another's inspection. What a medical student needs instead is a framework within which to inspect any particular organ.

In this book, I propose a different approach in which the normal characteristics of the anatomical structure and the physiologic function of the organ are defined, and the examiner is asked to use whichever subjective modality is appropriate to assess that feature. A combination of the use of subjective modality of the physician and the objective features of normality should make physical examination more accurate.

For example, while describing the examination of the head, first describe the normal dimensions and characteristics of the head. This should include a description of its size, shape, and continuity. These can again be logically divided into subheadings. For example, the size of the head can be normal or abnormal; if abnormal, it has to be larger or smaller (than normal). The shape has to be even and symmetrical or uneven and asymmetrical. If it is asymmetric, it may be longer (from front to back), broader (side to side), or conical (vertical). Continuity can be described as intact, and a loss of continuity as a projection on the surface (dermoid) or a depression below the surface (depressed fracture).

Of the components of the normal head listed above, shape is available for inspection. Size is assessed using inspection and measurement. Continuity is available for inspection and palpation.

Thus, once the normal characteristics of an organ are defined, the physician can use an appropriate subjective modality (such as inspection, palpation, or auscultation) to define them. This description of the normal anatomic and physiologic components of any organ makes it easy to teach medical students what they should be looking for. In addition, a constant reminder of the normal characteristics of an organ and its functions will make it easier for the learner to recognize an abnormality.

# DEFINING NORMALITY: WHAT IS NORMAL?

Many of us intuitively know what normality is for a particular part of the body, but cannot describe it. A medical student can recognize the face of a child with trisomy 21 (Down) syndrome, but cannot describe the variations of the facial structures that generated the gestalt. To teach abnormal physical findings, we must be able to understand and communicate a description of normality.

Students and trainees seem to be more aware of normality of physiological functions than of normal anatomic characteristics. This may reflect in part the emphasis on the physiologic basis of disease in modern medicine. In pediatrics, there is an additional problem of age-dependent variations in physical, behavioral, intellectual, emotional, physiologic, and biochemical characteristics.

The clinician interprets laboratory abnormalities on the basis of normal values. Unless the clinician knows that the normal value for blood urea nitrogen is 8 to 18 mgm%, recognition of an abnormal value is impossible. Similarly, one cannot recognize an abnormality of the ear, the eye, or the gum unless one knows the characteristics of the normal structure of these parts of the body. For example, knowing that the ear makes an angle of 10 degrees or less with the scalp will help identify a protuberant ear. Knowing that all the metacarpophalangeal joints should be in an almost straight line when the hand is fisted should help identify a short fourth metacarpal.

A qualitative observation is not adequate by itself. Being a good clinician requires a sense of pattern recognition. Pattern recognition demands formation of mental images of normal features of various parts and organs of the body, so that if a pattern with minor variation appears, it is quickly recognized. This has to be confirmed, whenever possible, with actual measurement using available normative data. Murray Feingold made the following comments in a 1983 editorial: "It is no longer acceptable to describe dysmorphic physical findings without using proper measurements. Claims, such as low-set ears, wide-spaced eyes and long fingers, should not be made unless they are accompanied by accurate measurements. Incorrect clinical impressions, because of lack of measurements, have been responsible for persistent misinformation about specific syndromes. For example, many clinicians are still under the false impression that children with Turner's syndrome have widespread nipples and an increased carrying angle. Studies using proper measurements have shown that these observations are not correct." He also said, "The only measurements that should be used are those that have a significant number of normal controls."

These comments introduce the importance of knowing what is normal. They also emphasize the importance of observation and measurement. One has to apply this knowledge at every opportunity. To systematize our observations of normal structures and functions, the variables have to be defined under the following headings:

- Anatomic Variations
- Physiologic Variations

# DESCRIBING ANATOMIC STRUCTURES

The following variables must be considered in describing an anatomic structure: size, number, shape, position in relation to itself, position in relation to other structures, color, texture, continuity, and alignment.

Let us take the eye as an example and define the descriptors. The eye can be small or large (size). The very rare cyclops is recognized by answering the question on number. Hypotelorism and hypertelorism are recognized as alterations in position in relation to the other eye. Proptosis and enophthalmos are recognized as alterations in position in relation to the eye itself (forward and backward). Any color change in and around the eye is the next descriptor. Texture of the eye may be firm as in glaucoma or soft as in phthisis bulbi. The item on continuity is not applicable, but the alignment of the eye on the face in relation to other structures defines conditions such as slant. Recognition of abnormality in the structural components of the eye according to the descriptors given above is more useful and practical than remembering words such as microphthalmia, macrophthalmia, cyclops, hypotelorism, hypertelorism, proptosis, exophthalmos, and phthisis bulbi. *Instead of trying to remember Latin and Greek names, try to remember the anatomic basis of variations.*

An anatomic description of normality (**Table 1-1**) as described above gives a logical basis for describing abnormality. This is applicable to all anatomic structures and can be taught easily. For example, a normal finger can be described as follows:

*Size:* Small or large in relation to the hand and to other fingers.

*Number*: Extra fingers or fewer than five fingers? If fewer than five, is it because fingers are fused (as in Apert syndrome) or lost because of an accident?

*Shape*: Does the finger look fusiform or tapered?

*Position:* Is one finger placed more proximally or distally than others?

*Color*: Are the fingers blue, red, pale, or mottled?

*Texture*: Is the finger stiff? Is the skin soft, coarse, or peeling?

*Continuity*: Is there any disruption of continuity (e.g., fracture of phalanx)? Is there a rash or a nodule? Is there any other swelling?

*Alignment*: Is the finger straight or curved? Is it curved in a front-back direction (flexion contracture) or in a side-to-side direction (clinodactyly)? Are the fingers aligned normally in relation to the forearm and wrist (ulnar deviation-radial deviation-volar subluxation)?

An explanation is needed about continuity and alignment. As indicated in **Table 1-1**, extra growth as a descriptor is used under "continuity" to define the characteristics of rash, swellings, and other projections. Every extra growth has to be described under subheadings such as location, size, margin, shape, or surface. Continuity also is used to describe the skin and mucous membrane because ulcers signify loss of surface continuity. Displaced fractures are to be described under this heading as well. Alignment as a subheading is included to describe deformity of extremities but can be applied to other organs, as shown earlier in describing the normal eye.

# DESCRIBING PHYSIOLOGIC FUNCTION

Alteration in physiologic functions can be explained in a logical fashion using the characteristics listed in **Table 1-2**. For example, a function such as movement of an extremity may be present, lost, or only partially present. Complete loss of ability to move an extremity is called "paralysis" and a partial loss is called "paresis." Instead of focusing on the meanings of words (paralysis and paresis), the learner can focus on the logical possibilities and their precise descriptions.

To explain this example further, a function may be present, but painful or difficult. For example, passing of urine may be painful (as in dysuria) or difficult (as seen after surgery). Finally, function may be present but abnormal in frequency, intensity, or rhythm. For example, a patient may have normal micturition, but it may occur too often or too infrequently; the stream may be poor with dribbling, and there may be hesitation.

**Table 1-1. Possible Alterations in Anatomic Structures**

| Descriptor | Variables |
|---|---|
| Size – Normal, Large or small in relation to itself | |
| | Large or small in relation to other structures |
| | Abnormal rate of growth in size |
| Number – Normal | Fewer (absent or fused) |
| | More (extra or split) |
| Shape – Normal/uniform | Irregular (describe) |
| | Concave or convex |
| Position    – right/left | In relation to other structures: far off, elevated, depressed, |
|    – anterior/posterior | moved in, moved out, rotated |
|    – superior/inferior | In relation to itself: forward, backward, inward, outward, |
| | and combinations |
| Color – Normal | Less or more of normal color |
| | Abnormal color – blue, red, yellow, dark, etc. |
| Texture/consistency – Normal | Soft, firm, hard |
| Alignment – Normal | Abnormal in relation to itself |
| | Abnormal in relation to other structures |
| Continuity – Normal | Loss of continuity – such as fractures, ulcers |
| | Extra growth – not normally present includes skin rash, |
| | and swellings (see below) |

Extra growths should be described under: location, size, shape, rate of growth, flat or elevated, margins regular or irregular, surface smooth or rough, consistency soft, firm or hard, color as listed above, temperature (warm, hot, or cold), tenderness, pulsations, and attachment to skin and surrounding structures.

A function such as the rate of breathing or the heart rate may be less than normal or more than normal, just as volume of urine per day may be more than or less than normal. The depth of respiration may be shallow (decreased) or deep (increased). One may have a combination of these characteristics.

When describing functions with a rhythm (respiration, heart rate, etc.) look for regularity or irregularity. If irregular, one has to know whether it is regularly irregular or irregularly irregular.

When describing sounds heard with or without a stethoscope, describe whether the sounds are present or absent; if present, whether they are normal or abnormal, and if abnormal, whether it is the pitch, intensity, or frequency that is abnormal.

## Table 1-2. Possible Alterations in Physiologic Functions

Present

Loss of

Partial loss of

Function present—painful

Function present—difficult

(All symptoms due to difficulty in functions like dysphagia, dypnea, etc.)

Function present—abnormal

(applicable to rate, volume, size, depth)

Reduced  (slow)     (short)     (less)       (small)

Increased (fast)      (excess)   (large)

Combination of slow and fast rhythm

Irregular:  regularly irregular

           irregularly irregular

Sounds:   normal sound

       absent sound

       abnormal sounds and murmur

| Voluntary movements: | contraction | smooth |
| --- | --- | --- |
| | relaxation | irregular |

| Involuntary movements: | At rest— twitch |
| --- | --- |
| | tremor |
| | writhing |
| | fasciculation |
| | convulsions |

| Abnormal sensations (specific types): | Pain—intensity, characteristics, aggravating factors, relieving factors, frequency, spread, etc. |
| --- | --- |
| | Dizziness |
| | Vertigo |
| | Parasthesias |

Voluntary and involuntary movements may be described under various subheadings. Involuntary movements that present spontaneously are described, not those elicited by special stimuli such as muscle stretch reflexes. This classification does not lend itself to describing elicited responses.

The final heading in **Table 1-2** describes abnormal sensations such as pain or paresthesias.

Additional examples of descriptions of abnormality defining the anatomic or physiologic characteristics and their variations are given in **Table 1-3**.

**Table 1-3. Examples of Logical Description of Symptoms and Signs by Defining Characteristics**

| Traditional Term | Structure/Function | Alteration(s) |
| --- | --- | --- |
| Dyspnea | Respiration | Difficult |
| Hyperpnea | Respiration | Rate—fast |
| | | Depth—increased |
| Tachypnea | Respiration | Rate—increased |
| Diarrhea | Bowel movement | Rate—increased |
| | Bowel movement | Consistency—decreased |
| | Bowel movement | Volume—increased |
| Polyuria | Urine | Volume—increased |
| Melena | Bowel movement | Color—black |
| Hematochezia | Bowel movement | Color—red (bloody) |
| Hypertelorism | Eyes | Position—far off (in relation to each other) |
| Proptosis | Eyes | Position—forward (in relation to itself) |
| Ulcer | Skin | Continuity—loss of |
| Jaundice | Skin | Color—yellow |
| Papule | Skin | Extra growth—elevated—smooth |
| Purpura | Skin | Extra growth—flat—red (blood) |

# BIBLIOGRAPHY

Feingold M. Proper measurements in physical diagnosis. Am J Dis Child. 1983;137:828.

Feinstein AR. Clinical Judgment. Baltimore: Williams & Wilkins; 1967.

Murphy EA. The Logic of Medicine. Baltimore: The Johns Hopkins University Press; 1976.

Chapter 2

# GENERAL ASPECTS OF HISTORY TAKING AND INTERVIEWING

## GENERAL CONCEPTS

A detailed history of the presenting symptoms is the best lead to a proper diagnosis. In addition, a thorough and detailed history of the child's development, family history, social and economic conditions of the family, level of understanding of the parents, cultural background, support systems, and the strengths and weaknesses is necessary to formulate a management plan.

History-taking is an art. Skills in interviewing techniques, history-taking, and empathic communication can be learned by observing expert clinicians at work, by reading available literature, and by PRACTICE. Ideally these skills should be learned from working with good clinicians in action. Newer methods of learning such as simulation exercises and interactive modules are next best to learning from role models. Before going into the details of history- taking, some general remarks about useful concepts will be given.

Physicians gather and give information routinely in their daily practice. Together these become part of communication skills. Information gathering has traditionally been called history- taking. Until recently, the emphasis in history-taking has been on the content. Now, there is much needed emphasis on the process of obtaining the information required by the physician to make a diagnosis and plan management.

The content in history-taking has three components: biomedical or disease perspective, the patient's or illness perspective, and the psychosocial or the context perspective (**Table 2-1**). The physician is expected to gather information on all three components although the depth and details will vary depending on the setting. For example, in the emergency room, the focus has to be on the most urgent issue. In an office visit, the history has to be more thorough.

Unless the clinician has developed good communication skills, he or she cannot obtain adequate details of the content. He or she certainly will not be able to present his or her diagnostic and management recommendations effectively to the patient. Therefore, the process and style of gathering and giving information are as important as the content to be discovered.

There is increasing emphasis on teaching information gathering and information giving techniques to medical students as part of effective communication skills. Several models have been proposed and tried. The Calgary-Cambridge guide is one such model that defines the components of effective physician-patient communication skills and also provides a structure to teach these skills. (The complete guide is available on the internet at www.skillscascade.com).

Initially, this guide focused on the process of the medical interview. More recently, the authors of this guide have combined and enhanced the content and the process, and have provided a framework for a comprehensive clinical method (**Figure 2-1**). The figure presents the entire concept visually and emphasizes that even as the physician is gathering data on the content, he or she is developing a relationship with the patient. It emphasizes the interrelationship between the content and the process during the medical interview. Some of the skills required of a physician during this encounter are listed in **Table 2-2**.

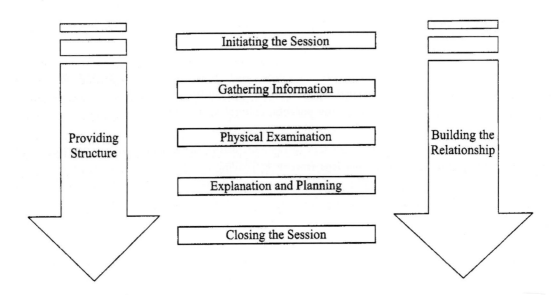

**Figure 2-1.** Objectives to be achieved during medical interview. (Modified from Kurtz S, Silverman J, Benson J, Draper J. Marrying content and process in clinical method teaching: Enhancing the Calgary-Cambridge guide. Acad Med 2003; 78(8):802-9. With permission from Wolters Kluwer Health)

### Table 2-1. Gathering Information: Content to be Discovered

| The biomedical perspective (disease) | The patient's perspective (illness) | Background information—context |
| --- | --- | --- |
| Sequence of events | Ideas and beliefs | Past medical history |
| Symptom analysis | Concerns | Drug and allergy history |
| Relevant systems review | Expectations | Family history |
| | Effects on life | Personal and social history |
| | Feelings | Review of systems |

*Modified from: Kurtz S, Silverman J, Benson J, Draper J. Marrying content and process in clinical method teaching: enhancing the Calgary-Cambridge guide. Acad Med. 2003;78(8):802-9. (With permission from Wolters Kluwer)*

The emphasis in this chapter is on the content. But the process is extremely important. It is important to look for non-verbal cues from patients and also use appropriate non-verbal approaches (such as use of voice, facial expression) to make the patient feel welcome and relaxed. Acknowledging the patient's problems with compassion and without judgment, and expressing concern and willingness to help will enhance rapport with the patient.

Make sure to introduce yourself to the child and to the parents and explain your role. Find out the proper way to pronounce the name and address the patient. Let the patient know that you are interested in what he or she has to say. The opening questions should concentrate on the chief complaint and primary problems the patient and the parent(s) want to address. The next step would be to explain what to expect during that visit and set an agenda (**Tables 2-3 and 2-4**).

One of our professors once said, "Go after the symptoms like a hound dog." Clinicians should go after the scent, dashing out occasionally, but getting back on the trail without getting lost. Failure to keep on track is responsible for many errors in diagnosis and unnecessary laboratory procedures. Take for example, a patient who is seen primarily for constipation, but who on review of systems, gives a history of his hands getting blue on exposure to cold. The clinician has to dart off the track and ask leading questions to establish whether or not the patient may have Raynaud's phenomenon. However, the clinician should decide how this symptom fits into the whole picture and how serious this symptom is before starting elaborate investigations.

Present day patients often give the name of a disease-designation (a diagnosis) when asked about their primary complaint. Instead, ask the parents/child about the original symptoms and signs that led to that diagnostic conclusion. It is important to do so even if another physician has given that diagnostic label. It is a good clinical habit to verify the accuracy of the diagnosis. Keep an open mind and follow the scent, detective style.

## Table 2-2. Gathering Information: Process Skills for Exploration of the Patient's Problems

Patient's narrative

Question style: open to closed cone

Attentive listening

Facilitative response

Picking up cues

Clarification

Time-framing

Internal summary

Appropriate use of language    Additional skills for understanding the patient's perspective

*Modified from: Kurtz S, Silverman J, Benson J, Draper J. Marrying content and process in clinical method teaching: enhancing the Calgary-Cambridge guide. Acad Med. 2003;78(8):802-9. (with permission from Wolters Kluwer)*

For example, if a parent says that her child had arthritis, ask for a history of swelling, pain and tenderness, and limitation of movement of the joint. If there was only joint pain, and there is no documentation of a swelling, the symptom designation should be arthralgia and not arthritis. In children with periodic fever syndromes, the parent often will give a history of the child having been treated with antibiotics for several ear and throat infections. Detailed history and review of old records may show that the child had fever but no well-documented infection.

During a visit for an acute problem in a busy office, make maximal use of your time by focusing on history taking and combining it with the preliminary steps of the physical examination. Establish confidence. Take a relevant history. For example, suppose a six-year-old whom you have followed in your office for well-child care presents with fever. Observe the child's alertness and sensorium and look for rashes and petechiae while you are asking the parent about the fever and associated symptoms, such as pain, coughing, vomiting, and diarrhea. Gently palpate the abdomen, as you continue to question the parent about any other recent illness. Ask if anyone else in the family is sick as you watch the respirations and softly flex the neck; ask about specific sites of pain-sore throat, earache, headache--as you soothingly run your hand over the neck and palpate the cervical nodes. Then you can perform a focused examination.

When evaluating a child with chronic complaints, it is important to ask about the factors that precipitated the visit. This has to be done gently and with proper choice of words. The timing of the visit may reveal precipitating factors, such as stress in the family, anxieties, or a new symptom that the child has never had before. This can in turn lead to questions about the real concerns of the parents. Very often you will find the parental concerns are far removed from the presenting complaint and from those of the physician's concerns (**Table 2-5**).

Another good question to ask parents is, "What do you wish this is not?" Usually, this question provides them with an opening to express their hidden fears and anxieties.

The first contact is the most important contact in human relations. Getting the interview started in a positive way is therefore essential. The techniques will have to vary depending on the setting and the time available. In an emergency room, the focus should be on the most important and urgent problems requiring immediate care. When seeing a child for developmental problems or behavior problems, however, the atmosphere should be relaxed and there should be no time pressure.

In addition to taking the history from the parents, it is important to talk with the children directly using language appropriate to their stage of development. However, early in the interview, it may be better not to approach the child too quickly. One should remember to have periodic communication with the child even though the parents may be talking. The physician also should be able to request the parent's permission to talk to the child separately, if indicated. This is particularly important when examining an adolescent.

It is important to use both open-ended questions and leading questions. To arrive at a medical diagnosis, it is necessary for the physician to lead the way and ask specific questions to clarify the details. Patients do not know the importance of specific details of their symptoms or may have forgotten unless specific questions are asked. This is one reason I disapprove of letting patients talk without interruption and free-associate early in the interview. I prefer to let them free-associate after I have defined the illness. Asking questions to clarify specific details of symptoms are not interruptions and will demonstrate to the patients that the physician is listening to their complaints carefully.

It is important to ask open-ended questions and allow time for the family to respond to questions on developmental and psychosocial issues. Once again, remember to use words that lay persons can understand and do not use words that can be misinterpreted. Also, remember that the way the questions are asked is as important as the questions themselves.

Listen carefully to the answers that are given and also to the way they are given. Be alert to the body language of the patient and parent but without over-interpretation. If a parent does not look in your eyes directly, it may mean evasion. On the other hand, this is an appropriate behavior in certain cultures. You should be alert to remarks made in passing for clues and follow through with leading questions. For example, if the child says "not now," ask about the last time the symptom was present.

Physicians ask the right questions always, but often hurry in listening. Constant interruptions with phone calls and paging systems will leave the parents wondering whether their history is being listened to. You can show the parents that you are listening by using various techniques: turning your pager off, looking at their faces if appropriate, asking questions that clarify the statements they make, and periodically summarizing what they said. This in turn will help them provide a better history. Other good listening habits are listed in **Table 2-6**.

When talking with the child, begin with easy subjects and use words the child can understand. Talk about the child's name and those of brothers and sisters, and about the family pets. It is good to find out where the child hurts so you can avoid touching that area until the latter part of the physical examination. The child's speech, affect, and position during these talks will give many clues to diagnosis. Ask the child to draw a picture of a person or anything else. Though one should be cautious about over-interpretation, children's drawings can give clues to their mental age and to the presence of problems in visual-motor integration. Also, when the child picks up a crayon or a pencil, some clinical clues may be available such as handedness and any abnormal patterns of holding the pencil suggestive of cerebral palsy or chorea. Handwriting itself may give clinical clues (the unsteadiness of chorea, reversing of letters, mirror-image writing).

## Table 2-3. Essential Elements of Communication in Medical Encounters— The Kalamazoo Consensus Statement

Build a relationship: strong, therapeutic, trusting relationship.

Open the discussion: elicit the patient's full set of concerns.

Gather information: listen actively; structure, clarify, and summarize; use open ended and closed ended questions, as appropriate.

Understand the patient's perspective.

Share information: use language patient can understand; check understanding.

Reach agreement: on problems to be addressed and plans.

Provide closure: ask for additional concerns, summarize, discuss follow-up plans.

*From: Makoul G. Essential elements of communication in medical encounters: the Kalamazoo consensus statement. Acad Med. 2001; 76(4):390-3. (with permission from Wolters Kluwer)*

Asking children about their wishes, if it were possible to get those wishes, will reveal their concerns and priorities, though this may not be related to their primary complaints. Asking about good and bad dreams, with reassurance that dreams do not come true, will help determine the child's level of anxiety and fears. Another very interesting question I have found useful to ask is, "What does Mommy say to you often?"

Some of the known pitfalls in interviewing and history taking are: lack of a systematic process, taking superficial history, not obtaining precise details of presenting symptoms, not clarifying vague symptoms and sequence of symptoms, accepting prior diagnosis without questioning, not following up on verbal and non-verbal clues, not asking specific questions to jog the memory of parents and children, allowing parents to wander without any control or too much control, lack of sensitivity, and use of technical language. Not providing adequate time and a place with adequate privacy are other major impediments.

# DETERMINING THE CHIEF COMPLAINT

Inquiry into the reason for the current visit starts with eliciting the chief complaint. Some parents will give a "diagnosis" instead of the complaints. It is necessary to ask what the actual symptoms and signs were that led to that particular diagnostic categorization. Accepting the diagnosis as given by the family may lead to a closed mind on the part of the physician and consequently to blind alleys, wrong diagnosis, and missed diagnosis.

### Table 2-4. Setting the Agenda for the Visit

**What are the patient's main concerns?**
- "What brings you to us today? Why this time as opposed to earlier or later (other than available appointment time)? What else do you want to take care of today?"
- "What concerns have you written down on your list?"
- "What is the one thing you want to make sure we address today?"

**What are my concerns for today? (These may be different from those of the patient, at least in priority)**
- What do I have to be sure of checking or discuss today?
- What are the issues most important to the patient?
- Go over my list with the patient.
- What items have to be addressed today and what can we postpone for future visits?

**How can we realign our priorities in terms of importance and discuss options?**

*Source: Baker LH, O'Connell D, Plat FW. "What else?" Setting the agenda for the clinical interview. Ann Int Med. 2005:143(10):766-80.*

Make note of the characteristics of the persons giving the history such as their ability to communicate properly (particularly if they are not able to speak the local language), their affect, and apparent reliability. Recognize that the stated reason for the visit may not be the same as the hidden reasons for the visit (**Table 2-5**).

Next, establish the *duration* and characteristics of onset of the chief complaint. A symptom that comes on very suddenly will be remembered clearly. The parent and the child may know exactly what they were doing and at what time of the day this symptom was noticed (e.g., headache of subarachnoid hemorrhage). This may not be true for symptoms of gradual onset. The next question should be about the intensity of the symptoms. For example, if a child has pain, find out how severe the pain is. Questions about the behavior of the child when the pain is experienced, and about interference with activity and sleep, will help to define the intensity. Question the periodicity and frequency of the symptoms. Recurrent bouts of fever once a month have a different connotation from daily fevers experienced for six to eight weeks. Find out what factors aggravate the main symptom and what factors relieve the symptom. An abdominal pain made worse by squeezing the abdomen is likely to be inflammatory in nature, whereas an abdominal pain relieved by holding the abdomen is probably due to colic. Note whether the illness has been getting worse or better (general trend or trajectory). Also know about other symptoms that have been added on to this chief complaint. If there are any, the description of those symptoms at onset, their course, chronology, and intensity should be obtained. On occasion, the child may have had a number of symptoms that were not of concern initially, but the appearance of a dramatic new symptom brought the child to medical attention. Details of these associated symptoms that brought the child to this visit should be obtained.

Find out where the child and the family were getting their medical care prior to this visit and what the reasons are for the change. Recent relocation, a need for specialty care, and cost are understandable reasons. A history of repeated dissatisfaction and changes of physicians should alert to potential problems in relationships. Always quiz gently, but carefully and firmly. If aspects of the history seem incongruous, try to verify the history. Be aware of the possibility of the pediatric version of the "Munchausen syndrome," particularly with a family that has been "doctor-shopping."

**Table 2-5. Actual Reason for Seeking Medical Attention**

---

1. Family history of serious, life-threatening illness
2. Fear of loss of vital functions of organs
3. Fear of death    Pressure from another family member for an answer
4. Feeling of inadequacy being a "good" parent and guilt
5. Media focus on a specific illness

---

*Source: Bass LW, Cohen RL. Ostensible versus actual reasons for seeking pediatric attention: another look at the parental ticket of admission. Pediatrics. 1982; 70(6):870-4.*

# SPECIFIC ASPECTS OF HISTORY TAKING

## Pregnancy and Delivery

What para? What gravida? (These questions relate to genetic and chromosome diseases and Rh incompatibility.) What was the mother's age at the time of the birth of this child? (Age is significant if the mother was an adolescent or over 40 years of age.) Did the mother have any illness during pregnancy? (There may be a possibility of congenital malformation and congenital infections.) Is there a history of sexually transmitted diseases and HIV infection? What drugs were taken during pregnancy? **Table 2-7** summarizes various diseases associated with maternal drug ingestion. Also ask about over-the-counter drugs and about drug abuse. Was there exposure to x-rays or injurious chemicals? Was there any emotional stress during pregnancy such as divorce, death, or change of location? A question such as "How did you feel when you found out about this pregnancy?" may give clues to family stresses.

Was the pregnancy full term, or premature, or over the full term? Was labor induced? If so, why? Was the delivery normal? Were forceps used? Was the baby delivered by C-section? Was the presentation normal? What was the total duration of labor and delivery (neonatal asphyxia, cerebral palsy)? Did the obstetrician report polyhydramnios (tracheoesophageal fistula) or oligohydramnios (renal agenesis)? Did the baby breathe spontaneously at birth? What was the Apgar score at birth? Was the cord around the neck? Was the baby meconium-stained? (This suggests asphyxia.) Were the cord and placenta reported to be normal in appearance? (This is to look for evidence of infection, postmaturity, abnormality of placental vessels.)

## Neonatal History

How long did the baby stay in the nursery? (If a good neonatal history is not available, prolonged stay in the nursery arouses suspicion of some problem.) Were there any infections? If so, what site? What organism? What antibiotics were used? Did the baby have convulsions? How severe was the jaundice? Did the baby receive blood transfusion? Were there any bleeding problems? Were there breathing problems?

### Table 2-6. Listening Habits of Good Clinicians

Let the patient talk without interruptions

Probe the hints and nonverbal cues

Acknowledge that you are listening

Do not prejudge

Check for accuracy

Know the expectations

Validate patient perspective

Maintain body and eye posture

*Modified from: Appleby C. Getting doctors to listen to patients. Managed Care. 1996; 5(12):28. (With permission from Managed Care Magazine)*

Nutritional Assessment (also see page 41; section on obesity and overweight)

Was the baby breast-fed or bottle-fed? If bottle-fed, what type of formula was used? How good an eater was the baby? When were solids introduced and in what sequence? How easy was it to introduce new food? Was there any food intolerance? What was the pattern of weight gain?

What are the current eating habits? What is the approximate intake of calories, vitamins, and protein? Does the child eat out or eat "junk" food too often? Is there family eating time? Does the child snack often? What kinds of snacks are in the house? Does the child eat fruits and vegetables? How many servings per day? Any allergies and associated food prohibitions?

A detailed dietary history is needed in patients with under-nutrition, overweight, and chronic illness. This will require a diet diary for three to five days.

## Past Medical History

Details of any prior illnesses, hospitalizations, infectious diseases, surgeries, accidents, allergies, and immunizations should be determined.

Most families will not remember details of minor illnesses. One should, however, ask for details of more serious illness, including the nature of the diagnosis, the age of the child at the time of the illness, the treatment given, and any complications that ensued. If the illness was considered serious, get details of the diagnosis, hospitalization, tests performed, treatment given, duration of illness, and complications. If possible, the records should be obtained and reviewed. Often the illness is considered serious, but the child may have been treated at home. The family's perception of the seriousness of the illness may not match the description. After a serious illness, the family may think that the illness is still present even if it has been cured. Also, after recovery from a serious illness, the family may consider that particular child as always vulnerable.

**Table 2-7. Examples of Drugs that, If Taken By the Mother During Pregnancy or Delivery, May Affect the Fetus or Newborn**

| Drug | Effect on | Type of Problem Encountered |
|---|---|---|
| Adrenal cortical steroids | Fetus | Cleft palate |
| Ammonium chloride | Newborn | Acidosis |
| Cyclophosphamide | Fetus | Malformations |
| Immunosuppressives | Fetus | Abortion/Malformations |
| Morphine (or other narcotics) | Newborn | Withdrawal |
| Potassium Iodide | Fetus | Goiter |
| Tetracycline | Newborn | Effects on skeletal growth and on teeth |
| Vitamin K | Newborn | Hyperbilirubinemia |
| Dilantin | Fetus | Cleft palate, lip and other malformations |
| Alcohol | Fetus | Facial abnormalities |
|  |  | Growth retardation |
| Thalidomide | Fetus | Phocomelia |

If any surgery was performed, find out the diagnosis, nature of the procedure done, when it was performed, the hospital in which it was performed, the pathology report, and complications, if any.

A history of accidents such as an automobile accident, sports-related injuries, and ingestions of poisons should be sought. A history of repeated accidents should alert the physician to problems, either in the child or in the family situation. A history of repeated ingestion of poison suggests problems with safety issues at home, social, and family problems. Injuries out of proportion to the accident may indicate a defect in the child, such as osteogenesis imperfecta or a bleeding diathesis, or child abuse (see Chapter 12D).

Obtain a history of allergies to medicines, food, and environmental agents with leading questions. This is one area where over-diagnosis and over-interpretations are common. The descriptions of symptoms considered indicative of allergy, time relationship to the allergen, experience with repeated exposures, response to treatment, and family history are important clues in establishing the accuracy of allergic history.

A history of immunization should include dates for primary immunization, completion of boosters, and the location where they were completed. It is important to review the past records or look at the immunization record the parent may carry.

It is important to talk to an adolescent directly with parental permission and obtain history of alcohol, experiment with over-the-counter drugs and chemicals, smoking or tobacco, sexual habits,

**Table 2-8. Excerpt from Questionnaire***

**Below are listed a number of common problems reported to us by other teenagers. Check yes or no for each, so that we may be in a better position to help you.**

|    |                                         | Yes | No |
|----|-----------------------------------------|-----|-----|
| 1. | Trouble falling asleep                  | ___ | ___ |
| 2. | Awakening during the night              | ___ | ___ |
| 3. | Being very tired during the day         | ___ | ___ |
| 4. | Occasionally wetting the bed            | ___ | ___ |
| 5. | Pain with menstrual periods             | ___ | ___ |
| 6. | Bothered by headaches                   | ___ | ___ |
| 7. | Bothered by stomach aches               | ___ | ___ |
| 8. | Bothered by dizzy spells                | ___ | ___ |
| 9. | Bothered by leg pains                   | ___ | ___ |
| 10. | Worrying about health                  | ___ | ___ |
| 11. | Concerned that I am too short          | ___ | ___ |
| 12. | Concerned that I am too tall           | ___ | ___ |
| 13. | Concerned that I am too thin           | ___ | ___ |
| 14. | Concerned that I am too fat            | ___ | ___ |
| 15. | Concerned that my breasts are too small | ___ | ___ |
| 16. | Concerned that my penis is too small   | ___ | ___ |

contraceptive use, pregnancies (completed or not), and venereal diseases. Answers to a standard questionnaire (**Table 2-8**) by the adolescent during the waiting period may be used as a starting point for discussion (see Chapter 12B).

## Developmental Milestones

Obtain a detailed history of milestones of development at every well-child visit. This is particularly important when evaluating a child with history of developmental delay, behavioral problems, school problems, and learning problems or for adoption. The usual questions are designed to establish the dates at which important milestones in various areas (gross motor, fine motor, language, and personal-social) of development were reached such as smile, vocalization, head control, sitting up unsupported, standing up and walking, and age at which the child attained full control over bladder and bowel for night and day (**Tables 2-9 and 2-10**).

## Behavioral and Emotional History

Behavioral and emotional history should be obtained during every well-child visit and whenever appropriate. Detailed history of developmental, behavioral, emotional, and social issues is particularly important when evaluating children with under-nutrition, recurrent physical symptoms, learning problems, school avoidance, enuresis, encopresis, and childhood behavioral disorders.

Details of history taking and physical assessment of children with developmental and psychosocial issues will be discussed in Chapter 12C, page 333.

|  |  | Yes | No |
|---|---|---|---|
| 17. | Worried that I might become pregnant before I am ready | ____ | ____ |
| 18. | Worried that I might make someone pregnant | ____ | ____ |
| 19. | Worried that I might not be able to get pregnant | ____ | ____ |
| 20. | Not yet ready for sex, but feel pressured | ____ | ____ |
| 21. | Worried about my parents relationship | ____ | ____ |
| 22. | Would you like to change something in your relationship with your parents? | ____ | ____ |
| 23. | Trouble getting to school | ____ | ____ |
| 24. | Worried about school | ____ | ____ |
| 25. | Troubled about future plans | ____ | ____ |
| 26. | Sometimes I'm so sad that I think about dying | ____ | ____ |
| 27. | Have other personal problems that I would like to discuss with the doctor but would rather not write down | ____ | ____ |

*From Stanford University Youth Clinic Medical History Form. From: Felice ME. Chapter 9A. Adolescence. In: Levine MD, Carey WB, Crocker AC, Gross RT, editors. Developmental-Behavioral Pediatrics. Philadelphia: WB Saunders; 1983. p. 141. (Copyright Elsevier 1983)*

## Social and Personal History

This should include history of developmental milestones, behavioral and emotional patterns, interpersonal relationships, habits, living arrangements, school performance, economic situations, strengths, and weaknesses. In obtaining a history of the child's personality characteristics, some sample questions might include: "How does the child compare with other children the same age?" "What are some of the child's strengths?" "What are some weaknesses?" "What are some items that scare the child or cause anxiety?" "How does the child show anger, fear, and anxiety?" "What are the usual

### Table 2-9. Emerging Patterns of Behavior During the 1st Year of Life
### *Neonatal Period (1st 4 Wk)

| | |
|---|---|
| Prone: | Lies in flexed attitude; turns head from side to side; head sags on ventral suspension |
| Supine: | Generally flexed and a little stiff |
| Visual: | May fixate face on light in line of vision; "doll's-eye" movement of eyes on turning of the body |
| Reflex: | Moro response active; stepping and placing reflexes; grasp reflex active |
| Social: | Visual preference for human face |

**At 1 Mo**

| | |
|---|---|
| Prone: | Legs more extended; holds chin up; turns head; head lifted momentarily to plane of body on vertical suspension |
| Supine: | Tonic neck posture predominates; supple and relaxed; head lags when pulled to sitting position |
| Visual: | Watches person; follows moving object |
| Social: | Body movements in cadence with voice of other in social contact; beginning to smile |

**At 2 mo**

| | |
|---|---|
| Prone: | Raises head slightly farther; head sustained in plane of body on ventral suspension |
| Supine: | Tonic neck posture predominates; head lags when pulled to sitting position |
| Visual: | Follows moving object 180 degrees |
| Social: | Smiles on social contact; listens to voice and coos |

**At 3 mo**

| | |
|---|---|
| Prone: | Lifts head and chest with arms extended; head above plane of body on ventral suspension |
| Supine: | Tonic neck posture predominates; reaches toward and misses objects; waves at toy |
| Sitting: | Head lag partially compensated when pulled to sitting position; early head control with bobbing motion; back rounded |
| Reflex: | Typical Moro response has not persisted; makes defensive movements or selective withdrawal reactions |
| Social: | Sustained social contact; listens to music and says "aah, ngah" |

**At 4 mo**

| | |
|---|---|
| Prone: | Lifts head and chest, with head in approximately vertical axis; legs extended |
| Supine: | Symmetric posture predominates, hands in midline; reaches and grasps objects and brings them to mouth |
| Sitting: | No head lag when pulled to sitting position; head steady, tipped forward; enjoys sitting with full truncal support |
| Standing: | When held erect, pushes with feet |

moods?" "What are favorite activities?" "How does this child relate to members of the family and to strangers?" "How does the child behave in a new situation?" "Who is the child's favorite person in the family and why?" "How is the child disciplined, and for what types of behavior?" "How does the child respond to these measures?"

In obtaining a history on personal habits one needs information on:

Feeding: What is the usual eating pattern? Are there any problems with feeding? What kinds of problems? Are there any favorite likes and dislikes? What is the eating pattern of the family?

---

| | |
|---|---|
| Adaptive: | Sees pellet, but makes no move to reach it |
| Social: | Laughs out loud; may show displeasure if social contact is broken; excited at sight of foot |
| **At 7 mo** | |
| Prone: | Rolls over; pivots; crawls or creep-crawls (Knobloch) |
| Supine: | Lifts head; rolls over; squirms |
| Sitting: | Sits briefly, with support of pelvis; leans forward on hands; back rounded |
| Standing: | May support most of weight; bounces actively |
| Adaptive: | Reaches out for and grasps large object; transfers objects from hand to hand; grasp uses radial palm; rakes at pellet |
| Language: | Forms polysyllabic vowel sounds |
| Social: | Prefers mother; babbles; enjoys mirror; responds to changes in emotional content of social contact |
| **At 10 mo** | |
| Sitting: | Sits up alone and indefinitely without support, with back straight |
| Standing: | Pulls to standing position; "cruises" or walks holding on to furniture |
| Motor: | Creeps or crawls |
| Adaptive: | Grasps objects with thumb and forefinger; pokes at things with forefinger; picks up pellet with assisted pincer movement; uncovers hidden toy; attempts to retrieve dropped object; releases object grasped by another person |
| Language: | Repetitive consonant sounds ("mama," "dada") |
| Social: | Responds to sound of name; plays peek-a-boo or pat-a-cake; waves bye-bye |
| **At 1 yr** | |
| Motor: | Walks with one hand held (48 wk); rises independently, takes several steps (Knoblach) |
| Adaptive: | Picks up pellet with unassisted pincer movement of forefinger and thumb; releases object to other person on request or gesture |
| Language: | Says a few words besides "mama," "dada" |
| Social: | Plays simple ball game; makes postural adjustment to dressing |

---

*Data are derived from those of Gessel (as revised by Knoblach), Shirley, Provence, Wolf, Bailey, and others. Knoblach H, Stevens F, Malone AF: Manual of Development Diagnosis. Hagerstown (MD): Harper & Row; 1980. From: Feigleman S. The First Year. Table 8-2. In: Kleigman RM, Behrman RE, Jenson HB, Stanton BF, editors. Nelson Textbook of Pediatrics. 18th ed. Saunders/Elsevier; 2007. p. 45. (Copyright Elsevier 2007)*

Sleeping: Is the child a good sleeper? Does the child share a bedroom or bed with someone else? If so, with whom? When does the child go to bed? When does the child go to sleep? What does the child do in bed? Is there a TV in the child's bedroom? What kind of TV shows does the child watch before sleep time? Is there any bed-wetting? Are there any bouts of night terror?

Toileting: When did the child attain bowel control? When did the child attain bladder control? Does the child have "accidents?" If so, under what conditions?

Games and Play: What are favorite toys and games? Does the child have friends? How does the child relate to them?

Living Arrangements: Is this a nuclear family, single parent family, or an extended family? Who are the current household members? What are their ages? What is their health status, both physically and emotionally? Who are the primary care givers? Is a baby-sitter or grandparent involved in this child's care? Obtain history on domestic violence, guns in the house, and safety hazards at home. Ask about the use of car seats. Obtain history of smoking, excess use of alcohol, and use of "drugs" by any members of the family. Does the child take part in sports or physical activities? Or is the child mostly sedentary?

## Table 2-10. Emerging Patterns of Behavior from 1 to 5 Yr of Age*

**15 mo**

| | |
|---|---|
| Motor: | Walks alone; crawls up stairs |
| Adaptive: | Makes tower of 3 cubes; makes a line with crayon; inserts raisin in bottle |
| Language: | Jargon; follows simple commands; may name a familiar object (e.g., ball) |
| Social: | Indicates some desires or needs by pointing; hugs parents |

**18 mo**

| | |
|---|---|
| Motor: | Runs stiffly; sits on small chair; walks up stairs with one hand held; explores drawers and wastebaskets |
| Adaptive: | Makes tower of 4 cubes; imitates scribbling; imitates vertical stroke; dumps raisin from bottle |
| Language: | 10 words (average); names pictures; identifies one or more parts of the body |
| Social: | Feeds self; seeks help when in trouble; may complain when wet or soiled; kisses parent with pucker |

**24 mo**

| | |
|---|---|
| Motor: | Runs well, walks up and down stairs, one step at a time; opens doors; climbs on furniture; jumps |
| Adaptive: | Makes tower of 7 cubes (6 at 21 months); scribbles in circular pattern; imitates horizontal stroke; folds paper once imitatively |
| Language: | Puts 3 words together (subject, verb, object) |
| Social: | Handles spoon well; often tells about immediate experiences; helps to undress; listens to stories when shown pictures |

**30 mo**

| | |
|---|---|
| Motor: | Goes up stairs alternating feet |
| Adaptive: | Makes tower of 9 cubes; makes vertical and horizontal strokes, but generally will not join them to make cross; imitates circular stroke, forming closed figure |
| Language: | Refers to self by pronoun "I"; knows full name |
| Social: | Helps put things away; pretends to play |

Use of Media: Is there TV in the child's room? What kind of TV shows does he/she watch? Who else watches TV shows with the child? Are there restrictions on the number of hours the child can watch TV per day? Are there other restrictions such as "no TV during meal time," "no TV until after home work is completed," etc. Ask similar questions about video games and use of cell phones.

What are the sources of support for the mother and father in physical, emotional, and financial areas? It is important to know about the family's religious affiliation, partly because of the emotional support religion plays in many lives. Also, the practices of certain religious sects may provide clues as to the etiology of disease and its management. For example, infants raised completely on breast-feeding without vitamin supplementation are susceptible to tetany, and those raised totally on an unsupplemented diet free of animal protein might have rickets. Some sects will not allow blood transfusions.

The sources of economic support, the nature of the parents' jobs, the availability of medical insurance, and any local or national government welfare aids the family receives are of great importance, particularly in the management of chronic and catastrophic illness. Therefore be aware of any agencies the families may be connected with already for counseling or supportive purposes. Obtain details of the agency involvement, years of contact, reasons for referral, and the name of the primary contact person.

---

**36 mo**

| | |
|---|---|
| Motor: | Rides tricycle; stands momentarily on one foot |
| Adaptive: | Makes tower of 10 cubes; imitates construction of "bridge" of 3 cubes; copies circle; imitates cross |
| Language: | Knows age and sex; counts 3 objects correctly; repeats 3 numbers or a sentence of 6 syllables |
| Social: | Plays simple games (in "parallel" with other children); helps in dressing (unbuttons clothing and puts on shoes); washes hands |

**48 mo**

| | |
|---|---|
| Motor: | Hops on one foot; throws ball overhand; uses scissors to cut out pictures; climbs well |
| Adaptive: | Copies bridge from model; imitates construction of "gate" of 5 cubes; copies cross and square; draws man with 2 to 4 parts besides head; identifies longer of 2 lines |
| Language: | Counts 4 pennies accurately; tells story |
| Social: | Plays with several children, with beginning of social interaction and role-playing; goes to toilet alone |

**60 mo**

| | |
|---|---|
| Motor: | Skips |
| Adaptive: | Draws triangle from copy; names heavier of 2 weights |
| Language: | Names 4 colors; repeats sentence of 10 syllables; counts 10 pennies correctly |
| Social: | Dresses and undresses; asks questions about meaning of words; engages in domestic role-playing |

*Data are derived from those of Gessel (as revised by Knoblach), Shirley, Provence, Wolf, Bailey, and others. After 5 yr, the Stanford-Binet, Wechsler-Bellevue, and other scales offer the most precise estimates of developmental level. To have their greatest value, they should be administered only by an experienced and qualified person. From: Feigleman S. The Second Year. Table 9-1. In: Kleigman RM, Behrman RE, Jenson HB, Stanton BF, editors. Nelson Textbook of Pediatrics. 18th ed. Saunders/Elsevier; 2007. p. 49. (copyright Elsevier 2007)*

The school history should include details of the name and address of the school, the grade level, the mode of transportation, any special emotional or physical needs at school, and any behavioral problems and learning difficulties. If appropriate, it is a good practice to call the school teacher, school nurse, or the gym teacher to get more details, after obtaining permission from the child and the family.

It is important to be aware of and follow local laws on privacy issues, reporting of designated diseases such as lead poisoning, suspected abuse, and dealing with adolescent issues. Be aware of HIPAA (Health Insurance Portability and Accountability Act) while trying to obtain health information from or give information to other sources.

## Family History

Family history has taken an increased importance in this era of genomic diagnosis. Many of the chronic diseases may have a genetic component, an environmental component, or both. Therefore, family history has become an important part of public health and preventive medicine.

It is best to start with a simple family history as outlined below and then proceed to a detailed history as outlined in the section on genetic history.

Obtain a history of siblings. How many brothers and sisters does the child have? What are their ages? What sex? Are there or has there been any illness in the siblings? If so, what and when? Did any sibling die due to any unknown or undiagnosed diseases?

What are the ages of the parents? Is there any consanguinity? (This is important in genetic history.) Are these the natural parents? Depending on the time available, get details of the parents' occupations, time spent by the parents at home, and a health history of grandparents and of baby-sitters. In a detailed workup of an undiagnosed or puzzling illness, details of health of close relatives of the mother and father are needed as well.

Are there pets in the family? If so, what and where is the pet kept? Was it acquired recently and from what source? Is there any illness in the pet?

Physicians are trained to look primarily for defects and weaknesses to help diagnose and treat. In the process, they forget that the resilience of the child and the family depend on their strengths. While trying to correct the defect and the weakness, physicians will have to identify and support the strengths. Physicians should look for strengths in the patients (inner, innate strengths) and in their support network, such as a strong grandparent or an involved school teacher. Obtaining a history of the strengths and weaknesses of the child and the family must become a part of the routine.

### Table 2-11. Web Resource Tools for Documenting Family History

American Medical Association: www.ama-assn.org/ama/pub/category/2380.html
US Surgeon General: My Family Health Portrait: www.hhs.gov/familyhistory
March of Dimes: www.marchofdimes.com/gyponline/index.bm2
Labcorp: www.labcorp.com/genetics/fha/genetic_questionnaire.html
Norwich Union Health Tree: www.norwichunion.com/healthtree/index.htm

# Genetic History

In certain situations a detailed genetic history is essential. A history of members of the maternal and paternal side of the family for up to three generations is necessary, although this may not always be available. This should include details about the spouses and the children of all the members. Start with screening tests such as FGENES (family history, groups of congenital anomalies, extreme presentations of common conditions, neurodevelopmental delay or degeneration, extreme or exceptional pathology, and surprising laboratory values) and SIDE (any similar problem? inherited condition? unexplained deaths? extraordinary laboratory tests or reactions?). If there are suspicions based on screening, a more detailed history is necessary. There are several tools available over the web for documenting family history (**Table 2-11**). Parents may be able to create their own using these tools and keep as part of their medical record.

A pediatrician should be able to make a reasonable map of the family tree (**Figure 2-2**). There are several web-based tools that can draw a pedigree. In certain situations where genetic counseling is indicated, a more detailed history and subtle questioning is desirable, based on knowledge of patterns of inheritance of the suspected syndrome.

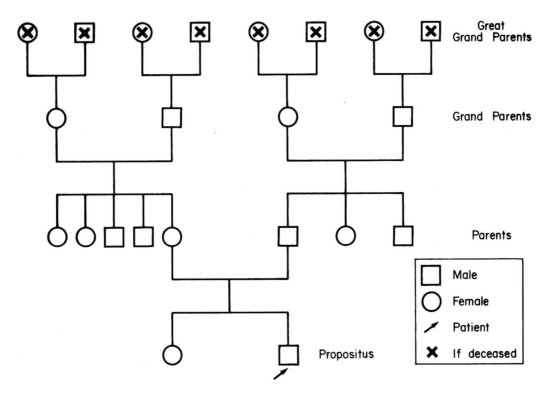

**Figure 2-2.** Genetic Family History

Dr. R. Juberg (1972) suggests a three-step approach to obtaining a genetic history depending on the clinical situation. The first step is applicable to all pediatric patients. In routine history taking, the following pieces of information on all first-degree relatives are to be obtained irrespective of the nature of the problem: given names, surnames, date of birth (or current age), age at death and cause of death, and presence of any disease or defect. The second step is designed to survey the family history for the occurrence of diseases or defects, particularly when the child has a set of symptoms and the diagnosis is not certain. This applies to most, but not all, situations. There are five questions designed to elicit the necessary information: 1) Is there a relative with any identical or similar trait? 2) Is there any relative with a possibly related trait? (For example, when taking a history from parents of an infant with anencephalus, ask about other central nervous system (CNS) malformations in the family.) 3) Is there any relative with a trait that is generally recognized to be genetically determined? 4) Is there any relative with an unusual disease or has any relative died of any unusual condition? 5) Is there any consanguinity in the pedigree?

The first two steps are adequate for most clinical situations. However, if there are questions about the patterns of inheritance of a defect or questions on possibilities of recurrence, maximal family history and construction of a pedigree are required. This includes details on as many relatives for as many generations as possible. This third step is reserved for those working in the genetic clinics.

## System Review

After getting the family and genetic history, it is appropriate to obtain a history on certain overlooked items and also to make sure that no associated related or unrelated problems are coexistent. A few crucial questions about each system should be adequate, but the interviewer should be flexible enough to pursue leads brought out during this review. Some examples are:

- General: weight loss, activity level, fever, appetite, poor weight gain, excess weight gain, delay in growth, delayed developmental milestones.
- Skin: rash, birthmarks, pigmentations, hair loss.
- Head and Neck: headache, any head injuries.
- Ears: past infections, hearing, drainage.
- Eyes: infections, injury, squint, visual problems, does the child wear glasses?
- Nose: infections, bleeding, nasal block, mouth breathing, snoring.
- Mouth, Teeth, and Throat: ulcers, caries, thumb sucking, sore throat, hoarse voice.
- Neck: stiffness, pain, glands.
- Respiratory System: cough, wheeze, dyspnea, chest pain.
- Cardiovascular System: cough, dyspnea, cyanosis, pallor, squatting, tolerance for physical activity.
- Gastrointestinal: vomiting, abdominal pain, diarrhea, constipation, jaundice, exposure to parasites, pica, food intolerance.
- Urinary Tract: usual habits, color of urine, burning, frequency, discharge, excess volume, thirst, enuresis, edema of hands and feet.

- Genital Tract: in prepubertal females, ask about discharge, itching, pinworms. In pubertal and adolescent females, get history of menstrual periods (onset, frequency, regularity, pain, etc.), date of the last period, sexual activity, contraceptive use, prior pregnancy, venereal diseases, history of vaginal discharge and itching. In males ask about history of sexual activity, discharge, pain or swelling of testes, and nocturnal emissions.
- Endocrine: breast development, asymmetry, pain or discharge, change in growth pattern, masses in the neck, nervousness, sleep habits, bowel habits, cold intolerance, delay or accelerated development of secondary sexual characteristics, loss of hair, excess hair, and acne.
- Central Nervous System: headache, visual disturbances, seizures, ataxia, paresthesia, personality changes, mental deterioration, school failure, speech problems, weakness.
- Blood: pallor, easy bruising, unusual bleeding, large nodes, bone pain.
- Musculoskeletal: pain in bone, joint, or muscle; swelling of bone, joint, or muscle; limping, stiffness, limitation of motion.
- Immunologic: recurrent infections, rash, under-nutrition.
- Travel: foreign travel.
- Pets: at home.
- Psychologic: memory loss, behavioral changes, sleep problems, eating problems, school failures, hallucinations, mood changes, temper outbursts, enuresis, encopresis.
- Any Current Medications: when started, for what purpose, what dosage, any side effects, any over-the-counter drugs?

## Symptoms of Unknown Origin

It is increasingly common to see children and adolescents with non-specific signs and symptoms with no identifiable disease pathology. Review of systems may yield multiple positive findings for every system. Unfortunately these patients often will be labeled as having a disease they do not have. Others will be called psychosomatic illness, functional disorders, or somatization disorders. It is important to remember that a diagnosis of psychosomatic illness need not be one of exclusion of all organic diseases. Also, one can have both organ pathology and psychosocial stresses contributing to the symptom complex. Physicians often operate with a strict biological model of disease and illness. This does not fit well with realities of medical practice. Some patients have many symptoms that do not fit into a neat biological entity called "disease." Clifton Meador groups these patients as having "symptoms of unknown origin" (SUO) thus avoiding labeling them with an organ pathology or psychosocial problem. These patients require follow-up and continuity of care by a sensitive physician. As pointed out by Dr. Meador, the condition of these patients may be due to one of the following, on long-term follow-up: 1) a rare illness no one thought of before; 2) identifiable psychosocial stress that produced the symptoms; 3) the patient was unknowingly (or knowingly) ingesting, inhaling, or in contact with a substance that caused the symptoms; 4) the symptoms are self-induced; 5) psychosocial stresses are causing the symptoms but the patient is unaware or refuses to acknowledge this.

It is, therefore, essential to take a very thorough history and listen carefully and with empathy to every verbal and non-verbal clue. Some of the clues to pay attention to are:
- symptoms that defy any anatomic or physiological explanation,
- positive history in every system,
- no objective findings on physical examination on several occasions,
- multiple consults and extensive laboratory and imaging studies all with negative results,
- school avoidance,
- taking multiple drugs in spite of lack of efficacy,
- someone else in the family with a similar illness or a serious illness,
- mental health problem in the parent.

# BIBLIOGRAPHY

Galanti G-A. Caring for Patients from Different Cultures. 4th ed. Philadelphia: University of Pennsylvania Press; 2008.

Garrett A. Interviewing: Its Principles and Methods. New York: Family Service Associates; 1970.

Hoekelman RA, Adam HA, Nelson NM, Weitzman ML, Wilson MH. Primary Pediatric Care. 4th ed. St. Louis: Mosby; 2001.

Kurta SM, Silverman J, Benson J, Draper J. Marrying content and process in clinical method teaching: enhancing Calgary-Cambridge guides. Acad Med. 2003;78:802-9.

Levine MD, Carey WB, Crocker AC, Gross RT, editors. Developmental-Behavioral Pediatrics. 3rd ed. Philadelphia: WB Saunders; 1999.

Meador C. Symptoms of Unknown Origin. Nashville: Vanderbilt University Press; 2005.

Olney RS, Yoon PW. Use of family history information in pediatric primary care and public health. Pediatrics. 2007;120:[Suppl 2].

Thomas A, Chess S. Temperament and Development. New York: Brunner/Mazel; 1977.

# SECTION II

# SPECIFIC ASPECTS OF HISTORY TAKING

Chapter 3

# THREE BASIC STEPS IN DIAGNOSIS

The word "diagnosis" means, "to know through." The word implies differentiation. In usage, however, the term diagnosis denotes an initial impression based on the presenting symptoms and signs, which is symptom-designation. The words that describe the process of establishing the specific cause of a symptom-sign complex are "differential diagnosis."

For example, when a child has generalized edema, the name given (symptom designation) is anasarca. There is one more step in arriving at the exact cause of this symptom/sign. That step is differential diagnosis. To proceed with the process of differential diagnosis , one needs a precise definition of the symptom. The three basic questions a clinician should ask when presented with a symptom, a sign, or a complex are:

1.  What is it?
2.  What is it not?
3.  How do you know?

Let us take two examples to explain the mental processes. A patient comes with pain in the joints (arthralgia). The first question is "what is it?" The obvious initial thought is "arthritis." However, this is not correct. The patient has arthralgia, but does this automatically mean "arthritis?"

Arthritis is defined as "non-bony swelling of the joint or the presence of two of the following three findings: limitation of passive movement of that joint, tenderness or pain on motion, and heat." If there is no swelling and only one of the other three features is present, the patient does not have arthritis.

Here is an example to show the importance of this step. A 12-year-old girl was diagnosed as having acute rheumatic fever. She was put on bed rest for two years. The diagnosis was based on a history of joint pains, elevated sedimentation rate, and a high anti-streptolysin O (ASO) titer. She had joint pain, but it was not the classical migratory kind. She did not have true arthritis. She did not have carditis either. If the physician had not used the word "arthritis" (as described above), but called it "arthralgia," the approach would have been different.

The first mental step assumes that the physician knows the definition of the condition he or she is naming. The first question therefore can be rewritten as:

1.  *"What is it?"* = "Define"

The second question about our hypothetical patient, assuming the presence of arthritis, is "What is it not?" In other words, what are the conditions that may mimic arthritis? Bone pain is one such condition. Tendon pain is another. Periarticular pain is a third. In this step, we are excluding conditions that may mimic the symptoms of the condition that the clinician thinks the patient has. You may, therefore, rewrite the second question as:

2. *"What is it not?"* = "Exclude"

The third step is, "How do you know that the initial impression is correct?" In this hypothetical case of arthritis, the ideal proof (though not necessary in every situation) is to show that the synovial fluid from the affected joint has all the characteristics of an inflammatory fluid. Also, one would like to see an increase in the level of acute phase reactants in the serum of the patient. If one or both of these factors are positive, we can infer that there is inflammation of the joint, that is, arthritis. We are now ready to proceed with the differential diagnosis of arthritis to establish the cause. In other words, the third step may be rewritten as:

3. *"How do you know?"* = "Confirm"

Let us take another example of a patient with yellow skin and highly colored urine. The initial question is "What is it?" The answer is "jaundice." The next question is "What is it not?" We have to exclude conditions that produce discolored conjunctiva (such as carotenemia) and ingestion of food or drugs that may discolor the urine. Finally, confirmation is obtained through urinalysis and blood tests.

# Chapter 4

# HISTORY TAKING BY SYSTEMS

In this chapter, symptoms and diagnostic labels are grouped according to the various systems of the body. Each symptom or diagnostic category is defined first, if appropriate. The definition (What is it?) is followed by a list of conditions that may resemble that particular symptom or diagnostic category. Following this list of "exclusions" (What is it not?) are questions that may help to obtain details of that particular symptom or diagnostic label. These questions are to be asked in addition to the initial questions about the duration, onset, severity, periodicity, aggravating factors, and factors that relieve the symptom. The significance of some of these questions is given within parentheses.

## GENERAL

### Cramps

*What is it?* Painful involuntary contraction of skeletal muscles due to motor unit hyperactivity, associated with sustained spasm. The average patient often confuses cramps with muscle pain.

*What is it not?* Tetany in which there is carpo-pedal spasm, hyperexcitability of the peripheral nerves, and paresthesias. Nor is it dystonia due to sustained contraction of the agonists and antagonists causing contortions of portions of the body.

*Important questions to ask:* Does this occur mostly at night, at rest, and is it asymmetric (ordinary cramps)? Is there a history of antecedent exposure to heat (outdoor games with excess sweating and inadequate fluid intake)? Is there a history of taking diuretics or calcium-channel blockers? Are there associated neurological problems such as muscle wasting (polyneuropathies) or mental status changes (hyponatremia)? Do they come on after general physical activity (McArdle disease)? Is there history of colored urine with these episodes (myoglobinuria)? Does the child use a particular group of muscles for prolonged period, as in playing musical instrument or video games? Are there evidences of hypothyroidism?

### Crying

Descriptions of the natural cry in newborns and infants are available in the book "The Infant Cry" by Wasz-Hockert et al. (1968). A 45 rpm recording of various types of crying of newborns accompanies this book.

*Important questions to ask:* Does the child cry on handling (meningeal irritation, septic arthritis, fractures)? Is it a shrieking cry (CNS insult)? Does cuddling comfort the child? (If not, or if cuddling makes the crying worse, it is more ominous.) Is it a mewing cry (as in cri-du-chat syndrome)? Is it a weak cry (various debilitating conditions and neuromuscular conditions, lipoid proteinosis)? Is it a cry without noise (vocal cord paralysis, laryngitis, babies of diabetic mothers, babies born of mothers on "drugs," and respiratory distress syndrome)? Is it a hoarse cry (laryngitis, hypothyroid, congenital laryngeal stridor, epiglottitis, foreign body in larynx, vocal cord weakness, papilloma of larynx, congenital vascular ring)?

## Difficult to Feed

When a mother says that her infant is difficult to feed, the reason may be anything from simple maternal anxiety and lack of understanding on the part of the mother about developmental needs, to a major medical problem such as congenital heart disease or severe hypotonia.

Important questions to ask: What exactly is the problem? (Ask the mother to describe the problem in her own words.) Is the baby a slow feeder? Or does he or she feed so fast that he or she swallows air? Is he or she too sleepy to feed? Can he or she suck (neuromuscular weakness)? Does the baby have tongue thrust (cerebral palsy)? Can he or she move the tongue from front to back? Is there nasal regurgitation (palatal defects or weakness)? Does the baby tire easily and have to rest frequently during feeding (congenital heart or pulmonary disease)? Are there choking spells during feeding (tracheoesophageal fistula)? Are there maternal anxieties? Does the quantity the baby eats fall below what the mother expects in quality or quantity? Are the mother's expectations realistic?

## Dizziness

*What is it?* Patient complains of a "funny feeling" and a sensation of unsteadiness. This is a common symptom specifically in older children and adolescents.

*What is it not?* Syncope (momentary loss of consciousness and tone), seizure (involuntary movements and post ictal behavior), and vertigo (nystagmus, unsteadiness).

*Questions to ask:* Does it occur when standing (vertigo, decreased cerebral perfusion, or loss of equilibrium)? Does it occur when turning (vertigo) or on standing from a sitting or lying down position (poor cerebral perfusion)? Is there history of ear infection? What are the medicines the child is taking? Is there associated sweating or nausea before the event (syncope)? Is there loss of orientation after the episode (seizure)? Are there other neurological symptoms? Is there mental illness and is the child on medication for this illness (see also syncope)? Is there orthostatic hypotension?

*Evidence-based examination: Postural dizziness and an increment in the pulse rate of 30 beats per minute or more in response to change of posture are the best indicators of hypovolemia. Examine the patient for postural changes in pulse at least two minutes after the patient lies down or at least one minute after the patient stands up. Volume depletion describes a state of loss of sodium from the extracellular space (intravascular and interstitial fluid).*

*Hypovolemia:* In adults with suspected blood loss, the most helpful physical findings are postural dizziness and increase of pulse rate by >30 beats/minute on change of posture from lying or sitting to standing. The presence of dry axilla in adults (and adolescents) suggests hypovolemia (positive likelihood ratio of 2.8); moist mucous membrane and tongue argue strongly against hypovolemia (negative likelihood ratio of 0.3). Capillary refill time (sensitivity 11%, specificity 89%, positive likelihood ratio 1.0) and skin turgor are of no value as isolated findings.

## Edema

*What is it?* Soft tissue swelling of various parts of the body due to accumulation of fluid.

*What is it not?* Nonpitting, firm swelling due to other causes (tumors, inflammation, tissue infiltration).

*Important questions to ask:* What part of the body is affected? Is it generalized or localized? Does it involve only one side (venous or lymphatic obstruction)? Does it involve only the feet (exclude vascular causes)? Is it facial edema only (exclude angioneurotic edema, superior vena cava obstruction)? Is there abdominal distension (ascites)? It there scrotal and facial edema (nephrosis)? Is there anemia? What is the dietary history (nutritional)? Is there dyspnea and cyanosis (heart disease)? Does the child have jaundice (liver disease)? Is it confined to one eye or one ear lobe (insect bite, infection)? Is the edema localized and migratory (as in Henoch-Schonlein purpura)?

## Fatigue

"Feeling tired" is a common symptom. The causes may vary from tiredness due to excess physical activity or lack of sleep, to any disease process including depression; therefore, detailed questioning is necessary.

*Example:* We were consulted to evaluate fatigue in a boy whose main interest was music. His mother's interest was for him to go out and play. She interpreted her son's desire to stay home as being caused by fatigue. She ignored the fact that he stayed home to play the guitar, which he loved. This is an example to show why parents should be asked to elaborate on the symptoms, particularly vague symptoms such as "fatigue," "weak," "tired." This also shows the need to speak with the child directly.

## Fever

*What is it?* Temperature over 37.4°C (99.4 F) in the axilla and over 38 C (100.4 F) by sublingual and rectal measurements using a mercury or electronic thermometer and over 38 C (100.4 F) by tympanic thermometry is considered fever. There is disagreement about the best site for the measurement of temperature in children. Tympanic thermometry using infra-red measurements is most suitable for several settings. This is not accurate in infants because of the angle of the ear canal. *(Also see page.... For details of measurement of temperature)*

*What is it not?* Adults can have fictitious fever; this is rare in children.

*Important questions to ask:* Was the onset sudden (infection) or gradual (rheumatic disease)? Does the temperature curve show high fever (as in malaria, drug toxicity) or low grade fever (minor infections)? Are there associated chills (tuberculosis [TB], infections)? Are there convulsions with fever (CNS infection)? Does the temperature curve show remittent fever with fluctuations more than 1.5°F but not touching normal (various infections)? Is the fever intermittently touching normal for part of the day (malaria, rheumatoid arthritis)? Is it continuous fever with fluctuations less than 1.5°F (typhoid)? Does the child sweat when the fever subsides (any high fever, TB, malaria)? Has the fever been present for a short duration (infection) or has it been present for weeks and months (rheumatic disorders)? Is it episodic or periodic (malaria; brucellosis; periodic fever, aphthous stomatitis, pharyngitis, and cervical adenitis [PFAPA]; autoinflammtaory syndromes such as familial Mediterranean fever)? Is there a history of exposure to any drugs? Is there history of heat exposure? Is there lack of sweating (heat stroke, atropine poisoning, ectodermal dysplasia)?

## Headache

Headache can be due to simple common causes such as stress and anxiety or it can be due to a serious disease such as brain tumor.

*Important questions to ask:* Is it acute or chronic? Is it acute single (or first) episode (infections, CNS trauma, or tumors)? If so, is there a history of trauma or are there any associated symptoms such as urinary tract infection, sinusitis, or CNS symptoms? Is it acute and recurrent? If so, are these separated by periods of no symptoms (migraine)? Is it chronic and progressive? If so, this is serious and often indicates intracranial pathology. Is it chronic and non-progressive with frequent and constant headache? This is a common pattern and requires good history and physical examination, but is rarely due to a definable cause.

*Other questions to ask:* Is it frontal (eye strain, regular headache, brain abscess), temporal (migraine), or occipital (tension headache)? Does it start in one place and spread? (Spreading is more significant than if it stayed in one place.) Is it so bad that it makes the patient vomit (migraine, brain tumor/abscess) or is it a mild headache (most viral illnesses)? Does light precipitate an attack (cerebral irritation) or does cough make it worse (increased intracranial pressure)? Is it worse in the morning (brain tumor/abscess) or is it worse at the end of the day (visual problems/tension)? Are there any associated symptoms such as diplopia, noise in the ears, vertigo, paralysis? (These signify more urgent problems.) Is there pain in other parts of the body?

In adults, a mnemonic called the "POUNDing" criteria is used to diagnose migraine. In this mnemonic, the letters stand for **P**ulsatile quality, lasting for four to 72 h**O**urs, **U**nilateral location, **N**ausea and vomiting, and **D**isabling intensity. The presence of three or more of these items increases the likelihood of migraine as the etiology of the headache.

Remember that small babies with headaches cannot express pain and may only be irritable. Children with headache show frowning and tightening of the muscles of the eyebrows and forehead, whereas children with abdominal pain show grimacing and tightening of the muscles of the lower face.

## Jaundice (icterus)

*What is it?* A syndrome characterized by hyperbilirubinemia and deposition of bile pigment in the skin, conjunctiva, and mucous membrane with resulting yellow appearance of the patient. This can be a symptom, a sign, or both.

*What is it not?* Carotenemia or lycopenemia (sclera not colored in these two conditions). Also exclude other causes of colored urine, such as concentrated urine, hematuria, hemoglobinuria, or due to drug ingestion.

*Important questions to ask:* Was it present at birth (infectious and hemolytic problem)? What was the age of onset (acquired conditions, hemolytic, infections, and obstructions)? What color is the stool (jaundice with pale-colored stool suggests biliary obstruction)? What color is the urine? Is there itching (itching with jaundice suggests an obstructive cause for jaundice)? Is there abdominal pain (calculi)? Is there history of hemoglobinopathy in the family? Has there been any recent drug ingestion?

## Obesity/Overweight

*What is it?* Body mass index (BMI) is the preferred method for evaluating obesity in children between the ages of two and 19 years. Other methods such as skin fold thickness and waist circumference are not recommended for routine clinical use.

Body mass index is used as a screening tool to identify overweight children and adults. It is independent of height and is applicable to males and females. Although there may be racial and ethnic differences in body fat and lean mass distribution, at present, the same BMI reference standards are recommended for all children.

The BMI (kg/m2) is calculated using the formula of weight in kg divided by height in cm2 and comparing the value obtained with normative data for age and sex. If pounds and inches are used, the formula is weight in pounds divided by the square of the height in inches, multiplied by 704.5. (This factor may vary in some calculations.) Several BMI tables, nomograms, and calculator programs are available online ( www.cdc.gov/nccdphp/dnpa/bmi/calc-bmi.htm and http://nhlbisupport.com/bmi/bmicalc.htm). Normal values and graphs are given in **Figure 4-1**, overleaf.

Children with a BMI between the 85th and the 94th percentile are considered to be "overweight" (previously classified as being at risk for overweight), and those over the 95th percentile are considered "obese" (previously classified as overweight).

In addition, severe obesity is defined as BMI at the 99th percentile, which is 30-32 kg/m2 for 10- to 12-year-olds and >34 kg/m2 for youths 14 to 16 years of age.

By another definition, an absolute value for BMI of 25 to 29 is considered overweight and a BMI of over 30 is defined as obesity. For children less than two years of age, weight for length, and not BMI, is used to estimate overweight.

*Evidence base: Sensitivity of the 85th percentile mark is 75%-93% and specificity is 67%-96%. Sensitivity for the 95th percentile mark is 54%-100% and specificity is 96%-99%.*

*Important questions to ask:* What is the family history, dietary history, emotional, and behavioral history. Dietary history should be in detail, including early feeding history. Obtain a sample menu for three to five days including type of food, energy dense foods consumed, and volume consumed. Rapid assessment tools are available on the internet (e.g., WAVE childhood version: http://bms.brown.edu/nutrition/acrobat/wave.pdf). Is there dry skin and intolerance to cold (hypothyroidism)? History of physical activity (frequency, duration, and intensity of exercises) and time spent on television, computer, and video games should be obtained as well.

## CDC Growth Charts: United States

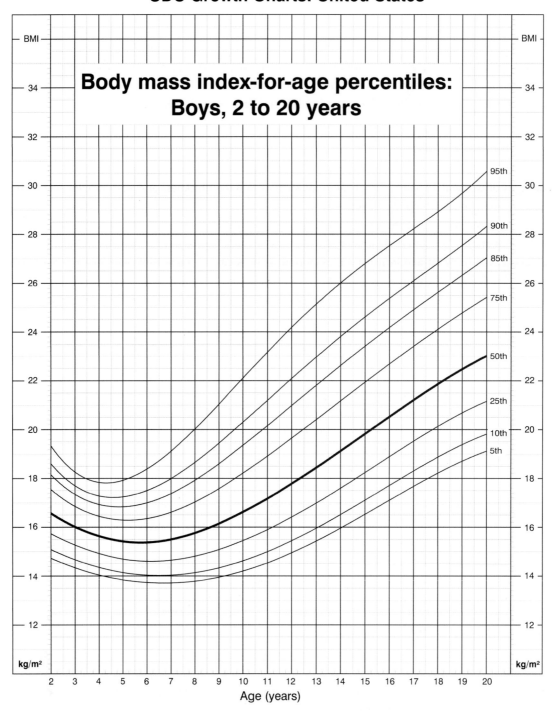

**Figure 4-1A.** BMI graphs (From Center for Disease Control and Prevention. Hyattsville, Md. 20782. USA. www.cdc.gov)

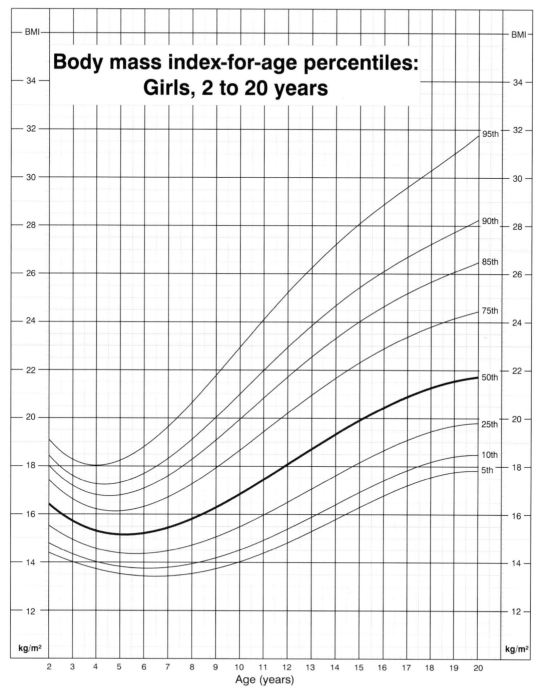

**Figure 4-1B.** BMI graphs (From Center for Disease Control and Prevention. Hyattsville, Md. 20782. USA. www.cdc.gov)

## Pain

Ascertaining the location of pain may be difficult in an infant. Usually pain in one area indicates some pathology immediately underneath. In some situations, pain is perceived away from the anatomic location where it originates. Certain locations of referred pain are very typical, e.g., retrosternal pain of pericarditis, shoulder-tip pain of gallstone disease, abdominal pain in lower lobe pneumonia, and knee pain in hip disease. Pain may be located strictly in one area, as in pancreatitis and peptic ulcer, or diffusely, as in appendicitis and colitis.

The spread of pain from one area to another may be characteristic and significant in adults (sciatica, angina) but not so common or useful in diagnosing illness in children.

Important questions to ask: What factors precipitate or aggravate the pain? For example, pain of pulp space infection or tenosynovitis in the hand gets worse with the limb held in the normal position, hanging by the side of the body. Pleural pain and pain of increased intracranial pressure get worse on coughing. Relief of pain is another important clinical clue. Moving relieves the pain and stiffness of juvenile idiopathic arthritis (JIA). Holding the abdomen with the hands may relieve pain due to colicky conditions, whereas it will worsen pain due to intraabdominal inflammatory process. Dramatic relief of pain with aspirin is characteristically seen in osteoid osteoma.

The severity of pain can be of help as well. In rheumatoid arthritis, the joint pain is not severe. In acute rheumatic fever and septic arthritis, the pain is very severe. Pain due to neurovascular dystrophy is the worst. Pain that keeps children awake at night is probably due to infectious processes (exclude emotional causes). But pain that wakes a child from sleep is seen commonly with septic arthritis, osteomyelitis, or osteoid osteoma. Periostitis also will cause night-time pain. Severe attacks of colicky intermittent pain are common in intussusception.

Children may not be able to give the details of the characteristics of pain. Dull aching pain of the joints is the usual picture in most rheumatic disorders. In reflex neurovascular dystrophy, the pain is of a burning kind. Throbbing pain is usual with acute abscesses. The pain of oxygen want is literally like someone tightening the chest with an iron chain. Timing is another important factor. Morning headache is of more serious significance than evening headache. Pain in the abdomen after eating is different from pain when the stomach is empty (gastric ulcer).

Severity of pain may be assessed by self-report in older children or by behavioral observation in infants and young children. Whenever possible, one of the visual analog scales should be used. There are several types of visual analog scales, some with figures of faces and some with metrics only. The metric scale is more appropriate for adults. Most childhood versions of visual analog scales depict drawings of human faces ranging in expressions from sad and crying to happy and smiling (**Figure 4-2**). The child is asked to select a face that represents the way he or she feels because of the pain. For younger children, an observational scale such as the one in **Table 4-1** may be used.

## Wong-Baker FACES Pain Rating Scale

0 = VERY HAPPY, NO HURT

1 = HURTS JUST A LITTLE BIT

2 = HURTS A LITTLE MORE

3 = HURTS EVEN MORE

4 = HURTS A WHOLE LOT

5 = HURTS AS MUCH AS YOU CAN IMAGINE
(Don't have to be crying to feel this much pain)

Explain to the person that each face is for a person who feels happy because he/she has no pain (no hurt) or sad because he/she has some or a lot of pain. Face 0 is very happy because she/he doesn't hurt at all. Face 1 hurts just a little bit. Face 2 hurts a little more. Face 3 hurts even more. Face 4 hurts a whole lot. Face 5 hurts as much as you can imagine, although you don't have to be crying to feel this bad. Ask the person to choose the face that best describes how he/she is feeling.

Rating scale is recommended for persons age 3 years and older.

**Brief word instructions:** Point to each face using the words to describe the pain intensity. Ask the child to choose face that best describes his/her own pain and record the appropriate number.

**Figure 4-2.** Wong – Baker Pain Scale from Wong's Nursing Care of Children. Hockenberry M, Wilson D (Eds) 8th Edition. St.Louis.2007. Mosby Publishers. pages 1876-1877. (Reproduced with permission from Elsevier)

## Table 4-1. Observation Pain Scale

| Observation | Scale |
| --- | --- |
| Laughing | 1 |
| Happy, smiling, playing | 2 |
| Asleep, calm (neutral) | 3 |
| Vocalizes pain, wrinkles brow, can be distracted (mild to moderate pain) | 4 |
| Crying inconsolably, screaming, expresses severe pain | 5 |

*Modified from: Tyler DC, Tu A, Douthit J, Chapman CR. Toward validation of pain measurement tools for children: a pilot study. Pain. 1993;52 (3):301-9. (Used with permission from International Association for the Study of Pain)*

## Pica

*What is it?* Is there altered appetite? Is there history of the child swallowing dirt, crayons, or any inedible objects?

*What is it not?* Mental retardation.

*Important questions to ask:* What was the age at onset of pica? What items are consumed? Is there any anemia? Is there history of worms? Is there evidence of lead toxicity? Explore family set-up for disorder.

## Polydipsia

*What is it?* Excessive thirst and drinking of water. This is a symptom with serious implications (diabetes). It is not unusual to see normal children (6 to 10 years) sip water many times a day even though the volume of water consumed is not high. The volume consumed (not the frequency) and the association with polyuria are important clues.

*What is it not?* Psychogenic polydipsia. (Children with psychogenic polydipsia will drink any water, including water from a toilet bowl, whereas children with polydipsia due to diabetes mellitus or insipidus will not do this).

## Recurrent Infections

It is common for children, particularly younger ones attending a nursery or preschool program, to experience repeated respiratory and gastrointestinal infections. Young children get three to six episodes of upper respiratory infection per year on average. In infants attending daycare, the numbers may be even greater. Therefore, it is important to recognize those with recurrent infections due to immunodeficiency or anatomical defects.

### Table 4-2 Classification of Protein-Calorie Malnutrition (Quantitative scale)

*Current Nutritional status* is best assessed by looking at the expected weight for a given height. This is a measure of under- or malnutrition. There are 3 grades of severity.

**Mild** – The current weight as a percentage of expected weight for height is between 80 and 90

**Moderate** - The current weight as a percentage of expected weight for height is between 70 and 80

**Severe** - The current weight as a percentage of expected weight for height is less than 70

*Past Nutritional Status* is best assessed by looking at the height at a given age. This may show a reduction in the rate of linear growth (growth retardation) or reduction in the final stature (stunting). There are 3 grades of severity.

Mild when the height as percentage of expected height for age is between 87.5 and 95

Moderate when the height as percentage of expected height for age is between 80 and 87.5

Severe when the height as percentage of expected height for age is less than 80.

*Source Reference: Waterlow JC. Classification and Definition of Protein-Calorie Malnutrition. BMJ 1972; 3: 566-569.*

Recurrent infection at the same site (other than upper respiratory infection) may point to a local anatomic defect. Recurrent infections with the same organism (pneumococcus, monilia) or infections due to unusual organisms may suggest congenital or acquired defects in the immune system including HIV infection.

## Swelling

Swellings can be due to trauma, congenital malformations, infection, or malignancy.

*Important questions to ask:* Was the onset acute or chronic (infection versus congenital)? Was it present from birth? Is it growing (abscess, tumor) or regressing (hematoma)? Is it fluctuating in size (infectious)? Are there any color changes? Does the swelling feel warm (infectious)? Was there any injury to the site? Is it painful? Has similar swelling occurred in other places (also see edema)? Is there fever?

## Syncope

*What is it?* Sudden loss of consciousness associated with loss of postural tone lasting for less than 10 to 20 seconds, followed by spontaneous recovery. It may be preceded by sweating and nausea. The patient will look pale and cold to touch during the episode. On recovery, there is no disorientation.

*Important questions to ask:* Causes of syncope can be grouped under four categories: cardiac (in children, primarily arrhythmia, not ischemia--consider drug-induced arrhythmia), neurologic (includes stroke and seizure), vaso-vagal or other (including orthostatic, medication-induced), and unknown. Therefore, ask for details of events before the attack (precipitating event such as change of position), description of the attack (loss of tone, seizures, color, muscle tone), and the mental status soon after the attack. A detailed medication history is important.

## Undernutrition (older terminology was Failure to Thrive)

This may relate to height (growth retardation, short stature), weight (failure to thrive, under-nutrition, wasting), or both (failure to thrive).

*What is it?* Under-nutrition is defined as weight (or weight for height) less than two standard deviations below the mean for age and sex AND/OR weight curve crossing more than two percentile lines on standardized growth charts. Waterlow recommended (**Table 4-2**) that clinicians differentiate between abnormal weight for height as a measure of the current nutritional status and abnormal height for age as a measure of past nutritional history. Waterlow also suggested that a quantitative classification (**Table 4-2**) be used in a community setting to grade the severity of protein-calorie malnutrition and that a qualitative classification be used to distinguish the severe forms of malnutrition (marasmus and kwashiorkor).

Weight for height can be used to differentiate stunting of growth (caused by chronic illness, genetic, and endocrine causes) from wasting (due to acute malnutrition).

Several different criteria have been used in studies on failure to thrive. These include 1) weight less than 75% of median weight for chronological age (Gomez criterion), 2) weight less than 80% of median weight for length (Waterlow criteria), 3) body mass index of less than 5th percentile for chronological age, 4) weight less than 5th percentile for chronological age, 5) length less than 5th percentile for chronological age, 6) weight loss trajectory crossing more than two major centile lines, and 7) conditional weight gain at the lowest 5%.

*Important questions to ask:* Since under-nutrition can result from medical and psychosocial and economic causes, a thorough history is essential. This should include questions about chronic medical conditions, history of medications, history of food allergies, premature birth, congenital anomolies, economic status, food habits, and social history.

## Vomiting

*What is it?* Forcible expulsion of gastric contents.

*What is it not?* Simple regurgitation in smaller babies or reflux.

Important questions to ask: How old is the child? (Certain conditions are characteristic of the newborn, such as congenital malformations.) What was the age of onset? What is the frequency? Is there associated diarrhea? Is there loss of weight (indicates severity)? What is the urine output (indicates level of dehydration)? What are the antecedent symptoms (pain in the abdomen indicating intestinal problems, and headache indicating meningeal or cerebral irritations)? Does fluid come through the nose during vomiting? (If it does, it indicates definite and severe vomiting, not regurgitation.) Is it projectile in nature (pyloric stenosis or CNS disease)? What is the relationship to feeding? (If it occurs soon after feeding, particularly in small infants, it may be because of faulty feeding techniques or acute gastrointestinal infections; if it occurs one half to one hour later, it often is caused by obstruction.) Is undigested food (delayed emptying or obstruction), bile (severity or obstruction distal to entry of the bile duct), or blood seen in the vomitus? Is there history of treatment with any drugs such as digoxin or aspirin? Is there history of accidental drug ingestion? Does the child regurgitate food into the mouth and chew on it (rumination)?

# CHEST (CARDIOPULMONARY)

## Abnormal Noisy Respiration

*What is it?* There are several kinds of noisy respiration. Stridor is a harsh, high-pitched sound heard during or at the end of inspiration. It is commonly heard in association with conditions characterized by narrowing of the upper air passages (laryngotracheobronchitis, foreign bodies, epiglottis, diphtheria, vocal cord paralysis). Croup is inspiratory stridor associated with barking cough and hoarseness. "Snoring" is a form of stridor that occurs during sleep.

Grunt is a short explosive sound at the beginning of expiration (produced by closure of the vocal cords). Rattle is a rapid succession of short, sharp sounds, usually heard in moribund patients, due to air going in and out through pooled saliva in the throat. It is heard at the beginning of inspiration or throughout respiratory cycle. Wheeze is a noisy musical sound occurring during expiration (heard in asthma) and may be heard even without a stethoscope.

# Cough

*What is it?* Paroxysmal forcible expirations.

*Important questions to ask:* Is it acute or chronic? How severe is the cough? Is it dry (pleurisy) or productive (pneumonia, TB)? What is the nature of the sputum (purulent as in lung abscess and cystic fibrosis or frothy as in heart disease)? Is there copious sputum (lung abscess)? What color is the sputum (blood tinged in mitral stenosis, greenish in cystic fibrosis)? Is there frank blood in the sputum (hemoptysis)? Does the sputum have a bad smell (lung abscess)? Is there associated fever? Is the cough worse in certain positions? (Postnasal drip gets worse on lying down.) Is there pain in the chest on inspiration or on coughing (fracture rib or pleurisy)? What is the character of the cough (hoarse as in laryngotracheobronchitis, whoop as in pertussis, or aphonic as in vocal cord paralysis)? Is the cough present all day or only while the child is awake (habit)? Is it worse when asleep or when awake (postnasal drip)? Is there respiratory distress?

# Cyanosis

*What is it?* Bluish discoloration of skin and mucous membrane due to excess deoxygenated hemoglobin in the superficial capillaries and venules. This is best looked for in areas with thin epidermis and rich supply of subepidermal vessels such as the lips, nose, ears, hands and feet, and mucous membranes of the mouth.

*What is it not?* Methemoglobinemia (the patient is blue without dyspnea), carbon monoxide poisoning (cherry colored lips).

*Important questions to ask:* Is it generalized, including the oral mucous membrane and tongue (central cyanosis)? Are the extremities warm (central cyanosis)? Are the oral mucous membranes and lips spared and are the extremities cold (peripheral cyanosis)?

# Dyspnea

*What is it?* Difficulty in breathing or labored breathing. (In newborn infants, dyspnea is characteristically associated with inability to breast-feed or suck continuously and by grunting respiration.)

Orthopnea is defined as difficulty in breathing (dyspnea) that appears when the patient lies down and is relieved by sitting. Trepopnea is dyspnea that appears when the patient lies down on one side (lateral decubitus) and gets better when lying on the other side. This occurs in unilateral lung or pleural disease. Platypnoea is dyspnea when the patient is sitting up that gets better on lying down, as in severe right-to-left shunting.

*Important questions to ask:* Is the onset acute (foreign body or anaphylaxis) or is it chronic (heart and lung disease)? Was there an episode of choking on food before the onset? Is there difficulty in feeding? Does the child get tired easily during feeding (heart disease)? Is there fever? Is there cough (infectious pulmonary problems)? What is the nature of the sputum (frothy in heart problems, purulent in pulmonary infections, pink in mitral stenosis)? Is there pain in the chest (pleural)? Does the patient have orthopnea (heart disease)? Is there cyanosis? Does the child have generalized edema? What is the urine output (heart failure)? Does the patient have dyspnea at rest or only on exertion (to indicate severity)? What position makes it worse?

## Hemoptysis

*What is it?* Blood in the sputum.

*What is it not?* Swallowed blood from epistaxis. Hematemesis (frothy material with bright red blood) is seen in hemoptysis; the blood is darker and non-frothy in hematemesis).

*Important questions to ask:* Is there history of cough? Is there history of TB in the family? Is there history of rheumatic fever or other rheumatic diseases? Are there any bleeding diatheses? Is there bad odor in the breath? Is there history of foreign body ingestion?

# GASTROINTESTINAL (GI)

## Blood in Stools

*What is it?* Hematochezia is fresh blood in stool. Melena is altered blood in stool.

*What is it not?* Dark stool due to ingestion of iron compounds or colored drinks such as grape juice or Hawaiian Punch.

*Important questions to ask:* When did it start? How often? How much blood? Is it frank blood (indicating bleeding from lower end, near rectum) or is it dark (bleeding from higher up)? Is there only blood or is there blood with mucus (amebiasis, inflammatory bowel disease)? Does the child have pain in the abdomen before passing blood (intussusception, anaphylactoid purpura) or is it painless (Meckel's diverticulum)? Is there a history of constipation (fissure) and severe pain during defecation (fissure)? Does the child have tenesmus (inflammatory bowel disease, amebiasis)? Tenesmus is painful contraction of the rectum with the sensation of wanting to evacuate bowels but no evacuation.

## Bulky Stool

Important questions to ask: Is the volume large for the age and the size of the child? What is the frequency? Is it foul smelling (cystic fibrosis)? Does it float (malabsorption syndrome)? Is it greasy (cystic fibrosis)? What color is the stool (pale in liver disease)? What is the food intake? (In starvation the stool may look fat and bulky, in malabsorption syndromes, there is voracious appetite.) What is the weight pattern? Is there prolapse of the rectum (cystic fibrosis)? Does the child complain periodically of pain in the abdomen (surgical malabsorption)? (In difficult to diagnose malabsorption syndrome, don't forget surgical lesions of the gut such as malrotation.)

## Constipation

*What is it?* Constipation is infrequent or difficult evacuation of the feces. Normal bowel movement has three variables, namely frequency, consistency, and volume (see page 10). When each variable is considered within a range of normality, it is easy to misinterpret this symptom. Add to these variables the usual maternal concerns about the functions of the baby's bowel movements, and it is easy to over-diagnose this common symptom.

*Important questions to ask:* How many stools per day or per week? What is the consistency? Is blood present? If so, is it around the stool (as in fissures or hemorrhoids) or mixed with the stool? Is it present from birth (Hirschsprung's disease)? Did it start around 10 to 18 months of age (during toilet-training pressures)? Did it start around certain changes in family life (arrival of new baby)? What is the dietary history (too much non-bulk food)? Is there any periodic diarrhea or encopresis? Is there any vomiting? Is there any loss of weight? In addition to the above questions, obtain complete family and emotional histories.

## Diarrhea

*What is it?* Diarrhea is characterized by increased frequency and decreased consistency of bowel movements. Increased volume of bowel movements may or may not be part of this picture.

Important questions to ask: Is it acute (infectious) or chronic (functional, parasites, malabsorption)? What is the frequency? Are the stools large and watery (severe diarrhea as in cholera) or is the volume small? What is the color (green indicates rapid peristalsis, pea soup color in typhoid, rice water color in cholera)? Is there vomiting? Is there pain in the abdomen? Is there blood and mucus (indicates dysentery)? Is there any history of ingestion of unusual food (toxin)? What is the urine output (to estimate severity)? (The number of wet diapers will give an idea of urine output in infants.) Is there weight loss? (In young children, this is a very important question.) Is the child well in every other way, afebrile, active, and alert (functional)?

## Dysentery

*What is it?* Blood and mucus in the stool.
*Important questions to ask:* Same as for diarrhea.

## Dysphagia

*What is it?* It is difficulty in swallowing. This may be associated with pain, in which case, it is called odynophagia.

*Important questions to ask:* Duration of the disease (is it present from birth [congenital] or acquired later)? Is there any history of lye ingestion? Does the food seem to stop in the upper portion (palatal paralysis) or lower portion (scleroderma)? Is there nasal regurgitation (palatopharyngeal paralysis)? Is there trouble with solids (strictures) or with liquids (muscle weakness)? Is there a history of reflux or gastroesophageal reflux disease? Is it associated with pain (candida or reflux esophagitis) or without pain (mechanical or neuromuscular)?

### Hematemesis

*What is it?* Blood in the vomitus.

*What is it not?* Swallowed blood in the vomitus (e.g., blood from epistaxis that was swallowed), colored drinks ingested recently (very common).

Important questions to ask: Is there prior history of "stomach upsets?" Is there history of bleeding diathesis? Is there history of drug ingestion (aspirin)? Is there history of liver disease? What color is the blood? Is there bleeding elsewhere?

# SKIN

## Rash

Described in Chapter 9, page 189.

# MUSCULOSKELETAL

## Arthritis

*What is it?* Swelling of a joint or the presence of two of the following three: pain or tenderness on motion, limitation of range of passive movement, and warmth of the affected joint.

*What is it not?* Bone pain or swelling, periarticular pain or swelling, tenosynovitis.

Important questions to ask: Is there a history of trauma? Is there fever (septic arthritis)? Does it involve a single joint (septic) or many joints (JIA)? Is it migratory (acute rheumatic fever)? Is it nonmigratory? What is the duration (short duration in trauma and septic arthritis, long duration in rheumatic disorders)? Are there any gastrointestinal symptoms (inflammatory bowel disease, salmonellosis with reactive arthritis)? Are there any low-back symptoms (ankylosing spondylitis)? Have there been any eye problems (uveitis of JRA/JIA and ankylosing spondylitis)? Is there history of bleeding diathesis in the family (hemophilia) or hemoglobinopathy (sickle cell)? Are there any oral lesions (systemic lupus, Behcet)? Is there any rash? If so, what kind (erythema marginatum of acute rheumatic fever, macular evanescent rash of juvenile rheumatoid arthritis [JRA/JIA], butterfly rash of systemic lupus erythematosus [SLE])?

# CENTRAL NERVOUS SYSTEM

## Ataxia

*What is it?* Failure of coordination of muscles. In practice, however, ataxia is equated with unsteady gait. It is best to differentiate between the causes of acute ataxia and recurrent ataxia.

*Important questions to ask:* Is this the first attack (drug reaction, infection) or has the child experienced prior attacks? Is there a history of fever and headache or history of recent viral illness? Is there a history of taking medicines for any reason? Is there history of access to or ingestion of drugs and poisons (with a history of alcohol too)? Is there history of any metabolic disease (e.g., hypoglycemia in a diabetic child)? Is there any history of migraine, seizure, or double vision? Is there history of ear infections or vertigo?

## Athetosis

*What is it?* Slow, writhing movements of the distal portions of the extremities.

*What is it not?* Dystonia in which there are involuntary twisting movements mostly of the proximal portions of the body including the neck.

## Chorea

*What is it?* Purposeless, **non-repetitive** involuntary movements of the extremities and face, which interrupt a normal activity.

*What is it not?* Tics, which are purposeless and **repetitive stereotypic** movements. They are absent during sleep.

## Coma

*What is it?* Loss of consciousness from which the child cannot be aroused even with noxious stimuli.

*What is it not?* Seizures (of which loss of consciousness is a part), syncope (momentary loss). Important questions to ask and the proper recording of the level of consciousness will be discussed in Chapter 11, page 241.

## Convulsions (also see seizures)

*What is it?* Convulsions are violent, involuntary movements or a series of movements of the voluntary muscles with or without loss of consciousness.

*What is it not?* Tetany (spasm with typical posturing of hands and feet). Hysterical movements (no patterns, occurs only during the day when being seen. Patients fall gently without getting hurt).

Important questions to ask will be discussed in Chapter 11, as part of the discussion of seizures.

## Delirium

*What is it?* An acute and fluctuating alteration of mental state characterized by confusion and lethargy. Major features are 1) acute onset with fluctuating mental status; 2) inability to focus and maintain attention; 3) disorganized thinking with incoherence and rambling conversations; and 4) lethargy, stupor, or irritability. Of these, items **1 and 2 must** be present together with **either 3 or 4.**

*Important questions to ask:* May be indicative of head injury, toxic infectious states (particularly typhoid fever), drug toxicity (atropine group), cerebral vasculitis (SLE). Therefore, ask about head injury and recent ingestion of drugs. Is there any fever? Are there any other systemic symptoms?

## Diplopia *(also see page 262)*

*What is it?* Double vision.

*Important questions to ask:* Is it monocular (problem with contact lens or diseases of the eye such as cataract, astigmatism, keratitis, drooping lid) or is it binocular (several causes)? Is there associated headache and vomiting (increased intracranial pressure)? Does the child have strabismus? Is there history of head injury? Does the child have buzzing in the ears (labyrinthine involvement)? Is the hearing normal (eighth nerve involvement)? Does the child have weakness of any part of the body? Is diplopia present all day (as in tumors and multiple sclerosis) or at the end of the day (eye strain, myasthenia)? Is there associated ptosis (suspect third nerve palsy)? Is diplopia present only during the movement of the eye in certain directions (lateral rectus paralysis, for example)?

## Seizure

*What is it?* A sudden attack or recurrence of a disease. This term is preferred by neurologists to describe the general category of epilepsy and convulsions.

Important questions to ask will be discussed in Chapter 11, as part of the discussion of seizures.

## Tremors

*What is it?* Fine rhythmic involuntary oscillations of equal amplitudes of a part of the body (usually of hands) due to movements of agonists and antagonists.

*Important questions to ask:* Is tremor present at rest (static tremor as in Parkinsonism) or only in certain postures (postural tremor as in when a limb is extended against gravity)? Static tremor is present in old age as exaggerated physiologic tremor. Tremor of thyrotoxicosis, cerebellar lesions, and asterixis of hepatic failure also belong to this group. Asterixis is irregular flapping movements of the fingers and hand when the patient holds his or her arms outstretched with fingers spread apart. The main problem is inability to maintain a fixed posture. Kinetic tremor occurs during voluntary movements as when writing. This is characteristic of essential tremor. Is the tremor brought about by active movement toward an object (intention tremor), as in diseases of the superior cerebellar peduncle? Is the tremor precipitated by anxiety or tension (functional physiological tremor)? Is there a family history of tremor (essential tremor)? Is there a history of thyroid disease? Is the child taking any medications (neuroleptics, antidepressants, bronchodilators, metoclopramide, caffeine)? Is there any history of substance abuse? Are there associated symptoms in other systems, for example, weight loss and heat intolerance as in hyperthyroidism or psychiatric manifestations as in Wilson disease?

## Vertigo

(Children often cannot describe vertigo. Frequent falling to one side, unexplained crying episodes, or suddenly closing the eyes as if in terror may be indicative of vertigo.)

*What is it?* A sensation as if the surrounding objects are revolving around (objective vertigo) or the patient him- or herself is revolving (subjective). Patients may use the word "dizziness."

*What is it not?* Dizziness,which is a "funny" feeling within one's head; a sensation of unsteadiness.

Important questions to ask: Is it present at rest (tumors) or on movement (labyrinthine)? Is it on looking to one side (labyrinthine)? Is it associated with diplopia and vomiting (more serious)? Is it acute (infection or toxin) or chronic? Is there a past or recent history of head injury or meningitis? Did the child have recent respiratory or ear infection (labyrinthitis)? Are these recurrent attacks (Meniere's)?

# DEVELOPMENTAL (ALSO SEE CHAPTER 12C)

## Developmental Delay

*What is it?* "A condition in which a child is not developing and/or achieving skills according to the expected time frame." Synonyms are "delayed development," "developmental abnormality," and "disordered development." Any child who fails to complete a developmental step (e.g., sit, stand) that is completed by 90% of children of the same age may be considered "slow" and delayed in development.

## Mental Retardation (MR)

"A disability characterized by significant limitations both in intellectual functioning and in adaptive behavior as expressed in conceptual, social, and practical adaptive skills" as defined by the American Association of Mental Retardation (AAMR). This disability originates before age of 18 years." "Significant limitation" is defined as "an intelligence quotient (IQ) standard score at least two SD below the mean of an individually administered assessment instrument."

The Diagnostic and Statistical Manual of Mental Disorders, 4th Edition (DSM IV-TR) uses the cut off score of 70 on an individually administered IQ test. It further classifies MR at four levels based on the values on IQ.

Mild: 50/55 to 70

Moderate: 35/40 to 50/55

Severe: 20/25 to 35/40

Profound: less than 20/25

Exclusions: Although any of the following conditions may lead to developmental delay, these have to be excluded:

- Environmental Deprivation. This is defined by a history of poor socioeconomic conditions, broken home, or inadequate parent-child interactions. Demonstrations of definite improvement of the child in a neutral and nurturing environment after a short time period suggests environmental deprivation rather than primary mental deficiency.
- Cerebral Palsy. In an infant, developmental delay often is recognized by delay in motor development such as head control, turning over, walking, and talking. Although cerebral palsy and mental retardation can coexist, one has to differentiate these conditions.
- Sensory Defects. Developmental delay or deficit in vision or hearing can lead to delay in language and communication development.

- Primary Personality Disorder (e.g., autism). Failure to relate to the environment appropriately and failure in development of interpersonal relationships are indicative of this diagnosis.
- Metabolic Diseases. Family history, other findings such as failure to thrive, diarrhea, and jaundice are clues pointing to metabolic disease as a cause of developmental delay in the differential diagnosis.
- Syndrome. Presence of other physical stigmata suggests the presence of a chromosomal abnormality or a nonchromosomal syndrome.
- Isolated Areas of Delayed Development. This is not mental retardation. A child may be normal in every area except one, for example, confusion with right and left. If this is not part of a global delay, it is not mental retardation.
- Variation in Maturation. One should be able to compare the trajectory of the development of any particular child with the rate of development of an "average" child of the same age, sex, and socioeconomic conditions. As a child's development deviates further and further away from the average, the child is less likely to be normal. (Normal milestones of development are presented in Tables 2-9 and 2-10 and can be followed in the Denver Developmental Reference Chart in Figure 12C-1, page 344).

*Important questions to ask:* Is the child premature? If so, by how much? Was there illness during pregnancy? Is there family history? What was the parental age at birth of patient? Was this a multiple pregnancy? Was there toxemia? Was there antepartum hemorrhage? What are the details of delivery--how prolonged, use of anesthesia, forceps, presentation? Were there neonatal problems? Were there neonatal infections? Is there history of emotional deprivation? What are the socioeconomic conditions? When did the child smile for the first time? When did the child turn over? At what age could the child hold the head steady? When did the child sit? When did the child take the first step with help? When did the child walk without help? When did the child speak the first meaningful word? When did the child speak in sentences? How old was the child when dry at night? When was the child toilet trained? (Also see pages 24 & 51).

## Enuresis

*What is it?* Involuntary discharge of urine, occurring during sleep at night in a boy who is older than six and in a girl, older than five years of age.

*What is it not?* Polyuria from any cause.

*Important questions to ask:* Does it occur during the day (more serious) or at night only? Did the child ever achieve bladder control and then lose it? Or did the child never achieve bladder control (needs more investigation)? What is the urine volume (diabetes insipidus)? Was there any recent stress in the family? Is the child a very sound sleeper?

## Hyperactivity

*What is it?* There are variations in the levels of activity of children. Some are more active than others; boys in general are more active than girls. Also, cultural factors, the irritability quotient of the parents, and mismatch between the personalities of the parents and the child may determine how hyperactivity is interpreted and acted upon.

There are clear objective criteria to define children who need intervention. Hyperactivity may imply an attention deficit disorder (ADHD), but most hyperactive children are not to be classified as having ADHD (see page 348 for more discussion).

## Learning Disability

*What is it?* According to the Interagency Committee on Learning Disabilities, this is a generic term and includes "significant difficulties in the acquisition and use of listening, speaking, reading, writing, reasoning, or mathematical abilities or of social skills." Some children may have no neurologic disorder or mental retardation but still have problems in learning. In others, there may be a concomitant handicapping condition, psychosocial problem, or an attention deficit disorder.

*What is it not?* Mental retardation, visual problems, cerebral palsy, neurological disorders, hearing difficulties, behavioral problems, psychiatric illness, and environmental and social deprivation.

# BIBLIOGRAPHY

American Academy of Pediatrics--Committee on Nutrition. Pediatric Nutrition Handbook. 5th ed.
Kleinman RE, editor. Elk Grove Village (Il): American Academy of Pediatrics; 2004.
Hall M. Principles of Diagnosis. 2nd ed. New York: D. Appleton; 1835.
Knobloch H, Pasamanick B. Developmental Diagnosis. 3rd ed. Hagerstown, MD: Harper & Row; 1974.
Shapiro B, Batshaw M. Mental retardation. In Behrman RE, Kleigman RM, Jenson HB (Editors).
Textbook of Pediatrics. 18th ed. Philadelphia: Saunders/Elsevier; 2007.
Wasz-Hockert O, Lind J, Vuorenkoski V, et al. The infant cry: A Spectrographic
and Auditory Analysis. Clinics in Developmental Medicine, No. 29. London: Heinemann Medical Books; 1968.

# SECTION III

# PHYSICAL EXAMINATION

Chapter 5

# GENERAL PHYSICAL EXAMINATION

## GENERAL COMMENTS

Every physician should be able to examine every system of the body and recognize common physical findings. The first step is to learn how to conduct a proper examination of infants and children from books, audio-visual aids, and experienced clinicians. However, one tends to forget without repeated application of what was learnt.

It is obvious that a cooperative patient is essential for a good physical examination. In the pediatric age group, however, one does not always get a cooperative patient. Even the best of us will face a "tough customer" occasionally. Children's needs, fears, and behavior differ depending on their age, prior experience, and developmental level. Therefore, the physician's approach to examining a child has to vary depending on the child's developmental level and needs, acuteness of the illness, and other circumstances. However, there are certain useful approaches.

During the initial contact, pay peripheral attention to the child, particularly the young ones, until you have had a nice relaxing talk with the parents. Let the child play around, sit on a chair, or sit on a parent's lap. You may want to avoid looking at the child directly. The fact that the parents are talking to you freely may relax the child.

On the contrary, it is better to deal directly with adolescents. Gently remind the parents, if necessary, to let the boy or girl tell his or her own story. This approach is often applicable to even younger children.

Any sudden movements may frighten the young ones. Beginning the physical examination without any instruments helps allay the child's anxieties. Allow the child to play with the stethoscope, flashlight, or reflex hammer during examination of the skin, abdomen, or the limbs. Examine whatever part is available first and do not insist on going from head to foot in an orderly fashion. Examine in whatever position the child is in and do not insist, at least initially, on the child lying down on the examining table. Examine the most painful parts last and look into the throat and the ears at the end of the examination. Allow the child to cling to a parent or sit on a lap for as much of the examination as possible.

In spite of all of these tricks, many points may be missed. If there is urgency, be firm but gentle, and complete the examination of the most important systems as quickly as possible. In non-acute situations, the child may have to be seen more than once before getting a satisfactory, thorough examination. The ability to discover the key findings in the initial examination of a difficult child is one of the hallmarks of a skilled clinician.

Each physician develops personal tricks to elicit and increase the cooperation of children during the examination. Here is a partial list:

1. Let the child play with the examining instruments.
2. Explain the procedures, particularly the painful ones.
3. Tell firmly what is expected; do not ask "Can you please open your mouth?" (That question gives the child an option to say "no!")
4. Have a colorful examining room with cartoon characters or toys.
5. Come down to their level, even if they are on the floor, both mentally and physically.
6. Never tell them that "It won't hurt" if, in fact, the procedure will hurt.
7. With young children, allow as much parent contact as possible.
8. Another interesting approach to help relax the children and make them share some of their hidden fears and anxieties is the Winnicott Squiggle Game. In this game, the physician draws a squiggle and asks the child to complete it, to make a picture. Next, the child is asked to draw a squiggle and the physician completes a picture out of it. Even if no impressions can be made out of these pictures, certainly they will improve the physician-child communication and the child's cooperation during the physical examination.
9. Make a game out of the examination (see pages 241 & 242 for Three Penny Neurological).
10. Several observations can be made while talking with the parents. These, in turn, can help focus on some areas for formal examination (as in a child who has torticollis) and postpone examination of some areas (as with a child who is able to get up from a sitting position without any help).

When ready to examine the child, start with the child sitting or standing. When ready to examine the abdomen, lay the child on the table. If there is no one to help restrain the child for examining the throat or ears, use one of the techniques shown in **Figures 5-1** and **5-2**.

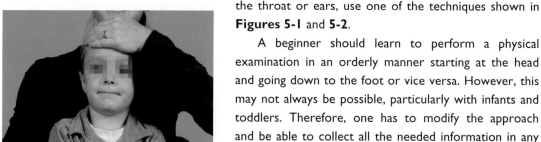

A beginner should learn to perform a physical examination in an orderly manner starting at the head and going down to the foot or vice versa. However, this may not always be possible, particularly with infants and toddlers. Therefore, one has to modify the approach and be able to collect all the needed information in any available sequence. A comedian used to say "What you see is what you get." This is true with some children. A good clinician should be able to aim for the major problem very quickly in an emergency room setting, and perform a thorough examination when more time is available.

**Figure 5-1.** Proper method to restrain the child for physical examination. Note that the mother is able to restrain the child's legs with her legs, and the child's arms and the head with her two hands.

# SOURCES OF ERRORS

Before discussing the details of physical examination, let us consider common sources of errors and how to minimize them. Errors may be due to *faulty techniques in examination* or in *interpretation*.

Weiner and Nathanson classified the errors in physical examination under the following headings: 1) errors in *techniques of examining* various parts of the body, 2) errors of *omission* (failure to examine certain areas), 3) errors owing to failure to recognize signs that were present, and 4) errors because of *incomplete and poor recording of examination*. These errors can be corrected only by the combined efforts of the clinical teachers who teach proper techniques of physical examination, and of the physician-students who apply them methodically.

Experience is essential for the proper interpretation of physical findings. Even after one gets the experience, the following common pitfalls must be avoided. All clinical findings must be interpreted within the context of the whole patient. It is easy, but erroneous, to accept those findings that confirm our suspicion and ignore those findings that seem contrary to our clinical judgment. The specific significance of a clinical finding depends on the probability of the patient having a particular disease (given the rest of the clinical picture) and the probability of occurrence of that particular physical finding in that disease. For example, the presence of jaundice in a three-year-old child in India has a higher specificity for hepatitis than for congenital hemolytic anemia. The reverse may be true in Mediterranean countries.

When a physician makes an initial diagnosis based on symptoms and signs, he or she has developed a working hypothesis, which explains certain facts. This working diagnosis needs confirmation. In this respect, the clinician is a scientist trying to prove a hypothesis. The clinician is liable to make the same mistakes that scientists are warned against, with even more serious consequences. Beveridge describes these pitfalls as follows: 1) clinging to ideas that have been proved useless or untrue, 2) inability to subordinate ideas to facts, 3) inability to submit hypotheses to most careful scrutiny, and 4) inability to recognize that false hypotheses interfere with progress.

Ingle listed fallacies in reasoning under the following headings: 1) fallacies that concern associated or correlated events, e.g., *post hoc, ergo propter hoc* (after this, therefore, because of); 2) fallacies of generalization, e.g., judging an individual on the basis of the general characteristics of the group; 3) fallacies of oversimplification, e.g., assuming that our "hypothesis must be true because there is no proof that it is not true"; and 4) fallacies that beg the question, e.g., the fallacy of hiding behind untestable hypotheses.

Good clinicians have to guard against all these errors in observing, interpreting, and reasoning.

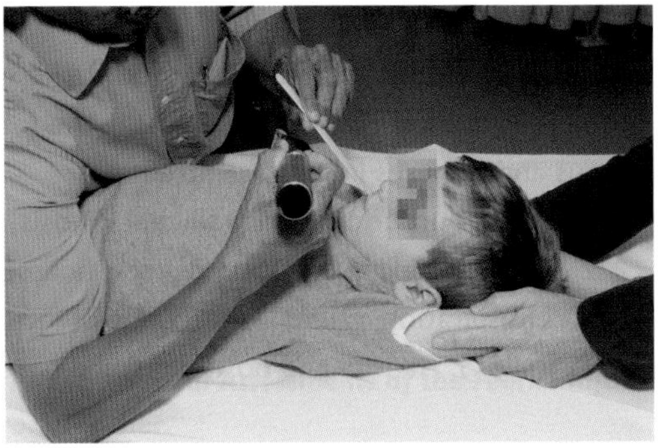

**Figure 5-2.** Proper method to restrain the child for physical examination. Note how the examiner leans over the abdomen without pressing on the abdomen to prevent the legs from allowing the child to roll over. Also, the mother holds the arms of the child held in extension and the head with both of her hands.

**Table 5-2. The Yale Observation Scale***

| Observation Variable | Normal (1) | Moderate Impairment (3) | Severe Impairment (5) |
|---|---|---|---|
| Quality of cry | Strong with normal tone or content and not crying | Whimpering or sobbing | Weak or moaning or high pitched |
| Reaction to parent stimulation | Cries briefly then stops or content and not crying | Cries off and on | Continual cry or hardly responds |
| State variation | If awake, stays awake or if asleep and stimulated wakes up quickly | Eyes close briefly when awake or awakes with prolonged stimulation | Falls to sleep or cannot be aroused |
| Color | Pink | Pale extremities or acrocyanosis | Pale or cyanotic or mottled or ashen |
| Hydration | Skin normal, eyes normal and mucous membranes moist | Skin, eyes normal and mouth slightly dry | Skin doughy or tented and dry mucous membranes or sunken eyes |
| Response (talk, smile) to social overtures | Smiles or becomes alert | Brief smile or becomes alert briefly | No smile, anxious, dull, expressionless or cannot be alerted |

*Total score ranges from 6 to 30.*
*Reprinted with permission from: Bonadio WA. The History and Physical Assessments of the Febrile Infant. Pediatr Clin N Am. 1998;45(1):65-77. With permission from Elsevier.*

# Position/Posture

The position taken by the patient gives valuable clues to diagnosis. Dyspnea that gets worse on lying flat may indicate congestive heart failure. During a severe asthmatic attack, children sit on the edge of the bed with legs dangling, leaning forward with hunched shoulders, with hands supporting the body weight and placed slightly behind the midline. They may have a barrel chest and active accessory muscles of respiration. If children have colicky pain in the abdomen, they are restless and roll about, holding their hands over the abdomen; but if there is peritoneal irritation, they lie still and do not want their abdomen touched. The decerebrate posture is characterized by extended neck, extended shoulders and elbows, pronated forearm, with lower limbs in extension (**Figure 5-3**). Decorticate posture is flexion at the elbow and wrist, with thumb adducted into the palm, with lower limbs extended (**Figure 5-4**). Patients with spinal cord injury and hypotonic conditions have flail limbs and they lie in a "pithed frog" position. A child who wants to lie still in one position with eyes shut may have vertigo.

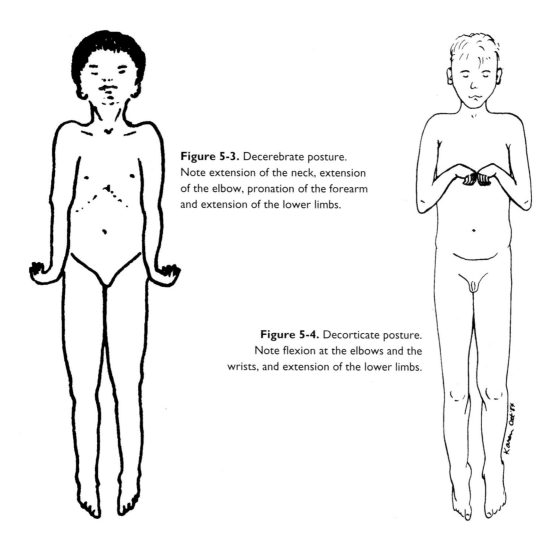

**Figure 5-3.** Decerebrate posture. Note extension of the neck, extension of the elbow, pronation of the forearm and extension of the lower limbs.

**Figure 5-4.** Decorticate posture. Note flexion at the elbows and the wrists, and extension of the lower limbs.

# Cry *(also see Chapter 4 for how to obtain history)*

Listening to the cry may give clues to several diagnoses. The irritable cry of a sick newborn is recognized easily with experience. Normal fussiness becomes less if a baby is picked up and handled. In contrast, the crying of children with cerebral irritation gets worse with handling. In painful conditions of the skeletal system and joints, the child cries on handling. The cry is shrill, shrieking, and high pitched in diseases of the central nervous system. It is very weak in neuromuscular paralysis. It is voiceless in vocal cord paralysis and in the presence of tracheostomy. The cry sounds like a cat in cri-du-chat syndrome. It is hoarse in laryngotracheobronchitis and recurrent laryngeal paralysis.

## Alertness

A febrile child who is alert and responsive is less of a concern than one who is lethargic or irritable. A blind child is often extra sensitive to noise and startles easily when there is sudden noise. On the other hand, a child who is overly alert visually may be deaf. A blind child may exhibit one or more of the following features: 1) a vacant distant look, 2) oscillations of the eyeball, or 3) unusual alertness to sound. Children with autism make no eye contact.

## Odor

During this early observation period, be alert to recognize characteristic odors in the patient that may aid in the diagnosis. For example, smell of acetone in the breath of diabetes mellitus, fruitish smell of diphtheria, or smell of ingested toxin (kerosene), are well known. Other smells of diagnostic significance are given in **Table 5-4**. In addition, experienced clinicians can smell the characteristic odor of E. coli diarrhea and the stool of cystic fibrosis.

### Table 5-3. Simple Tests of Mental Proficiency

| Age | Numerical Skill | Other Concepts |
|-----|-----------------|----------------|
| 6 | Counts forward to 30 | Tells right from left |
| | Repeats 4 digits | Tells AM from PM |
| | | Draws a man with head, neck, hands, and clothing |
| | | Defines objects in terms of how they are used |
| 7 | Counts by 2s and 5s | Copies a diamond |
| | Repeats 5 digits forward; 3 backwards | Recognizes parts left out of a drawing |
| 8 | Makes change from a quarter | Knows days of the week |
| | Counts backward from 20 | Has an idea about distant places |
| | | Can give similarity and difference between simple objects |
| 9 | Can do simple multiplication and division | Knows correct date |
| | | Can arrange weights in order of heaviness |
| 10 | Uses fractions | |
| | Knows numbers over 10 | |
| | Repeats 6 digits forward | |
| 11 | | Defines abstract terms such as honesty, fair play, deceit |
| | | Can give themoral of fables |

*From: Blake FG, Wright FH, Waechter EH. Nursing Care of Children. 8th ed. Philadelphia: Lippincott; 1970, p. 442. (Reprinted with permission from Wolters Kluwer)*

# Gait

Careful observation of a child's gait as he or she enters the room may give clues to the diagnosis of several neurological and musculoskeletal diseases. Abnormal gait has been classified traditionally as antalgic, ataxic, paralytic, and spastic.

Looking at the worn-out portions of the shoe may give clues to gait abnormalities. A shoe worn out in front without any marks on the heels indicates a tight heel cord (as seen in cerebral palsy) or a foot drop. In foot-drop, the box of the shoe will also show marks of scraping on the floor. Children with arthritis and pain at the metatarsophalangeal joints learn to bear weight on the outside so that the shoe is worn off on the outer side.

Gait cycle consists of the activity that occurs between heel strike of one foot and subsequent heel strike on the same foot (**Figure 5-5**). Heel strike occurs at the moment the heel touches the floor. During one gait cycle, each limb goes through two phases: 1) stance phase, beginning from the moment the heel touches the floor (heel strike) and ending when the toe leaves the floor (toe off); and 2) swing phase, beginning with toe off until the heel strikes the floor.

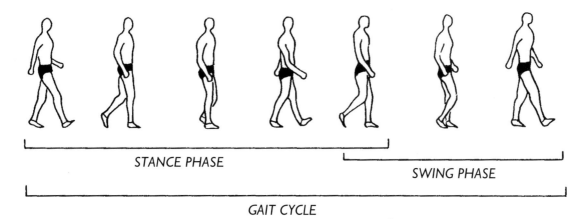

STANCE PHASE                    SWING PHASE

GAIT CYCLE

**Figure 5-5.** Normal gait cycle.

## Table 5-4. Conditions Distinguished By Characteristic Odor of the Patient (Breath, Skin, or Urine)

| Disease | Odor |
| --- | --- |
| Diabetes Mellitus | Acetone |
| Diphtheria | Fruity |
| Maple Syrup Urine Disease | Caramel-like (maple) |
| Phenylketonuria | Musky ("mousy") |
| Oasthouse Urine Disease | Dried malt (brewery) |
| Fatty Acid | Sweaty foot |

Whenever it is indicated, ask the child to walk about 12 to 24 steps and observe each limb in the stance phase and in the swing phase. Look at the gait from front and back. Look at the ankle, knee, hip, and spine during the stance and the swing phases. If one does this systematically, one can observe many important clues.

Some abnormalities that can be detected during the stance phase include:

1.  Lateral trunk bending during stance phase toward the side bearing weight suggests gluteus medius weakness on that side. The cause of this can be diseases of the hip, such as dislocation, or diseases of the muscles, such as dermatomyositis or muscular dystrophy.
2.  Posterior trunk bending suggests gluteus maximus paralysis.
3.  Excess lordosis suggests hip flexion contracture or severe hypotonia.
4.  Hyperextended knee suggests weakness of quadriceps.
5.  Slapping contact of the forefoot with the floor, where the toe touches the floor before the heel does, indicates anterior tibial weakness.
6.  Excessive lateral foot contact suggests evertor weakness (peroneus) or pain on medial side of the foot.
7.  Excessive medial foot contact suggests weakness of invertors of the foot or tightness of the evertors (peroneus) or knock-knee.

Some abnormalities that are observed during the swing phase are:

1.  Lateral bending, away from the side which is in swing phase, denotes weak gluteus medius on the side that is bearing weight.
2.  Hip hiking (lifting the hip vertically) suggests that the lower limb is longer on the side with hip hiking or shorter on the opposite side. Hip hiking also may indicate hip flexor spasticity or hamstring weakness.
3.  Circumduction gait is seen in hemiparesis due to weakness of hamstring or flexors.
4.  Anterior trunk bending suggests weakness of quadriceps.
5.  Bobbing up and down with too much vertical movement of the hip above and below an imaginary line going through the umbilicus is seen in hip flexor weakness and hamstring weakness. This is different from hip hiking where the vertical movement is only upwards above the umbilical line from clearing the floor but no bobbing down.
6.  Dangling flail foot suggests anterior tibial weakness which may be isolated, as in peripheral nerve disease, or part of a generalized weakness of muscles of the leg, as in polio or myelomeningocele.
7.  Insufficient push off. This is characterized by the entire foot leaving the floor simultaneously instead of the heel first, then the middle of the foot, and finally the toes. This is seen in gastrocnemius weakness and painful foot syndromes.

When the length of step and period of time spent on one side are different from that on the other, look for pain anywhere in the limb, fear of falling, or cerebellar dysfunction.

# Face and Facial Expressions

Facial expressions give valuable clues to the child's emotions and facial features may aid in diagnosis of various syndromes. Facial expression is a composite of movements of various muscles of the face, the opening of the eyelids, and of the color and size of the pupils. Anxious, angry, and happy faces are easy to recognize. Muscles of the upper part of the face are wrinkled in painful conditions of the head and neck, whereas the lower part of the face is also wrinkled when the pain is in the chest or abdomen. Spasm of the muscles of the jaw and of the face in tetanus gives rise to a facial expression characterized by clenched teeth, tightly pursed tips, and the drawing up of perioral muscles (risus sardonicus). The prominent eyes of hyperthyroid, the wide eyes with prominent forehead of Cruzon disease, whistling face in Freeman-Sheldon syndrome, and the chubby cheeks of Cushingoid facies are typical examples of how facial appearance can help in making a diagnosis.

Flattening of the face on one side, with wide palpebral fissure, enophthalmos, and ptosis is seen in Horner syndrome. Blue face, petechiae, and subconjunctival hemorrhage indicate thoracic outlet obstruction due to whatever cause, for example, cord around the neck or whooping cough. Flame-shaped nevus on one side of the face is seen in Sturge-Weber syndrome. Heliotrope (amethyst-violet) discoloration of eyelids is seen in dermatomyositis. An expressionless, flat, mask-like face is seen in overdose of the phenothiazine group of drugs.

The cheek is pink in normal and healthy children. Pale cheek is often an indication of fear, anemia, or aortic regurgitation. In systemic lupus, one may see the butterfly rash (**Figure 5-6**) characterized by discoloration, dryness, scaling, and follicular plugging, resembling acne, on either side of the bridge of the nose.

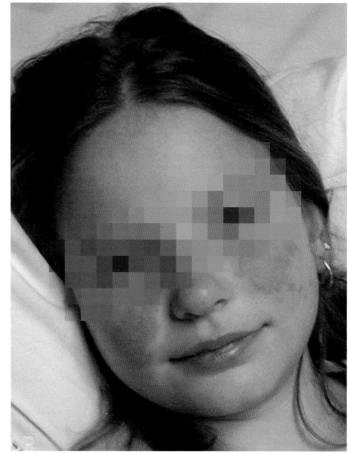

**Figure 5-6.** Macular rash in "butterfly" distribution in a girl with Systemic Lupus Erythematosus. Reproduced with permission from 1972-2004 American College of Rheumatology Slide Collection.

Other well-known facies described in the literature include the elfin facies, mask-like facies, and old-man's facies. These terms are used to give the description of a composite image of the face. If one has to give the details of abnormalities of the face, one has to take each component and give a description. For example, the appearance in Down syndrome is determined by the set, the slant, and the epicanthic folds of the eyes. Bilateral parotid swelling gives a "chipmunk appearance" to the child's face, as seen in mumps and Sjogren syndrome. (The best way to look for parotid swelling is to look from behind the patient and observe the elevation of the lobule of the ear away from the cheek.)

Appearances can be deceiving. For example, true hypertelorism (wide-set eyes) and hypotelorism (eyes set too close) are abnormal. However, a broad nasal bridge in a child may give the impression of wide-set eyes. Similarly, the association between Turner syndrome and widely spaced nipples was found to be wrong when actual measurements were made. Therefore, special graphs have been constructed based on actual measurements for inter-pupillary distance, length of the ears, etc. These graphs with age-related values have to be used for accuracy in cases where clinical observation alone is not adequate (**Figures 5-7, 5-8, 5-9, and 5-10**).

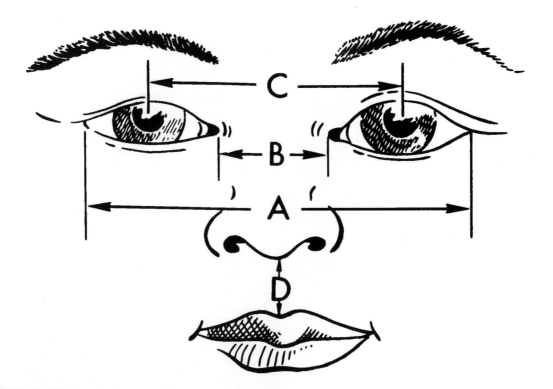

**Figure 5-7.** Measurement of the face. (A) Outer canthal distance. (B) Inner canthal distance. (C) Interpupillary distance. (D) Height of philtrum.
From Feingold M, Bossert WH. Normal values for selected physical parameters. An aid to syndrome delineation. Bergsma D (ed). White Plains, NY. The national Foundation, Birth Defects:OAS X(13): 1-16, 1974. (Reproduced with permission from the March of Dimes Foundation)

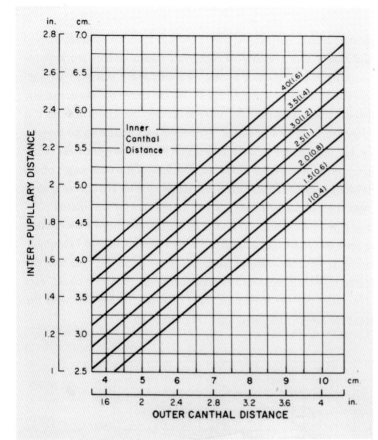

**Figure 5-8.** Relationship between outer canthal distance, interpupillary distance, and inner canthal distance. From Feingold M, Bossert WH. Normal values for selected physical parameters. An aid to syndrome delineation. Bergsma D (ed). White Plains, NY. The national Foundation, Birth Defects: OAS X(13): 1-16, 1974. (Reproduced with permission from the March of Dimes Foundation)

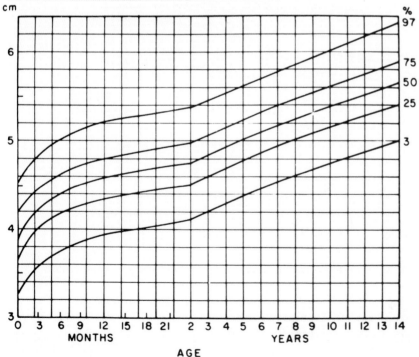

**Figure 5-9.** Normal values for interpupillary distance at various ages. From Feingold M, Bossert WH. Normal values for selected physical parameters. An aid to syndrome delineation. Bergsma D (ed). White Plains, NY. The national Foundation, Birth Defects:OAS X(13): 1-16, 1974. (Reproduced with permission from the March of Dimes Foundation)

The position of the ears and axial rotation of ears are features contributing to the total composite called "facies." Though relatively large ears and absent ears are easy to recognize, measurements are available to define low-set ears, small ears, and protuberant ears. Using a measuring instrument that goes through medial canthi and measuring the total length of the ear, the percentage of the ear above the horizontal line connecting medial canthi can be calculated. Lateral canthus is not used as a reference point because this may vary in children with upward and downward slants of the eyes. Whenever ears appear to be low-set, nomograms should be used for accuracy, but one can get a clinical impression by observing the helix of the ears in relation to a horizontal line passing through the medial canthi. At least 20% of the total height of the ear should be above this line in normal children. Ears may appear to be low-set (when they are not) whenever the neck is short or the cranial vault is high, the mandibular ramus is short, or the auricles are rotated.

There are no available definitions of a prominent ear. When the ear sticks out more than usual, it is called "prominent ear" and may be seen in syndromes associated with Trisomy-13 and Trisomy-8. Occasionally one sees loss of supporting structures, such as absence of the superior crus and the antihelix, resulting in a "lop ear." This also may be interpreted as prominent ear. "Railroad track" ears are seen in fetal alcohol syndrome. Normally the ear makes an angle of about 10 degrees with the mastoid. There are nomograms for total ear length at various ages (**Figure 5-10**).

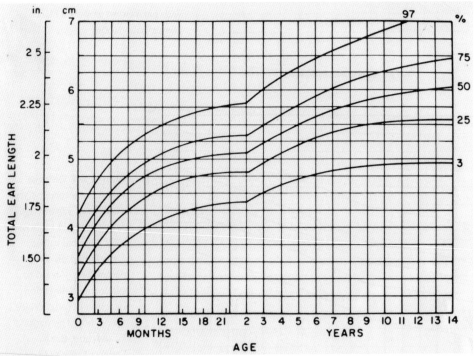

**Figure 5-10.** Ear length: Normal values at various ages. Total ear length is the distance between the most inferior and superior portions of the ear. Also refer to Figure 6-8 on page 129.
From Feingold M, Bossert WH. Normal values for selected physical parameters. An aid to syndrome delineation. Bergsma D (ed). White Plains, NY. The national Foundation, Birth Defects:OAS X(13): 1-16, 1974. (Reproduced with permission from the March of Dimes Foundation)

The shape of the nose gives clues to a number of syndromes. For example, the nose is unusually small or short in Apert syndrome and Trisomy-18 syndrome, and prominent in trichorhinophalangeal syndrome. The characteristics of the nose are determined by the length of the nasal bridge, height at the root of the nose, height of the septum, and the angle the septum makes to the coronal plane of the face. For example, the root of the nose may be sunken (flat nasal bridge) as in achondroplasia or Down's syndrome, or broad as in Trisomy-8 syndrome. The length may be long as a familial characteristic, in which case the septum makes a downward angle (as in Pfeiffer syndrome). In addition, the alae nasi may be well-formed or broad and flat bilaterally (as a familial characteristic) or flat on one side (cleft palate). The nasolabial distance (philtrum) is another part of the "facies" for which normal values for age are available. Smooth, flattened philtrum may be seen in fetal alcohol syndrome.

A vertical line drawn from the medial border of the pupil should touch the angles of the mouth. If the angle of the mouth lies lateral to this line, the mouth is probably large (macrostomia) and if it lies medial, the mouth is probably small (microstomia). A partially opened mouth in a child with nasal voice suggests adenoidal hypertrophy. When viewed in profile, a line drawn vertically from the glabella downward should touch the upper and lower lips and the chin. In cleft lip, the upper lip is behind the line. In micrognathia the chin is too far behind the line (**Figure 5-11**).

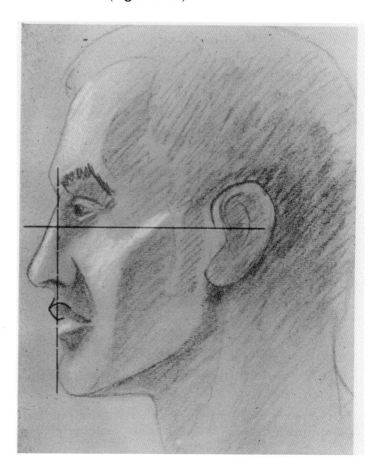

**Figure 5-11.** Idealized face in profile. Note the vertical line touching the lips and the chin. Also, note that the longtitudinal axis of the ear is parallel to that of the bridge of the nose. (Figure courtesy of Dr.Linton Whittaker)

# Skin

The details of skin examination will be dealt with later in Chapter 9. Only those observations that can be made during general evaluation of the patient, such as color and skin eruptions will be discussed in this section.

*If an infectious disease is suspected, one should take precautions quickly before other children in the clinic or office are exposed.*

Look for edema of the dependent parts, particularly over the anterior aspect of the leg and feet. Unilateral edema is seen in obstruction of venous flow. Bilateral edema denotes generalized disease such as heart failure, kidney disease, anemia, or hypoproteinemia. In a bedridden patient the dependent part is the sacrum, not the legs. Edema of the scrotum signifies severe edema, as in nephrosis. The impressions made by socks and clothes on the body are good indicators of edema. Recurrent bouts of facial edema with or without edema elsewhere indicate angioneurotic edema. Facial edema may be seen in thoracic/superior vena cava obstruction. Presternal and scalp edema may be seen in hemorrhagic edema of infancy and Henoch-Schonlein purpura. Presternal edema used to be seen in mumps.

The time it takes for pitting of an edematous area to recover (pit-recovery time) may help differentiate between conditions associated with low albumin and those associated with increased venous pressure and capillary leak. Edema due to conditions with low serum protein levels (congestive heart failure, nephrosis) pits easily on pressure and also recovers quickly compared with the edema of conditions with elevated serum protein levels (lymphedema or inflammatory edema). The method to elicit this sign is to press the pretibial skin with the thumb for about a second or two and determine the time it takes to refill. In adults, the recovery time is less than 40 seconds in patients with low albumin, and over 40 seconds in patients with other causes. No such study is available in children.

If the neck and chin appear swollen, feel for crepitus, which signifies subcutaneous emphysema. Occasionally, if crepitus is not palpable, one can place the diaphragm of the stethoscope on the skin and press gently, eliciting a crackling noise.

Poor skin turgor may help recognize children with dehydration (loss of intracellular water). This is elicited by pinching a fold of skin over the lateral abdominal wall between the thumb and index finger, releasing it promptly, and noting the time it takes for the fold to return to the normal position. (This is also called "tenting.") No normative data are available. It is best to describe whether the skin returns to normal immediately, with a slight delay, or long delay. Loss of water content markedly alters the viscoelastic properties of elastin and prolongs the recoil time.

Capillary refill time is measured by applying moderate pressure over the pulp of the middle or index finger for five seconds and measuring the time in seconds for the return of color to baseline. Ideally a stopwatch should be used, the room temperature should not be too cold, and the arm should be held at the level of the heart. The upper limit of normal for children is two seconds.

*Evidence based medicine: A meta-analytic report summarizing the reliability of signs and symptoms of dehydration in children showed that the most useful signs for predicting five percent dehydration in children are abnormal capillary refill time (likelihood ratio [LR] 4.1; 95% confidence interval [CI] 1.7 to 98), abnormal skin turgor (LR 2.5; 95% CI 1.5-4.2), and abnormal respiratory pattern (LR 2.0; 95% CI 1.5-2.7).*

# Hand

During general examination, observe the hand for clues such as pallor and jaundice, which are noted on the palmar aspect, and cyanosis, which is noted at the fingertips (also see Chapter 9).

*Clubbing* can be observed during this initial observation period. The nail bed is thicker in a clubbed finger and the angle at which the nail takes off is altered. It is usually painless except in hypertrophic osteoarthropathy. There are several methods of observation and one method of palpation to identify clubbing. On inspection the shape, width, and thickness of the terminal phalanx is altered. The angle at which the nail takes off from the nail bed (nail-fold angle), and the angle the nail makes with the dorsum of the terminal phalanx (hyponychial angle), have been used as evidence of clubbing. However, I found the description of the methods confusing. The best clinical method is to look at the finger in profile (**Figure 5-12**). The vertical height at the proximal edge of the nail (base) should be equal to or just less than the height at the distal interphalangeal joint in normal children. In true clubbing, the height at the base of the nail is taller than at the distal interphalangeal joint.

Hyponychial angle is measured as shown in **Figure 5-13**. The normal is 180 degrees +/- 4.2 degrees. Any angle over 190 degrees is abnormal.

Another sign described by a South African physician (Dr. L. Schamroth) on himself is elicited by apposing the dorsal surfaces of the terminal phalanges of corresponding fingers (**Figure 5-14**). Normally, there is a diamond-shaped space at the base of the nail bed. In clubbing, the diamond-shaped space is lost.

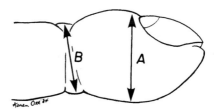

**Figure 5-12** Clubbing of the finger. (A) Height at the base of the nail. (B) Height at the distal interphalangeal joint.

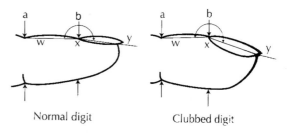

Normal digit                Clubbed digit

**Figure 5-13** Hyponychial angle. The middle of the distal inter-phalangeal joint is marked a. The junction of the nail and skin is marked b. The hyponychial angle is the angle wxy , which is 185 degrees for the normal digit. Hyponychial angle of over 190 degrees indicates clubbing.

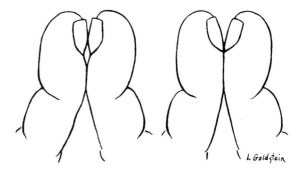

**Figure 5-14.** Schamroth sign. The diamond-shaped space at the base of the nail-bed seen in normal fingers (left) is lost in the presence of clubbing (right).

A beaked nail also will appear clubbed, but the height at the proximal edge of the nail will not be taller than the height at the distal interphalangeal joint. In hyperparathyroidism, though the finger is described as clubbed, it is a rounded, spatulous finger, not a clubbed finger.

In the palpatory method, the proximal edge of the nail feels like it is floating on a bed of water. *Evidence based data: Interobserver agreement between clinicians varies widely in recognizing clubbing at the bedside (k score 0.39-0.9). Accuracy of physical examination for clubbing is difficult to determine for want of an external standard. However, the presence of clubbing in adults is associated with LR of 3.9 for lung cancer and 2.8 for Crohn's disease.*

Tremor of the hands, flexion deformities, and unequal grip strength can be observed easily at this stage. Hand dominance also can be determined during this early stage by offering things to the child and seeing which hand comes out first. If a child can write, give the child a paper and pencil and see how the paper and the pencil are held.

## Hip

Barlow's maneuver is used to identify dislocated hip and Ortolani's maneuver to identify dislocatable hips. These tests should be done on all newborns and infants routinely, one hip at a time.

*How to Test for Developmental Dysplasia of the Hip*

1) Ortolani's maneuver: Place the infant in the supine position on the examining table. Take a grip over the slightly flexed hip with the thumb over the femoral triangle and the long middle finger over the greater trochanter (**Figure 5-15**). Flex the hip to 90 degrees in the neutral position and then bring it to the midabduction position. (This may be difficult to do and unilateral limitation of abduction suggests congenital dislocation of the hip.) With the thigh in midabduction position, press gently over the greater trochanter in a forward direction using the middle finger. A "clunk" is felt if the femoral head moves anteriorly into the socket with this maneuver, suggesting that it was out of place (dislocated) before pressure was applied.

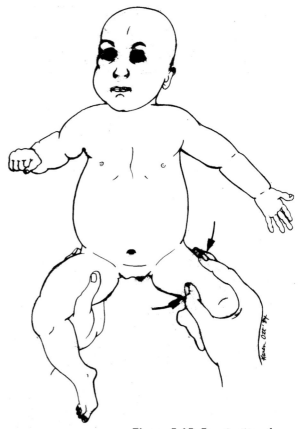

**Figure 5-15.** Examination of the hip joints for Developmental Dysplasia of the Hip (DDH).

2) Barlow's test is a provocative test to look for a dislocatable hip. Place the infant in the supine position and flex the hip to 90 degrees. Gently adduct the flexed hip and give a gentle posterior pressure over the medial aspect of the thigh using the thumb. If the femoral head moves out of the acetabulum with this pressure and returns back when the pressure is released, the hip is probably unstable. This is the original Barlow sign. During this procedure, whenever the femoral head moves into or moves out of the acetabulum, or when the flexed hip is abducted, you may feel a sensation of "clunk." This is different from the normal variant "click" that may be elicited during flexion and extension of the hip in newborn infants.

In untreated developmental dysplasia of the hip, one also may find the following: 1) the gluteal and thigh folds are asymmetric; 2) there is leg length discrepancy, with shortening of the affected limb; 3) there is limitation of abduction of the affected hip; and 4) with the child supine, if the knee joints and the hips are flexed and the feet are held flat on the table, the knee on the affected side is at a lower level. This is called the Allis sign (**Figure 5-16**).

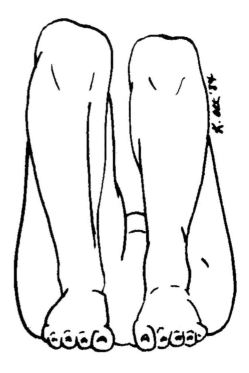

**Figure 5-16.** Allis sign. Note the lower level of the knee on the affected side.

# MEASUREABLE OBSERVATIONS

## Height

In infants and children below two years of age, height should be measured in a lying position (recumbent length) and older children should be measured in a standing position (stature). Two people may be needed to measure infants, with one holding the head in proper position and the other holding the feet and ankles. The head has to be aligned against the headboard so that a line connecting the external auditory meatus and the lower margin of the orbit is perpendicular to the table. The recumbent length should be recorded to the nearest 0.1 cm. For infants born prematurely, the chronological age should be corrected by the gestational age till 40 months of age.

When measuring stature in children older than two years, the feet should be bare with the child standing erect such that the occiput, shoulders, buttocks, and the heels touch the measuring board. The eyes should be looking straight ahead so that a line joining the external auditory meatus to the lower border of the eye socket is parallel to the floor. The readings are recorded to the nearest 0.1 cm. Normal values for height in American children are given in **Figures 5-17** to **5-20**.

## CDC Growth Charts: United States

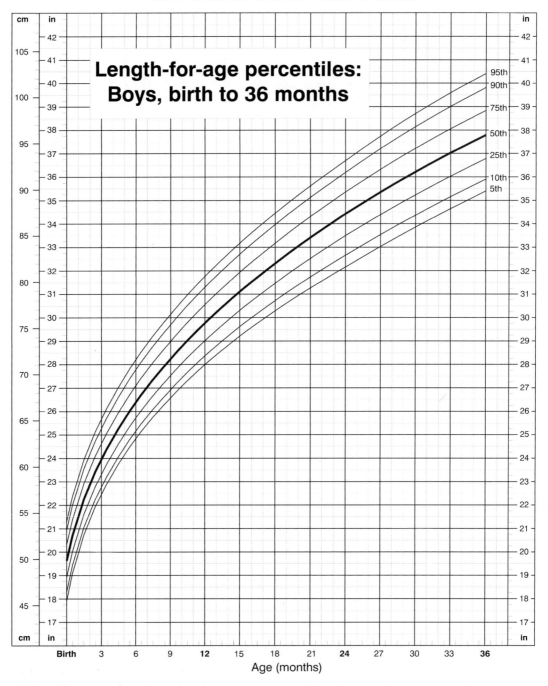

**Length-for-age percentiles: Boys, birth to 36 months**

**Figure 5-17.** Boys length in percentiles by age: from birth to 36 months.
SOURCE: Developed by the National Center for Health Statistics in collaboration with the National Center for Chronic Disease Prevention and Health Promotion (2000). http://www.cdc.gov/growthcharts Revised April 20, 2001

## CDC Growth Charts: United States

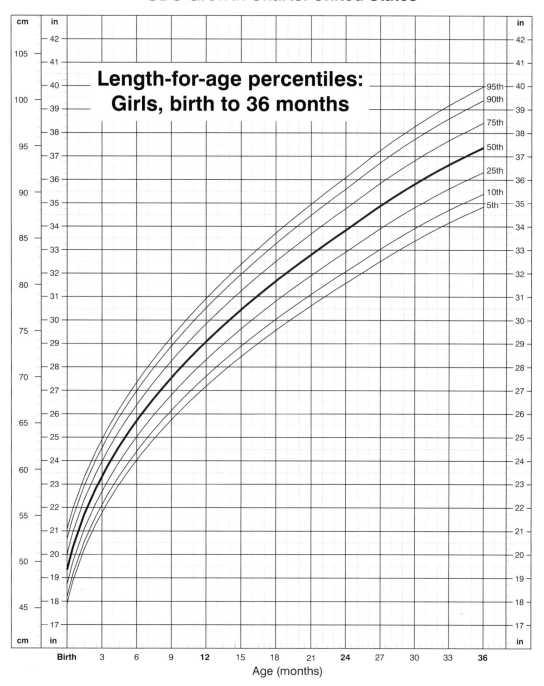

**Figure 5-18.** Girls length in percentiles by age: from birth to 36 months.
SOURCE: Developed by the National Center for Health Statistics in collaboration with the National Center for Chronic Disease Prevention and Health Promotion (2000). http://www.cdc.gov/growthcharts Revised April 20, 2001

# CDC Growth Charts: United States

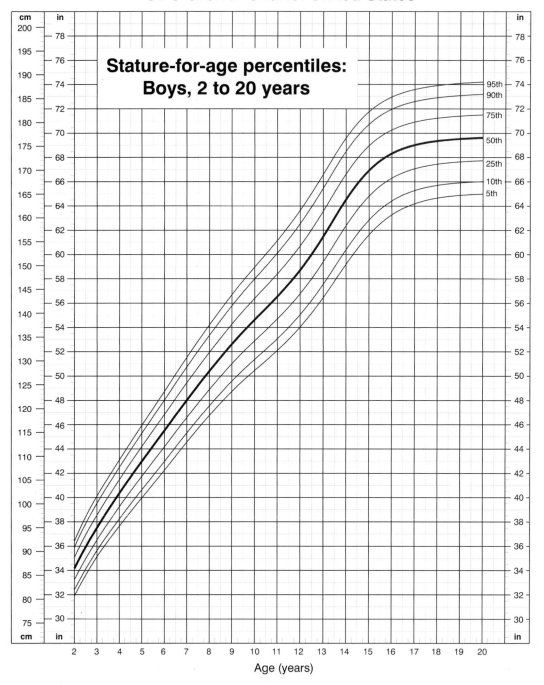

**Stature-for-age percentiles:
Boys, 2 to 20 years**

Age (years)

**Figure 5-19.** Boys stature in percentiles by age: from 2-20 years.
SOURCE: Developed by the National Center for Health Statistics in collaboration with the National Center for Chronic Disease Prevention and Health Promotion (2000). http://www.cdc.gov/growthcharts Revised April 20, 2001

# CDC Growth Charts: United States

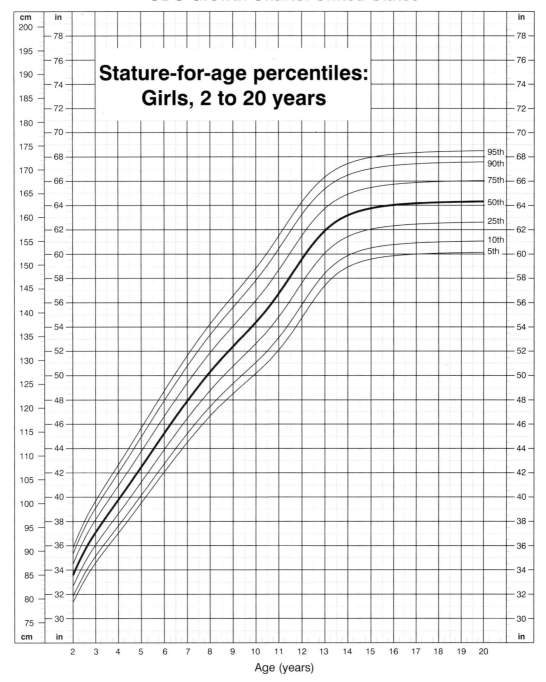

**Stature-for-age percentiles: Girls, 2 to 20 years**

**Figure 5-20.** Girls stature in percentiles by age: from 2-20 years.
SOURCE: Developed by the National Center for Health Statistics in collaboration with the National Center for Chronic Disease Prevention and Health Promotion (2000). http://www.cdc.gov/growthcharts Revised April 20, 2001

# Weight

Weight is taken preferably on the same scale at the same time of the day (before breakfast) with minimal clothing. Infants should be weighed preferably nude or with a dry diaper. Older children should be wearing light clothes and no shoes. There are different types of scales (infant scales, balance-beam, and read out) and they should be calibrated using standard weights every three to six months. Infants born prematurely should have their chronological age corrected by gestational age until 24 months of age.

Weight should be taken to the nearest 10 gm in infants and to the nearest 100 gm in older children. Pay attention to all details when accurate follow-up is essential, as in heart failure or in estimating dehydration. Normal values for weight in American children are given in **Figures 5-21** to **5-24**.

- A growth chart that can be modified to the needs of the country, both for home use and for primary care centers, was developed by the World Health Organization (WHO) and entitled "A Growth Chart for International Use in Maternal and Child Health Care" (World Health Organization, Geneva 1978). These were helpful only to document how infants and children grew in a particular geographical region and at a particular time. Since then, the WHO initiated a multicenter growth reference study and collected data from several countries including USA, Norway, Brazil, India, and Ghana. This data show clearly that growth up to five years of life is influenced more by nutrition, environment, and local practices than by genetics and ethnicity. These WHO child growth standards are available at www.who.int/childgrowth/en and as a supplement to Acta Paediatrica (2006;[Suppl]:450:5-101) (**Figures 5-25 and 5-26**). An initial set of graphs are available for weight, height, weight for length, and body mass index (BMI). It also includes windows of achievement in six key areas of motor development. Future publications of normative data on arm circumference-for-age, head circumference-for-age, subscapular skinfold-for-age, and triceps skinfold-for-age are planned.

WHO strongly recommends that these normative data be used worldwide since they will help parents, doctors, and policymakers know when the nutrition and healthcare needs of children are not being met. "The WHO child growth standards provide new means to support every child to get the best chance to develop in the most important formative years."

# Head Circumference

Head circumference is measured at the maximum point of occipital protuberance posteriorly and at a point just above the supraorbital ridge anteriorly. The tape is then moved slightly up or down to obtain the maximum circumference. Infants born prematurely should have their chronological age corrected by gestational age until 18 months of age.

Cloth tape is safer to use in uncooperative children but stretches easily. The cloth tape, therefore, should be periodically verified for accuracy by comparing it with a steel tape. Normal values for head circumference in boys and girls in the United States are given in **Figures 5-27** and **5-28**.

## CDC Growth Charts: United States

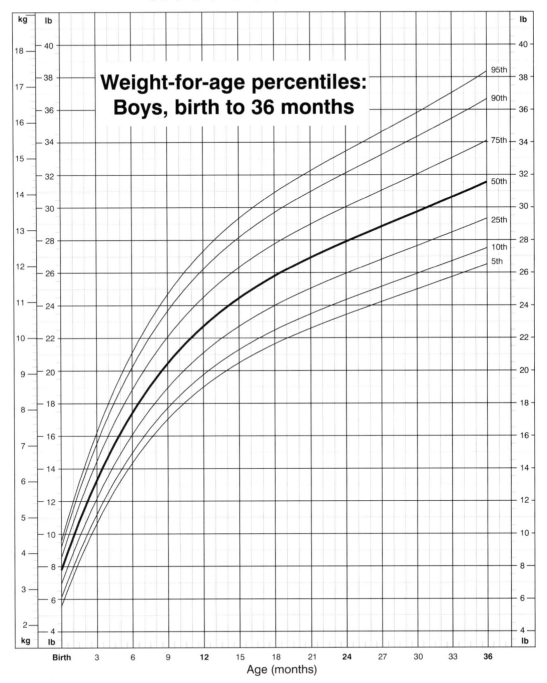

**Weight-for-age percentiles: Boys, birth to 36 months**

Age (months)

**Figure 5-21.** Boys weight in percentiles by age: from birth to 36 months.
SOURCE: Developed by the National Center for Health Statistics in collaboration with the National Center for Chronic Disease Prevention and Health Promotion (2000). http://www.cdc.gov/growthcharts Revised April 20, 2001

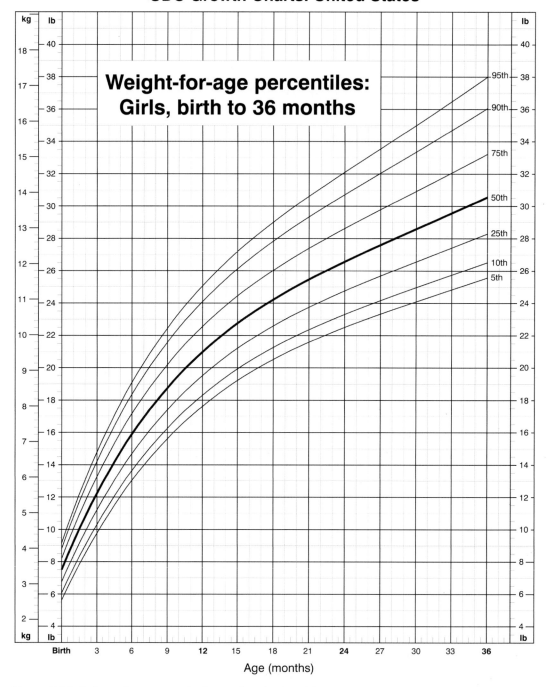

**CDC Growth Charts: United States**

**Weight-for-age percentiles:
Girls, birth to 36 months**

Age (months)

**Figure 5-22.** Girls weight in percentiles by age: from birth to 36 months.
SOURCE: Developed by the National Center for Health Statistics in collaboration with the National Center for Chronic Disease Prevention and Health Promotion (2000). http://www.cdc.gov/growthcharts Revised April 20, 2001

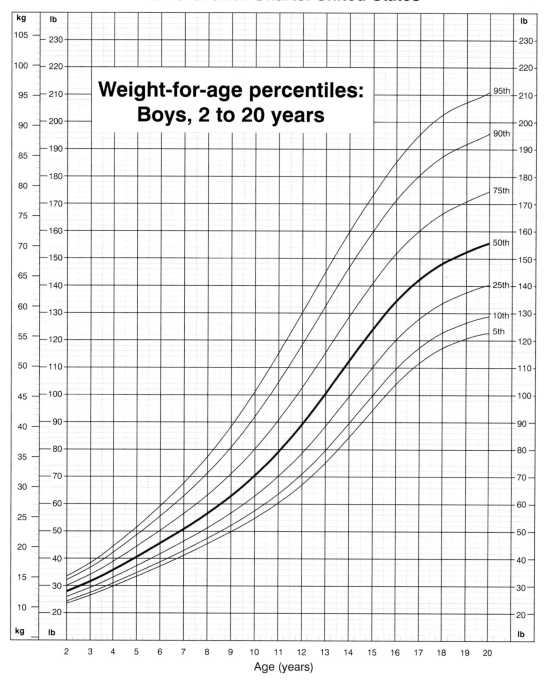

**CDC Growth Charts: United States**

Weight-for-age percentiles: Boys, 2 to 20 years

**Figure 5-23.** Boys weight in percentiles by age: from 2-20 years.
SOURCE: Developed by the National Center for Health Statistics in collaboration with the National Center for Chronic Disease Prevention and Health Promotion (2000). http://www.cdc.gov/growthcharts Revised April 20, 2001

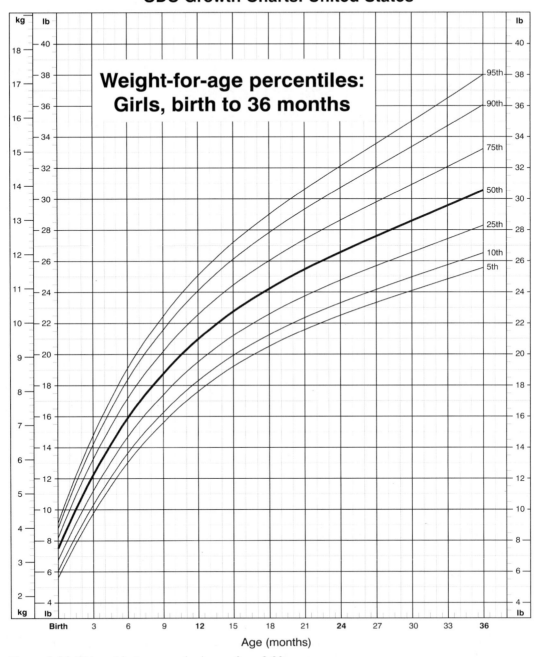

**Figure 5-24.** Girls weight in percentiles by age: from 2-20 years.
SOURCE: Developed by the National Center for Health Statistics in collaboration with the National Center for Chronic Disease Prevention and Health Promotion (2000). http://www.cdc.gov/growthcharts Revised April 20, 2001

**Figs. 5-17 to 5-24** SOURCE: Developed by the National Center for Health Statistics in collaboration with the National Center for Chronic Disease Prevention and Health Promotion (2000). http://www.cdc.gov/growthcharts Revised April 20, 2001

## Height-for-age BOYS

5 to 19 years (percentiles)

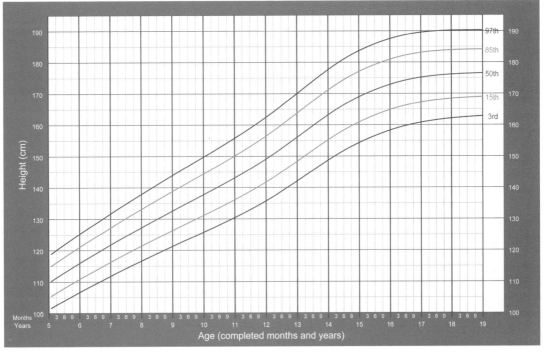

**Figure 5-25 A.** Height for age: Boys 5 to 19 years in percentiles.
Source: World Health Organization. http://www.who.int/childgrowth/standards/ chts_lhfa_girls_p/en/index.html

## Chest Circumference

Different studies have used different landmarks for the measurement of chest circumference. Some authors recommend placement of the tape at the level of the substernal notch (xiphoid process) anteriorly with the tape below the angle of the scapula posteriorly, in "mid-respiration." Others recommend placement of the tape across the nipple line and measurement midway between inspiration and expiration. Rheumatologists use the fourth intercostals space as the landmark. The examiner can choose one of these methods and be consistent with it, so that the values are comparable.

Normally at birth, head circumference is larger than chest circumference and remains so until six months of age. Later, chest circumference is larger than that of the head, except in the presence of malnutrition. However, in the presence of malnutrition, head circumference and chest circumference do not become equal until the first birthday.

*Evidence based examination: The mean absolute differences in the measurement of head circumferences of infants by two examiners were small (interobserver 0.37 and 0.36 cm; intraobserver 0.29 and 0.29). For chest circumference, the mean differences were more prominent (interobserver 0.59 and 0.72 cm; intraobserver 0.50 and 0.78 cm). (Measurement of chest expansion will be described in the section on examination of the chest, page 145).*

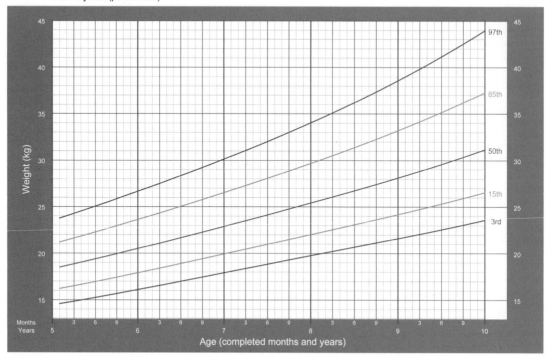

**Figure 5-25 B.** Weight for age: Boys 5 to 10 years in percentiles.
Source: World Health Organization. http://www.who.int/childgrowth/standards/ chts_lhfa_girls_p/en/index.html

## Other Measurements

1. *Arm span* is measured from the tip of the middle finger of one hand to that of the other hand with both shoulders abducted to 90 degrees and the palms supinated. Normally arm span equals total height. (Arm span is significantly less than total height in skeletal dysplasia syndromes. In Marfan syndrome, arm span is longer than the total height.)

2. *Sitting height* versus standing height: Sitting height is measured as described under the section on height (page 77), except the child is sitting close to the scale. Normally in a newborn, sitting height is approximately 70% of the total length. By age three years, it is 57% of total height, and at puberty it is 52% of total height. This may help identify skeletal dysplasia syndromes.

3. *Skinfold thickness* is a measure of adiposity and is no longer commonly used. Measuring skin fold thickness accurately and reproducibly is almost impossible in obese children. Skin fat fold thickness may not be a reliable indicator of total body fat. However, this measurement may be useful in following individual patient's response to nutritional therapy. There are varieties of calipers available for skinfold measurement such as Lange (Beta Technology, Santa Cruz,CA) and Harpenden (Baty International, West Sussex, UK). Measurements are made over the

# Height-for-age  GIRLS

5 to 19 years (percentiles)

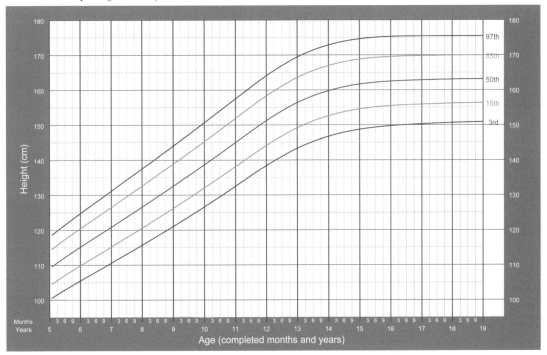

**Figure 5-26 A.** Height for age: Girls 5-19 years in percentiles.
Source: World Health Organization. http://www.who.int/childgrowth/standards/ chts_lhfa_girls_p/en/index.html

triceps and suprailiac crest on the left side as indicators of distribution of fat in the limbs and in the trunk. With the elbow in 90 degrees of flexion, a horizontal mark is made at a point midway between the tip of the acromion process and the tip of the olecranon process with the arm bent at a right angle. With the arm now hanging at the side of the body, a vertical line is placed to cross the horizontal line indicating the midpoint. A piece of skin is pinched between the left thumb and index finger, and the caliper is used to measure the thickness of fat. Details of proper techniques of measurement and software for calculation of body fat are available at the websites associated with the calipers. (http://www.beta-technology.com/lange and www.baty.co.uk)

4.  Muscle bulk is estimated by measurement of the mid-upper arm circumference and is very useful in following children with malnutrition on treatment, combined with measurement of skinfold thickness (which measures fat). Mid-upper arm circumference may help determine the proportion of fat to muscle. The area to be measured is marked on the left side as described in the section on skinfold thickness. With the arm hanging by the side, a steel tape is passed around the circumference of the arm (the tape should not be held tight enough to produce an indentation) and the measurement noted in centimeters.

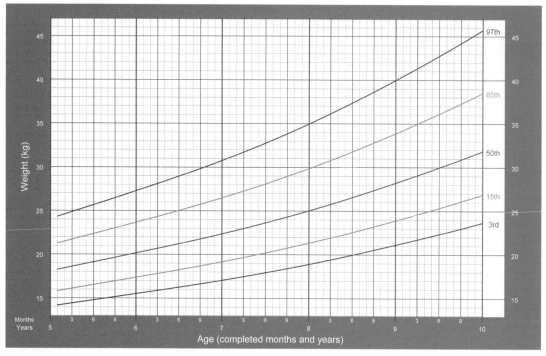

**Figure 5-26 B.** Weight for age: Girls 5 to 10 years in percentiles.
Source: World Health Organization. http://www.who.int/childgrowth/standards/ chts_lhfa_girls_p/en/index.html

## Temperature

In 1868, Carl Reinhold August Wunderlich firmly established that body temperature is constant within a specified range in healthy persons, and variation in temperature is evidence of a disease process. He defined what constitutes subnormal temperature, fever, and high fever. Based on recent studies, fever is considered to be present if the temperature is over 37.6°C by tympanic thermometry and over 38°C by rectal measurment. A body temperature of over 42°C suggests hyperthermia and below 35°C is considered hypothermia.

Although physicians and mothers are more often interested only in the presence or absence of fever, it is one of the vital signs and accurate measurement of temperature is necessary in the neonate, hospitalized patients (particularly in the ICU), febrile seizures, in immunocompromised children and in hypothermic conditions. Changes in body temperature have to be documented during anesthesia and in conditions associated with hyperthermia and hypothermia.

The temperature of deep body tissues, called the core temperature, is maintained at 37° C (+/- 0.6) through homeostatic mechanisms. Core temperature is defined as temperature measured within the pulmonary artery. Temperature measured with special probes at the lower end of the esophagus, in the bladder and over the anterior, inferior quadrant of the tympanic membrane gives an indication of the body's core temperature. However, these are neither practical nor necessary in clinical practice.

## CDC Growth Charts: United States

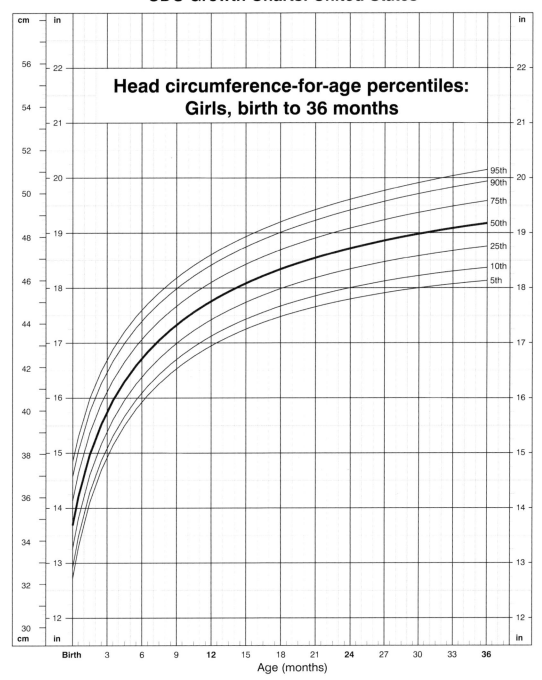

**Head circumference-for-age percentiles: Girls, birth to 36 months**

**Figure 5-27.** Head circumference in Girls in percentiles: from birth to 36 months.
SOURCE: Developed by the National Center for Health Statistics in collaboration with the National Center for Chronic Disease Prevention and Health Promotion (2000). http://www.cdc.gov/growthcharts Revised April 20, 2001

## CDC Growth Charts: United States

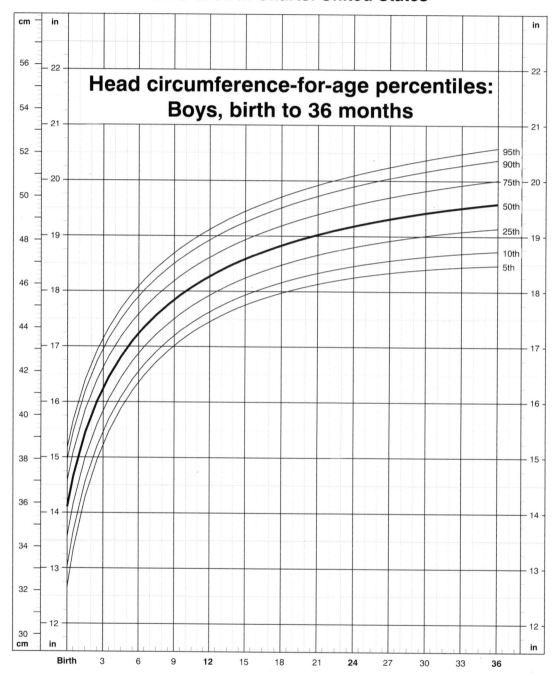

**Head circumference-for-age percentiles: Boys, birth to 36 months**

**Figure 5-28.** Head circumference in Boys in percentiles: from birth to 36 months.
SOURCE: Developed by the National Center for Health Statistics in collaboration with the National Center for Chronic Disease Prevention and Health Promotion (2000). http://www.cdc.gov/growthcharts Revised April 20, 2001

## Table 5-5. Normal Body Temperatures at different sites *

**AXILLA:** Range: 34.7° to 37.3° C

Advantage: easily accessible site; safe

Disadvantage: takes longer contact time; poor sensitivity; poor correlation with core temperature.

Comment: Useful in neonates.

**SUBLINGUAL:** Range: 33.2° to 38.2°

Advantage: Easily accessible; convenient; relatively safe.

Disadvantage: Accuracy affected by several factors such as proper placement of the thermometer under the right or left sublingual pockets (not under the tip of the tongue), mouth breathing, recent ingestion of hot or cold liquid, tachypnoea; co-operation of the child is needed; oral laceration and cross infections have been reported.

Comments: Useful in children over 5 years of age who can cooperate; more reliable than rectal when there is rapid alterations in body temperature.

**RECTAL:** Range: 34.4° to 37.8°

Advantage: Has been in use for a long time; good sensitivity; reasonable correlation with core temperature; arguable status as the gold standard.

Disadvantage: Inconvenience, discomfort and embarrassment to children and also frightening to the very young; hygiene and transmission of infection are issues; perforation of rectum has been reported; relative contra-indication in neutropenic patient and in patients with rapid changes in temperature.

Comments: Routinely used in children under 3 to 5 years of age; lubrication of the instrument and proper and gentle placement and use of gloves by the examiner are necessary.

**TYMPANIC:** Range: 35.4° to 37.8°

Advantage: easy to use; fast; clean and safe.

Disadvantage: Operator dependent; not reliable in neonates; beam has to be directed at the ear drum; cerumen in the ear and otitis will give false readings. Sensitivity is questionable. Too many false negatives.

Comments: It is the most commonly used method. However, when failure to detect fever can have serious consequences, an alternate, appropriate method has to be used.

*Several sources*

Different types of thermometers are available for routine use in children: oral (mercury in glass or electronic), rectal (mercury in glass or electronic), ear canal (infra red) and skin (thermophototropic crystals). The skin strip method is inaccurate with both false-positive and false-negative results. Mercury-in-glass thermometers are still popular and in use in many parts of the world, although they are being replaced by digital electronic thermometers. The oral thermometer has a long mercury section and a blue tip for identification. The bulb of the rectal thermometer is round, and there is a red identification on the tip. In very active and frightened children, trying to put a glass instrument into the rectum can be a traumatic experience and can be dangerous. There are reports of broken thermometers with rectal perforation, and they are not used in some countries. Electronic thermometers avoid this complication and give digital read-outs of temperature, some in both the Centigrade and in Fahrenheit scales. (**Table 5-5**)

There are several problems with taking oral temperature in children although it is more accurate than axillary temperature. Generally, oral temperature cannot be taken in children who are young and cannot understand instructions. Therefore, most of the time, the temperature is measured in the axilla. This is inaccurate compared with core temperature. If axillary temperature is to be taken, remember to hold the thermometer for longer duration ( about 4-5 minutes for the mercury type and 1 to 1 ½ minutes for the digital types), and also remember that axillary temperature is at least 0.5°C lower than the oral temperature.

Tympanic membrane temperature gives a close approximation of the core temperature and is currently the most popular method at home and in the clinics. The thermometer used most commonly in routine clinical practice is the external ear thermometer. It works on the principle of infra red reflections from the tympanic membrane and its accuracy is operator dependent. Cerumen in the ear, direction of the ear canal and the presence of otitis media may give false values. There are several in the market with wide variations in the range and accuracy. External ear thermometry may not give accurate results particularly in children younger than three years of age.

Patterns of fever may have some diagnostic value. However, they are difficult to document since the fever patterns are altered by the early, frequent, and universal use of antipyretics in children with fever. Some of the known patterns are 1) continuous fever when daily fluctuations do not exceed 1°C (1.5°F) as in typhoid, 2) hectic fever as in Kawasaski disease, and 3) intermittent fever when the temperature touches normal for several hours in a day. The intermittent fever is called "quotidian" if it occurs daily (as in JRA or JIA), "tertian" if it occurs every other day (malaria), and "quartan" when it occurs every third day (malaria). Daily rise of temperature in the evening is seen in TB and JIA. In JIA, the temperature returns to normal and actually goes subnormal the next morning. Double rise of temperature also is seen in JIA and typhoid fever, but in typhoid it does not reach normal at its low point.

Fever with chills is seen in all infectious processes, but particularly in urinary tract infections, TB, and malaria.

## Table 5-6. Normal Pulse Rate

| Age | Pulse Rate/Minute (Range) |
|---|---|
| Newborn | 70-170 |
| Up to 1 year | 80-160 |
| 2 years | 80-130 |
| 4 years | 80-120 |
| 6 years | 75-115 |
| 8 to 10 years | 70-110 |
| Adolescent years | 65-110 |
| 18 years and over | 55-95 |

# Pulse

Sir John Floyer invented a watch with a second hand and published his article on "Physician's Pulse Watch" in 1707. If the older method of feeling the radial artery is used, data on the following characteristics of the pulse should be noted: 1) rate, 2) rhythm, 3) volume, and 4) tension. Normal pulse rates for various ages are given in **Table 5-6**.

The rhythm is either regular or irregular. Regular rhythm does not necessarily indicate a normal heart. Actually, it is a good practice to always listen to the heart when counting the pulse to appreciate missed beats. One can have an arrhythmia in which every other beat is not carried to the periphery as a pulse, so that the pulse rate is 50% of the heart rate. Thus, a regular rhythm may be perceived peripherally, even though a serious arrhythmia exists.

Sinus arrhythmia is characterized by a rapid pulse during inspiration and a slower pulse during expiration. This is normal. A regularly irregular pulse may be observed when there are extra systoles at fixed intervals (every fifth beat or tenth beat). Irregularly irregular pulse is seen most often in auricular fibrillation.

Volume of the pulse is appreciated by the lift of the fingers as the pulse wave passes through. It is a composite of the force with which the fingers are lifted and the duration for which the force is maintained. Large volume pulse is seen in fever, thyrotoxicosis, anemia, patent ductus, and aortic regurgitation. Small volume pulse is seen in shock and aortic stenosis.

Estimate tension by noting the force required to obliterate the pulse; however, this is an unnecessary procedure. Measurement of blood pressure is more exact and will be dealt with later.

Certain types of pulse are diagnostically important. In sinus arrhythmia, the pulse rate gets fast with inspiration and slow with expiration. This is normal. Collapsing pulse is best felt with the arm raised above the head and the pulse felt by the palmar aspect of your proximal interphalangeal joints. This type of pulse is felt in patent ductus and aortic regurgitation. Another method of feeling for collapsing pulse is to feel the superficial palmar arch as it crosses the metacarpal heads. Forceful pulsation of this arch is uncommon in infants below two years of age and, if present in the absence of fever and anemia, indicates patent ductus.

*Pulsus paradoxus:* Pulsus paradoxus is said to be present when the pulse volume gets lower and even disappears at the end of inspiration. The presence of pulsus paradoxus is best confirmed by listening to the Korotkoff sounds, while measuring blood pressure during inspiration and expiration. The patient should be sitting comfortably with the arm at the side. A proper size cuff should be used. Inflate the cuff until the pulse disappears completely. Then, deflate the cuff very slowly at approximately 2-mm of Hg per second while auscultating over the brachial artery. Note the pressure at a point when the first Korotkoff sounds are heard. Initially these are intermittent, audible during the expiratory phase of respiration. Now continue to deflate the pressure slowly until every Korotkoff sound is heard. Note the pressure at this point. This may have to be repeated three times with a pause between. In adults, normal mean difference is 0.6 mm with 95% confidence interval of 0.6 to 2.1 mm. A difference of over 10 mm between systolic pressure at a point when sounds are heard intermittently and at a point when every sound is heard indicates the presence of pulsus paradoxus. If pulsus paradoxus is present, the differential diagnosis includes pericardial effusion and severe airway obstruction (bronchial asthma).

An alternate method of measuring pulsus paradoxus using pulse oximeter has not been tested in children. The combination of distended neck veins, muffled heart sounds, and hypotension is called Beck's triad and suggests cardiac tamponade.

*Evidence based data: Dyspnea is the most sensitive symptom (87%-88%) for the presence of cardiac tamponade. The LR for a pulsus paradoxus of >10 mm Hg was found to be 3.3 (95% CI, 1.8-6.3).*

After feeling the radial artery, also feel the pulse in the temporal arteries, femoral arteries, and dorsalis pedis. The femoral pulse is felt at a point midway between the symphysis pubis and anterior superior iliac spine along the inguinal ligament. Feel the radial artery while feeling the femoral artery. Strongly felt pulse in the arm together with a delay between the pulse in the upper and lower limbs or a higher volume of the pulse in the upper limbs indicates coarctation of the aorta.

Another method for detecting coarctation of the aorta is to have the child lie prone, flex the knee joints, and place the palms of the child's hands close to the feet. In the presence of coarctation of aorta, the pale color of the feet will contrast markedly with the normal colored palms.

## Blood Pressure

There are different types of instruments to measure blood pressure. Accurate systolic measurements can be obtained using Doppler instruments. Mercury or aneroid variety of sphygmomanometers and oscillometric devices are the instruments commonly used in clinical practice. A sphygmomanometer with a mercury column is the most accepted instrument.

To obtain a proper blood pressure recording in older children, blood pressure cuffs of the following sizes are available: 3 cm, 5 cm, 8 cm, 12 cm, and 18 cm. The 18-cm cuff is for recording pressures in the lower limb and for obese adolescents. A narrower cuff will give spuriously high blood pressure and a broader cuff will give a lower blood pressure.

Other points to observe in taking blood pressure are:

1.  Mercury type manometers are superior to the aneroid variety.
2.  If an aneroid manometer is used, it should be checked for accuracy against a properly functioning mercury manometer.
3.  The mercury manometer should be checked for leaking and zero line.
4.  The bladder of the cuff should cover 80% to 100% of the circumference of the upper arm.
5.  The width of the cuff should be 40% of the circumference of the upper arm.
6.  The patient should be seated without crying or agitation for at least five minutes before the readings are taken.
7.  The arm should be at the level of the heart.
8.  The mercury column should be vertical and the blood pressure reading read at the observer's eye level to avoid parallax error.
9.  The cuff should be wrapped snugly around the limb with enough space at the antecubital fossa or popliteal fossa for the stethoscope.
10. Before auscultating for the blood pressure, it is a good habit to first estimate systolic blood pressure by palpation. This relaxes the child. One also gets an idea of how high one has to inflate the bag.

11. In the presence of dyspnea and arrhythmia, the readings at which the sounds disappear should be recorded for both the stronger sound and the weaker sound.

12. Systolic pressure in the lower limb is normally 10 to 40 mm higher than in the upper limb, but the diastolic pressure is the same.

13. If the blood pressure is found to be elevated, repeat the measurement, preferably outside of the hospital/office setting, before embarking on an expensive work-up (unless the elevations are significant with associated symptoms and signs).

For recording blood pressure, inflate the cuff rapidly for about 10 to 20 mm Hg above the point at which the pulse in the radial artery disappears. Place the stethoscope over the brachial artery. Slowly release the pressure (2 to 4 mm Hg per heartbeat), while listening until the first sound (Korotkoff sound) is heard. This point, at which the first sound is heard, is the systolic pressure. Now continue to slowly release the pressure. As the pressure is lowered, the sound suddenly becomes faint or muffled and finally ceases. Diastolic pressure is best measured at the point of complete disappearance of the sound. Normal values for boys and girls are given in **Tables 5-7** and **5-8**, respectively.

## Respiration

Count the respiration for a full minute when the child has been at rest for a few minutes or while sleeping. Even in sleep, the rate may vary depending on the sleep cycle. In the presence of fever, respiratory rate increases by 10 breaths per minute for each degree rise in temperature. Normal rates are given in **Table 5-9**. The other characteristics of respiration to be noted are rhythm, depth, positions of discomfort, and adventitious sounds.

Alternate periods of deep and shallow respiration with recurring periods of apnea occur in left ventricular failure and in cerebral edema. This is called "Cheyne-Stokes" respiration. Biot's breathing is characterized by periods of apnea alternating with four or five breaths of normal depth. This type of breathing is seen in association with increased intracranial pressure. Respiratory rhythm in the neonate is discussed in Chapter 12A.

Rapid, deep respiration is seen in metabolic acidosis (salicylate overdose, diabetes). (Tachypnea is rapid, but not deep, breathing.) This is also called "Kussmaul" breathing. Shallow respiration is seen in narcotic overdosage and shock.

Orthopnea is indicative of pulmonary edema. An asthmatic child likes to sit up at the edge of the bed and lean forward with the palms on either tide. The child with pleurisy or a fractured rib splints the side of involvement. This child feels more comfortable lying on the involved side. In the presence of massive effusion, the discomfort is increased if the child is made to lie on the opposite (uninvolved) side.

Adventitious sounds audible even without a stethoscope are due to pathology in the upper airway. (The only exception is the wheezing sound of an asthmatic.) The sniffling sounds of nasal obstruction, snoring noise of soft palate weakness, the rattling sound of mucus in the trachea, and the crowing inspiratory stridor of laryngeal obstruction are examples of adventitious sounds. Two interesting points to note are 1) all noises due to upper airway problems are inspiratory noises, and 2) children with upper airway obstruction cannot appose the alae nasi to the midline cartilage during deep inspiration.

## Table 5-7. BP Levels for Boys by Age and Height Percentile

| Age, y | BP Percentile | SBP, mm Hg Percentile of Height | | | | | | | DBP, mm Hg Percentile of Height | | | | | | |
|--------|---------------|------|------|------|------|------|------|------|------|------|------|------|------|------|------|
| | | 5th | 10th | 25th | 50th | 75th | 90th | 95th | 5th | 10th | 25th | 50th | 75th | 90th | 95th |
| 1 | 50th | 80 | 81 | 83 | 85 | 87 | 88 | 89 | 34 | 35 | 36 | 37 | 38 | 39 | 39 |
| | 90th | 94 | 95 | 97 | 99 | 100 | 102 | 103 | 49 | 50 | 51 | 52 | 53 | 53 | 54 |
| | 95th | 98 | 99 | 101 | 103 | 104 | 106 | 106 | 54 | 54 | 55 | 56 | 57 | 58 | 58 |
| | 99th | 105 | 106 | 108 | 110 | 112 | 113 | 114 | 61 | 62 | 63 | 64 | 65 | 66 | 66 |
| 2 | 50th | 84 | 85 | 87 | 88 | 90 | 92 | 92 | 39 | 40 | 41 | 42 | 43 | 44 | 44 |
| | 90th | 97 | 99 | 100 | 102 | 104 | 105 | 106 | 54 | 55 | 56 | 57 | 58 | 58 | 59 |
| | 95th | 101 | 102 | 104 | 106 | 108 | 109 | 110 | 59 | 59 | 60 | 61 | 62 | 63 | 63 |
| | 99th | 109 | 110 | 111 | 113 | 115 | 117 | 117 | 66 | 67 | 68 | 69 | 70 | 71 | 71 |
| 3 | 50th | 86 | 87 | 89 | 91 | 93 | 94 | 95 | 44 | 44 | 45 | 46 | 47 | 48 | 48 |
| | 90th | 100 | 101 | 103 | 105 | 107 | 108 | 109 | 59 | 59 | 60 | 61 | 62 | 63 | 63 |
| | 95th | 104 | 105 | 107 | 109 | 110 | 112 | 113 | 63 | 63 | 64 | 65 | 66 | 67 | 67 |
| | 99th | 111 | 112 | 114 | 116 | 118 | 119 | 120 | 71 | 71 | 72 | 73 | 74 | 75 | 75 |
| 4 | 50th | 88 | 89 | 91 | 93 | 95 | 96 | 97 | 47 | 48 | 49 | 50 | 51 | 51 | 52 |
| | 90th | 102 | 103 | 105 | 107 | 109 | 110 | 111 | 62 | 63 | 64 | 65 | 66 | 66 | 67 |
| | 95th | 106 | 107 | 109 | 111 | 112 | 114 | 115 | 66 | 67 | 68 | 69 | 70 | 71 | 71 |
| | 99th | 113 | 114 | 116 | 118 | 120 | 121 | 122 | 74 | 75 | 76 | 77 | 78 | 78 | 79 |
| 5 | 50th | 90 | 91 | 93 | 95 | 96 | 98 | 98 | 50 | 51 | 52 | 53 | 54 | 55 | 55 |
| | 90th | 104 | 105 | 106 | 108 | 110 | 111 | 112 | 65 | 66 | 67 | 68 | 69 | 69 | 70 |
| | 95th | 108 | 109 | 110 | 112 | 114 | 115 | 116 | 69 | 70 | 71 | 72 | 73 | 74 | 74 |
| | 99th | 115 | 116 | 118 | 120 | 121 | 123 | 123 | 77 | 78 | 79 | 80 | 81 | 81 | 82 |
| 6 | 50th | 91 | 92 | 94 | 96 | 98 | 99 | 100 | 53 | 53 | 54 | 55 | 56 | 57 | 57 |
| | 90th | 105 | 106 | 108 | 110 | 111 | 113 | 113 | 68 | 68 | 69 | 70 | 71 | 72 | 72 |
| | 95th | 109 | 110 | 112 | 114 | 115 | 117 | 117 | 72 | 72 | 73 | 74 | 75 | 76 | 76 |
| | 99th | 116 | 117 | 119 | 121 | 123 | 124 | 125 | 80 | 80 | 81 | 82 | 83 | 84 | 84 |
| 7 | 50th | 92 | 94 | 95 | 97 | 99 | 100 | 101 | 55 | 55 | 56 | 57 | 58 | 59 | 59 |
| | 90th | 106 | 107 | 109 | 111 | 113 | 114 | 115 | 70 | 70 | 71 | 72 | 73 | 74 | 74 |
| | 95th | 110 | 111 | 113 | 115 | 117 | 118 | 119 | 74 | 74 | 75 | 76 | 77 | 78 | 78 |
| | 99th | 117 | 118 | 120 | 122 | 124 | 125 | 126 | 82 | 82 | 83 | 84 | 85 | 86 | 86 |
| 8 | 50th | 94 | 95 | 97 | 99 | 100 | 102 | 102 | 56 | 57 | 58 | 59 | 60 | 60 | 61 |
| | 90th | 107 | 109 | 110 | 112 | 114 | 115 | 116 | 71 | 72 | 72 | 73 | 74 | 75 | 76 |
| | 95th | 111 | 112 | 114 | 116 | 118 | 119 | 120 | 75 | 76 | 77 | 78 | 79 | 79 | 80 |
| | 99th | 119 | 120 | 122 | 123 | 125 | 127 | 127 | 83 | 84 | 85 | 86 | 87 | 87 | 88 |

| Age, y | BP Percentile | SBP, mm Hg Percentile of Height | | | | | | | DBP, mm Hg Percentile of Height | | | | | | |
|---|---|---|---|---|---|---|---|---|---|---|---|---|---|---|---|
| | | 5th | 10th | 25th | 50th | 75th | 90th | 95th | 5th | 10th | 25th | 50th | 75th | 90th | 95th |
| 9 | 50th | 95 | 96 | 98 | 100 | 102 | 103 | 104 | 57 | 58 | 59 | 60 | 61 | 61 | 62 |
| | 90th | 109 | 110 | 112 | 114 | 115 | 117 | 118 | 72 | 73 | 74 | 75 | 76 | 76 | 77 |
| | 95th | 113 | 114 | 116 | 118 | 119 | 121 | 121 | 76 | 77 | 78 | 79 | 80 | 81 | 81 |
| | 99th | 120 | 121 | 123 | 125 | 127 | 128 | 129 | 84 | 85 | 86 | 87 | 88 | 88 | 89 |
| 10 | 50th | 97 | 98 | 100 | 102 | 103 | 105 | 106 | 58 | 59 | 60 | 61 | 61 | 62 | 63 |
| | 90th | 111 | 112 | 114 | 115 | 117 | 119 | 119 | 73 | 73 | 74 | 75 | 76 | 77 | 78 |
| | 95th | 115 | 116 | 117 | 119 | 121 | 122 | 123 | 77 | 78 | 79 | 80 | 81 | 81 | 82 |
| | 99th | 122 | 123 | 125 | 127 | 128 | 130 | 130 | 85 | 86 | 86 | 88 | 88 | 89 | 90 |
| 11 | 50th | 99 | 100 | 102 | 104 | 105 | 107 | 107 | 59 | 59 | 60 | 61 | 62 | 63 | 63 |
| | 90th | 113 | 114 | 115 | 117 | 119 | 120 | 121 | 74 | 74 | 75 | 76 | 77 | 78 | 78 |
| | 95th | 117 | 118 | 119 | 121 | 123 | 124 | 125 | 78 | 78 | 79 | 80 | 81 | 82 | 82 |
| | 99th | 124 | 125 | 127 | 129 | 130 | 132 | 132 | 86 | 86 | 87 | 88 | 89 | 90 | 90 |
| 12 | 50th | 101 | 102 | 104 | 106 | 108 | 109 | 110 | 59 | 60 | 61 | 62 | 63 | 63 | 64 |
| | 90th | 115 | 116 | 118 | 120 | 121 | 123 | 123 | 74 | 75 | 75 | 76 | 77 | 78 | 79 |
| | 95th | 119 | 120 | 122 | 123 | 125 | 127 | 127 | 78 | 79 | 80 | 81 | 82 | 82 | 83 |
| | 99th | 126 | 127 | 129 | 131 | 133 | 134 | 135 | 86 | 87 | 88 | 89 | 90 | 90 | 91 |
| 13 | 50th | 104 | 105 | 106 | 108 | 110 | 111 | 112 | 60 | 60 | 61 | 62 | 63 | 64 | 64 |
| | 90th | 117 | 118 | 120 | 122 | 124 | 125 | 126 | 75 | 75 | 76 | 77 | 78 | 79 | 79 |
| | 95th | 121 | 122 | 124 | 126 | 128 | 129 | 130 | 79 | 79 | 80 | 81 | 82 | 83 | 83 |
| | 99th | 128 | 130 | 131 | 133 | 135 | 136 | 137 | 87 | 87 | 88 | 89 | 90 | 91 | 91 |
| 14 | 50th | 106 | 107 | 109 | 111 | 113 | 114 | 115 | 60 | 61 | 62 | 63 | 64 | 65 | 65 |
| | 90th | 120 | 121 | 123 | 125 | 126 | 128 | 128 | 75 | 76 | 77 | 78 | 79 | 79 | 80 |
| | 95th | 124 | 125 | 127 | 128 | 130 | 132 | 132 | 80 | 80 | 81 | 82 | 83 | 84 | 84 |
| | 99th | 131 | 132 | 134 | 136 | 138 | 139 | 140 | 87 | 88 | 89 | 90 | 91 | 92 | 92 |
| 15 | 50th | 109 | 110 | 112 | 113 | 115 | 117 | 117 | 61 | 62 | 63 | 64 | 65 | 66 | 66 |
| | 90th | 122 | 124 | 125 | 127 | 129 | 130 | 131 | 76 | 77 | 78 | 79 | 80 | 80 | 81 |
| | 95th | 126 | 127 | 129 | 131 | 133 | 134 | 135 | 81 | 81 | 82 | 83 | 84 | 85 | 85 |
| | 99th | 134 | 135 | 136 | 138 | 140 | 142 | 142 | 88 | 89 | 90 | 91 | 92 | 93 | 93 |
| 16 | 50th | 111 | 112 | 114 | 116 | 118 | 119 | 120 | 63 | 63 | 64 | 65 | 66 | 67 | 67 |
| | 90th | 125 | 126 | 128 | 130 | 131 | 133 | 134 | 78 | 78 | 79 | 80 | 81 | 82 | 82 |
| | 95th | 129 | 130 | 132 | 134 | 135 | 137 | 137 | 82 | 83 | 83 | 84 | 85 | 86 | 87 |
| | 99th | 136 | 137 | 139 | 141 | 143 | 144 | 145 | 90 | 90 | 91 | 92 | 93 | 94 | 94 |
| 17 | 50th | 114 | 115 | 116 | 118 | 120 | 121 | 122 | 65 | 66 | 66 | 67 | 68 | 69 | 70 |
| | 90th | 127 | 128 | 130 | 132 | 134 | 135 | 136 | 80 | 80 | 81 | 82 | 83 | 84 | 84 |
| | 95th | 131 | 132 | 134 | 136 | 138 | 139 | 140 | 84 | 85 | 86 | 87 | 87 | 88 | 89 |
| | 99th | 139 | 140 | 141 | 143 | 145 | 146 | 147 | 92 | 93 | 93 | 94 | 95 | 96 | 97 |

*From: www.nhlbi.nih.gov/guidelines/hypertension/child_tbl.htm*

## Shape

Observe the skull from different angles: front, side (profile view), back, chin (worm's eye view), and top (bird's eye view). This will allow observation of the cheeks, orbits, and mid-face as well.

*Abnormal shapes* may be described under three headings: flattened, prominent, and specific shapes.

A flat occiput or parietal region may be seen in children who lie in one position for prolonged periods, as in some normal children and in children with mental retardation or severe muscle weaknesses.

Prominent occiput may be seen in Dandy-Walker syndrome and Trisomy 18. Frontal bossing is seen in rickets, Crouzon syndrome, and Hurler syndrome. Biparietal bossing may indicate subdural hematoma. Caput succedaneum may be seen in newborns.

Some of the abnormalities of shape of the head with descriptive names include oxycephaly (tower head), which is caused by premature closure of all the sutures resulting in the growth of the head in the region of the anterior fontanel (e.g., Apert syndrome); turricephaly in which the top of the head is pointed; brachycephaly, which is a short, wide, broad forehead (e.g., Down syndrome); plagiocephaly (one side rounded more than the other) due to unequal closure of cranial sutures as in craniostenosis; trigonocephaly in which the metopic suture is pointed (e.g., hyperphosphatasia-osteoectasia syndrome); scaphocephaly in which the head is elongated in the anteroposterior direction when seen in profile (e.g., craniostenosis, Sotos syndrome). Some normal children may have a slightly elongated head.

*The word normocephaly should be used only in reference to normal shape of the head, and not to denote absence of any abnormal findings.*

## Abnormal Swelling

Next, palpate for abnormal swelling (extra growth) which may be congenital (dermoid), traumatic (hematoma due to trauma), infectious such as abscess, or tumors. Describe these conditions using the standard *descriptors for swellings*: location, size, shape, characteristics of the margin and of the surface, consistency, color, heat, tenderness, pulsation as may be felt over vascular malformations (or absence of it), and attachment of the swelling to deeper and surrounding structures.

## Abnormal Depressions (Continuity)

Next, look for depressions and defects (continuity) in the skull which may be abnormal (as in fracture or burrhole) or normal (as in fontanel).

## Color

Patches of abnormal color may indicate a nevus, vascular malformation, or a bruise. Bruise over the mastoid process is called Battle's sign and is pathognomonic of fracture of the base of the skull. However, this may take several days to appear and is not a sensitive sign.

# Fontanels

There are six fontanels at birth, each of which may or may not be palpable (**Figure 6-1**). The two most important are the anterior and posterior fontanels. The anterior fontanel usually measures 2.5 cm by 2.5 cm at three months of age. The size then diminishes and closes between nine to 18 months of age. In some normal infants, anterior fontanels may close as early as four to five months of age. Boys seem to have earlier closure than girls. The posterior fontanel is small even at birth (usually the size of a finger tip) and closes rapidly by two months of age.

The *characteristics of fontanels* to be described are size, age at closure, fullness, and pulsation. Normal size has been described in the previous paragraph. An anterior fontanel that seems to close too early (before four months) is not abnormal per se, if the head circumference grows normally. In microcephaly and craniostenosis, the fontanel may be small or close early. The fontanels are larger than normal, or remain open for abnormally longer periods, in conditions such as hypothyroidism, hydrocephalus, rickets, and Trisomy18 syndrome. An abnormally full, tense, and elevated fontanel signifies increased intracranial pressure, whereas a depressed fontanel in a child with diarrhea and vomiting is a good indicator of severe dehydration. Normally, the anterior fontanel is pulsatile, but absence of *pulsation* may be normal. In the presence of increased intracranial tension, the fontanel may be tense without pulsations.

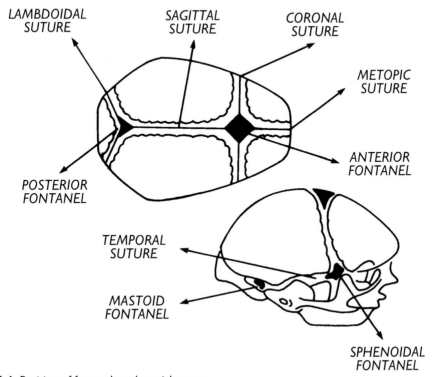

**Figure 6-1**. Position of fontanels and cranial sutures

## Additional Procedures

Remember that the skull behind the ears can be dented on pressure in rickets. Palpate the mastoid bones behind the ears. Normally, these bones are not well developed until a child is two or three years of age. Palpate for swelling, heat, and tenderness (evidence of mastoiditis).

Examine for characteristics of the *cranial sutures* (**Figure 6-1**). The sutures normally tend to overlap during the newborn period due to intrauterine molding. In a few older children, some of the suture lines may appear prominent (particularly the metopic suture). The suture lines should not be easily palpable after six months of age, although the ossification is not complete until about eight years of age. Easily palpable wide suture lines after five to six months of age may indicate hydrocephalus.

Three other procedures to be completed during the examination of the head are percussion, auscultation, and transillumination.

## Percussion

In children with increased intracranial pressure and closed fontanels, percussion of the skull with a finger may produce a resonant sound. It is called Macewen's sign.

## Auscultation

Auscultation of the skull, particularly over the occipital and frontal region, may be of value in infants with congestive heart failure of unknown etiology. Cranial bruit has been described in association with arteriovenous fistula or aneurysms of cerebral vessels, brain tumors, and coarctation of the aorta. However, cranial bruit is very common even in normal children, particularly in the very young. Therefore, routine auscultation of the skull is not necessary.

## Transillumination

Transillumination of the skull may help recognize infants with suspected subdural hematoma, hydrocephalus, and poor growth of the brain. Conduct the examination in a dark room. A rubber (non-translucent, black) ring should be fitted to a large flashlight and the ring applied firmly against the scalp. Move the flashlight to examine the back, the side, and the front. Normally, a small ring of light is seen around the rubber attachment. If the ring of light is over 0.5 cm wide, it denotes abnormality (e.g., subdural hematoma). In anencephaly and hydrocephalus, light may be transmitted directly across to the opposite side.

## SCALP

Examine the scalp for the following *abnormalities of the skin*: 1) congenital defects; 2) congenital masses, such as hemangioma; 3) infection, such as folliculitis, and abscess. Follow this up with examination of the scalp hair. The characteristics of hair to be observed are:

- Quantity (generalized increase, localized increase, generalized decrease, localized decrease)
- Color

- Texture
- Surface characteristics (straight, curled, or beaded)
- Strength (brittle)
- Pattern of distribution/parietal whorl

## Quantity

Abnormal increase (hypertrichosis) in scalp hair is difficult to appreciate, but facial hair may be more than usual in premature births, steroid toxicity, porphyria cutanea tarda, and various syndromes, such as de Lange and Hurler. Decrease in quantity of hair (hypotrichosis) with uniformly sparse distribution may be seen in hypothyroidism, drug toxicity, cytotoxic therapy, heavy metal toxicity, and cartilage-hair hypoplasia.

Areas of total loss of hair in the midst of normal hair (*alopecia*) may be seen in congenital conditions, fungal infection, SLE, or may be due to psychological hair-pulling (trichotillomania). In all of the acquired conditions with alopecia, stubs of hair may be seen in the area of hair loss.

## Color of Hair

The color may be black, brunette, red, or blonde depending on genetic and racial characteristics. If there are abnormalities of color, determine whether the hair color is uniformly abnormal, abnormal only in certain areas, or whether there are alternating normal and abnormal colors. (Remember that adolescents may bleach their hair or use artificial coloring.) The color of scalp hair may be uniformly abnormal, such as the blonde color in phenylketonuria, and white in albinism. Abnormal color may be seen only in certain areas, such as the white forelock seen in Waardenburg syndrome and Chediak-Higashi syndrome, or *alternately* pigmented and depigmented as in pili annulati.

## Texture

Dry coarse hair is common in hypothyroidism and fetal alcohol syndrome, whereas fine thin hair is seen in hyperthyroidism, homocystinuria, Weaver syndrome, and many other syndromes.

## Surface Characteristics

Curled hair is a normal racial characteristic (African) but twisted shape of the hair along its long axis (associated with increased fragility) is known as pili torti and is seen in Menkes syndrome. A beaded appearance of the shaft may be due to constriction at regular intervals (as in monilethrix) or caused by nodular swellings along the shaft (as in trichorrhexis nodosa). Cork-screw type hair (pig tail hair) in the midst of a shower of petechiae suggests scurvy.

Remember to look for lice and nits, which may give a beaded appearance to the hair.

## Strength

Fragile hair is characteristic of many congenital syndromes and fungal infections.

## Pattern of Scalp Hair

Aberrant scalp hair pattern is indicative of abnormal brain development in early fetal life. The normal pattern is characterized by a parietal whorl that is located anterior to the position of the posterior fontanel and from which the hair stream goes progressively outwards, sweeping anteriorly to the forehead. The whorl is usually unilateral and is to the left of the midline. Rarely, it is to the right of the midline or bilateral. Unruly hair over the scalp is often associated with various mental retardation syndromes. Parietal whorls may be absent or located centrally or posteriorly in microcephaly. The whorl also may be placed too far forward.

The frontal area and upper face have facial hair stream that seems to start from the ocular puncta and flows outward (affecting the direction of the eyebrow hair) and converges with the parietal hair stream of the forehead.

## Hair Line

One should look for abnormalities of hairline in the front, back, and the sides. The hairline may be abnormally low or high in each of these areas.

1. low hairline in the back often related to a short neck (Klippel-Feil syndrome) or webbed neck (Turner syndrome),
2. absence of hair on the sideburn area (as in anotia),
3. excess projection of hair into the sideburn areas as in Treacher Collins syndrome,
4. low beaked frontal pattern (widow's peak) as in nasal dysplasia,
5. frontal upsweep (cowlick) as in microcephaly,
6. abnormal hair over the lateral forehead associated with defective eye development.

# FOREHEAD

The characteristics to be described are:

- Size
- Shape
- Extra growth
- Hair pattern

The vertical height of the forehead is increased in hydrocephalus, Crouzon disease, and Apert syndrome. It is prominent in rickets, osteogenesis imperfecta, and Hurler syndrome. The forehead also may be prominent in chronic hemolytic anemia syndromes. The forehead is pointed in Apert, trigonocephaly, and midline brain defects. Extra growths in the form of dermoid cysts are located near the angles of the eye. Occasionally, an encephalocele or meningocele may present in the forehead. The frontal hairline is low in Hurler syndrome, de Lange syndrome, and in many cases of mental retardation. Inverted peak (widow's peak) of the frontal hairline is seen in frontonasal dysplasia.

# NECK

The points to look for in the neck are:

- Size
- Shape
- Position at rest
- Range of movement
- Anatomic structures:
- Cervical glands
- Muscles
- Thyroid
- Veins
- Arteries
- Swelling and defects

## Size and Shape

Severe swelling of the neck, obliterating all details, may be seen in severe diphtheria (bull-neck type), subcutaneous emphysema, and infection of the floor of the mouth. These conditions can be recognized easily, since the onset will be acute and the child acutely ill.

The neck may be *short* due to vertebral anomalies or may appear to be short due to webbing of the neck as in Turner syndrome. Obese individuals and patients with chronic obstructive lung disease often have short stocky necks. Webbing of the neck with low posterior line is seen in Turner and Noonan syndromes.

## Position

Normal position of the neck is in the midline. If the head is tilted, determine whether it is due to *torticollis or tilting of the neck*. This is best determined if the child is supine on his or her back, while you stand at the head of the table. In *torticollis, the occiput is tilted to one side and the chin tilted to the opposite side*. The child looks to one side all the time and cannot turn his or her neck to the opposite side. In long-standing torticollis, there may be atrophy of facial structures leading to facial asymmetry. *In head tilting, both the occiput and the chin are deviated to the same side*. This is seen when a patient is compensating for diplopia.

In severe atlantoaxial subluxation and weakness of extensors of the neck, the child may sit with the chin supported by the hand. In caries of the spine, the neck is held stiff, and the child walks very carefully to avoid jarring movements. In severe decorticate rigidity, meningeal irritation, and muscle spasm (as in tetanus), the occiput is tilted markedly backward, burrowing into the pillow (opisthotonus).

## Range of Movement

The range of movement of the cervical spine and testing for muscles are described on page 218.

Most of the flexion and extension takes place in the upper cervical spines. They are tested by first asking the child to touch the chest with the chin and then to look up at the ceiling. Rotation at the atlantoaxial joint is tested by asking the child to look over the shoulders. Lateral bending occurs in all the points along the cervical spine and is tested by asking the child to touch the shoulder with the ear.

## Various Anatomic Structures in the Neck

The cervical lymph nodes can be grouped into the horizontal and vertical groups (**Figure 6-2**). The preauricular, postauricular, and suboccipital nodes belong to the horizontal group. The suboccipital nodes are enlarged in scalp infections and in rubella. The submandibular nodes are also part of the horizontal group and are best felt with the examiner standing behind the patient and feeling the neck along the floor of the mouth while the patient is standing or sitting. The vertical groups of nodes are felt along the anterior and posterior margins of the sternomastoid muscle and most of them belong to the superficial groups of cervical lymph nodes. Deep cervical nodes are not palpable under normal circumstances.

Describe the characteristics of the palpable lymph nodes under the following headings: location, size, shape, consistency, temperature, tenderness, margin, and discreteness. Warm and tender nodes indicate infection. Acute unilateral swelling of a single cervical node is seen in Kawasaki disease. Painless swelling of the nodes in the posterior and lower cervical regions should increase the suspicion for malignancy. Soft fluctuant swelling indicates suppuration. Matted nodes indicate chronic inflammation. Discrete hard nodes (particularly a large hard node on one side only) may indicate malignancy.

When evaluating cervical adenopathy, it is important to examine lymph nodes in other parts of the body to determine whether this is part of a generalized adenopathy.

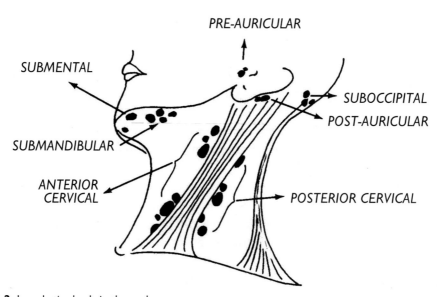

**Figure 6-2.** Lymphatic glands in the neck.

The *thyroid gland* should **not** be visible normally except during adolescence. Inspect for thyroid swelling from in front. Ask the child to swallow a drink of water or juice, since the thyroid is particularly visible during swallowing.

Stand behind the patient and palpate for the thyroid while the neck of the patient is slightly extended. Remember that the thyroid gland is located just below the thyroid cartilage (Adam's apple). Therefore, place your fingers on either side of the cricoid cartilage, just below the wings of the thyroid cartilage. Ask the patient to swallow and feel the gland as it moves upward. Evaluate both lobes for the following characteristics: swelling, symmetry, surface characteristics (smooth or nodular), and consistency. In addition, remember to auscultate for a bruit (often present in thyrotoxicosis).

The *jugular vein* gives a good indication about pressure changes and other hemodynamic events in the right atrium during the cardiac cycle. Evaluation of jugular venous pressure and its waveforms (**Figure 6-3**) may help evaluate intravascular volume status, valvular disease, and pericardial constriction. The right internal jugular vein is the preferred site for this evaluation since it acts as a manometer for the right atrium.

Examine the neck vein with the child sitting at an angle of about 45 degrees (not sitting erect) and in good light. It is often difficult to differentiate between the jugular venous pulse and the carotid arterial pulse. There are three differentiating points. 1) The jugular venous pulse has a clear upper level (absent in arterial pulse). 2) The venous pulse is more visible than palpable, and is diffuse and biphasic. The arterial pulse is more palpable than visible, sharply defined, and single. 3) Gentle manual pressure over the abdomen may increase the fullness in the vein and accentuate the venous pulse but will not alter the arterial pulse.

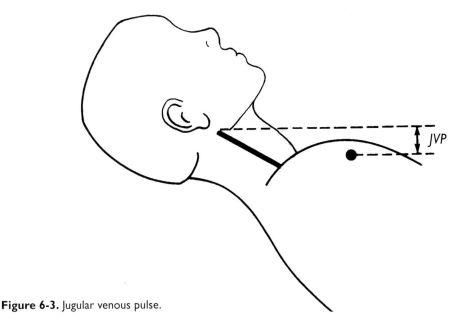

**Figure 6-3.** Jugular venous pulse.

edge of the eyebrow), infections, or tumors (also lacrimal gland swelling). Describe swellings using standard descriptors.

## Eyelids

The characteristics to be described are:
- Size
- Shape
- Position in relation to the lower (or upper) eyelid (palpebral fissure)
- Position in relation to the eyeball
- Color
- Continuity, which may be disturbed by a defect or a growth
- Hair along the lid margin
- Muscle movement

Lid swelling is seen commonly in allergy, trauma, insect bite, local cellulitis, and as part of generalized edema. Lids may be swollen in hypothyroidism and orbital venous congestion. The presence of pain on movement of the eyeball, proptosis, or decrease in visual acuity suggests periorbital cellulitis. Subcutaneous emphysema, as seen after a fracture of the orbit, also may cause swelling of the lids. If there is crepitus on gentle palpation, air under the skin should be suspected.

Remember to look for swelling of the lacrimal glands (as seen in obstruction of the duct and sarcoid) and also look at the puncta at the medial end of the upper and lower lids.

The lower lid may have a double pleat (Morgan's fold) in allergic children.

## Palpebral Fissure

The relation between the lower and upper lid defines the palpebral fissure. The vertical height of the fissure may be unusually narrow (as in ptosis, fracture of the orbit, edema of the eyelids) or wide (as in exophthalmos, hyperthyroidism). The horizontal length of the palpebral fissure may be short, as in Trisomy 18, or appear short because of lateral displacement of inner canthi, as in blepharophimosis syndrome. The palpebral fissure may be slanted upwards (so that the inner canthus is at a lower level) as in Trisomy 21 syndrome or slanted downwards (anti-Mongoloid slant with the outer canthus at a lower level) as in Treacher Collins. (See pages 70 & 73 for defining the direction of the slant.)

The palpebral fissure and epicanthic fold seen in East Asians have characteristics that are different from those seen in Trisomy 21 syndrome. Normally, the highest point of the palpebral fissure is at the junction of the outer two thirds with the inner third of the upper eyelid even in people from Eastern Asia. In contrast, the highest point of the palpebral fissure in Down syndrome is at the center of the upper eyelid.

The upper and lower lids become continuous with each other, giving a fold in people of Asian descent; whereas in Trisomy 21 syndrome, upper and lower lids meet medially behind a veil-like fold (**Figures 6-4** and **6-5**).

## Position in Relation to the Eyeball

Widening of the palpebral fissure is seen in patients with Graves' disease and in seventh cranial nerve palsy. Proptosis also causes widening of the fissure.

Drooping of the eyelid is called "ptosis" and may be unilateral or bilateral. Patients with bilateral ptosis appear to have narrow palpebral fissure and often tilt their heads back and furrow the forehead to see in front of themselves. Ptosis may obstruct vision and lead to amblyopia.

It is important to determine whether ptosis is unilateral, bilateral and symmetric, or bilateral and asymmetric.

Unilateral ptosis is seen in third cranial nerve palsy and in Horner syndrome. It also may be seen as congenital ptosis. Bilateral ptosis is seen in myasthenia gravis and neurological diseases. In infants, one should think of botulism as well.

Conditions that may mimic ptosis include enophthalmos and inappropriate lid retraction.

Ectropion is outward-folding of the lid as seen after burn injury to the face. Entropion is inward-folding of the lid, as seen in severe infections of the eye.

Marcus Gunn phenomenon is said to be present when a patient has unilateral ptosis and it corrects every time the patient opens the mouth (also called jaw winking phenomenon). This is due to congenital defects in innervation. Faults in seventh cranial nerve renervation may cause the lid to close every time the patient opens the jaw. This is called Amant's phenomenon.

## Color

The heliotrope coloration of the upper eyelid is characteristic of dermatomyositis (be aware of eye makeup in young girls). Bluish coloration of lower lid is common in allergic children (allergic shiner).

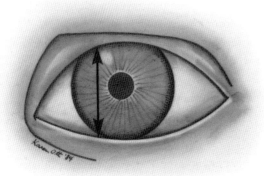

**Figure 6-4.** Left eye of an oriental male. Note that the upper and the lower lids are continuous and the maximum height of the palpebral fissure is close to the medial canthus.

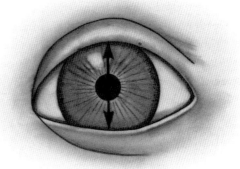

**Figure 6-5.** Left eye of a child with Trisomy 21 syndrome. Note the epicanthic fold behind which upper and lower lids meet. Also, the maximum height of the palpebral fissure is closer to the middle of the eye.

## Continuity

Interruption of the continuity of the lid margin is called "coloboma." Coloboma of the upper lid only is seen in Goldenhar syndrome, whereas coloboma of both upper and lower lids is seen in Treacher Collins syndrome.

The most common extra growths in the lid are 1) stye (hordeolum externum), which usually points along the edge of the eyelid at the root of one of the hair follicles, and 2) chalazion, which is seen on the inner aspect (tarsal aspect) of the lid.

## Hair Along the Lid Margins (Eyelashes)

The most common condition affecting the hair follicle is blepharitis, as seen by redness, scaliness, crusting, and ulceration. It is often associated with skin allergies and seborrhea. The eyelashes are unusually long in certain normal children (one of the features of an attractive child) and in children with any chronic illness. Syndromes associated with bushy eyebrows and long eyelashes include de Lange syndrome and Hurler syndrome.

A double row of eyelashes is called "distichiasis" and may be seen in association with congenital lymphedema.

Occasionally, lice may be seen along the eyelashes.

## Muscle Movement

The upper eyelid may droop because of edema or because of paralysis of the levator palpebrae superioris (see Ptosis on previous page).

Excess closure of eyelids due to tonic spasm of the orbicularis oculi muscle is called "blepharospasm" and is seen in the presence of a foreign body in the eye, corneal irritation, or photophobia from various causes. When examining small children, it is better not to force open the eyelids, since this is sure to make them close the lids even tighter. One can make newborns open their eyes by tilting them back and forth or by alternately turning them toward and away from a lighted window.

Inability to close the eyelids is seen in seventh cranial nerve injury resulting in everted lids, widened palpebral fissure, and dryness of eyes. Children with burn injuries to the face and scleroderma also may have difficulty with closing the eyelids.

Dystonia may present as tonic contraction of the lids and squinting.

## Eyeballs

The appearance of the eyeball may be described as prominent or recessed. Proptosis and exophthalmos are words used interchangeably when describing *prominent* eyeballs. Both mean an abnormal protrusion of the eyeball. This is most easily appreciated when you look at the patient's eye from above the top of the head with the patient seated or lying down. The palpebral fissure is wider and a larger proportion of the eyeball is seen in front of the lids than in normal individuals.

If the eye is prominent, the next question to ask is whether the eye is large in relation to the orbit (as in high myopia and buphthalmos) or if the eye has been pushed forward (as in trauma or a mass). But physical examination of the eyeball alone may not give clues.

Note whether the prominence is bilateral or unilateral. Bilaterally prominent eyeballs may be a familial characteristic (caused by a shallow orbit). True bilateral protrusion (exophthalmos) occurs in thyrotoxicosis, metastatic neuroblastoma, and many syndromes including Wegener's granulomatosis.

Other ocular features of hyperthyrodism (Graves Disease) include Graefe's sign and Stellwag sign. Lagging of the upper eyelid when the patient changes gaze from the ceiling to the floor is Graefe's sign. Infrequent blinking of the eyes associated with proptosis is Stellwag sign.

Another sign to remember is Colliers sign or the "sunset sign" of increased intracranial pressure. This is characterized by inability to look upwards together with excess exposure of sclera when the patient looks downwards.

Unilateral true exophthalmos usually indicates serious disease, such as orbital cellulitis or rhabdomyosarcoma. Rarely, it may be pulsatile. Asymmetry of the palpebral fissure, facial palsy, and unilateral problems with closure of cranial sutures may make one eye appear more prominent, but this is not true exophthalmos.

An eye may appear recessed either because it is truly small (microphthalmia), such as in "STORCH" complex, various congenital malformation syndromes, after severe ophthalmic infections with phthisis bulbi (as seen in severe vitamin A deficiency), or because of the contour of the orbit (enophthalmos), as in Horner syndrome.

## Tearing

Excessive tearing is seen in local irritation of the eye, allergies, or during crying. Even in the absence of excess production of tears, one may see tears running down the cheeks if the lacrimal puncta are closed (as in congenital occlusion or malformation of the duct) or if the eyelids are everted as seen after burn injury.

Dry eyes with lack of tears are seen in Riley-Day syndrome and Sjogren syndrome. The eyes may look dry even if the production of tears is normal if the eye is never closed, as in a comatose patient or in patients with ectropion.

## Conjunctiva

Remember to examine both the bulbar and palpebral or tarsal conjunctivae. Examination of the palpebral conjunctiva may be difficult in small children. Unless absolutely essential, there is no need to pull on the eyelids and lose a child's cooperation. In cooperative children, the lower lid can be examined by pulling the lower lid down with the patient trying to look up. To evert the upper lid, gently grasp the lid close to the lashes, and roll the lid up over a thin round stick, such as a pencil (non-sharp end) or cotton-tipped stick held horizontally over the lid.

Characteristics to look for in describing the conjunctiva are color, vessels, and secretion (described earlier under Tearing).

The color of the conjunctiva is pale in anemia and yellow in jaundice. It is important to know that the normal conjunctiva is pink at the anterior part and slightly pale posteriorly. In anemia, the anterior and posterior portions are equally pale.

Red eye ( **Table 6-1**) is one of the most common symptoms and may be due to conjunctivitis (**Figure 6-6**), scleral inflammation, corneal injury, foreign body, infection (keratitis), uveitis/iritis (**Figure 6-7**), or glaucoma. Transient, non-purulent conjunctivitis is an essential feature of Kawasaki disease.

The red eye of infection-related conjunctivitis is often, but not necessarily, unilateral and is not associated with pain. The redness may be mild to severe and often is associated with purulent discharge in bacterial conjunctivitis. The lids may be crusted, particularly in the morning when the child wakes from sleep.

Bilateral redness with itching and tearing is seen in allergic conjunctivitis. Redness of eyes with watery secretion, photophobia, and blepharospasm suggests corneal inflammation or corneal foreign body. Unilateral redness with pain, dilated pupil, and hazy cornea suggests acute glaucoma.

In conjunctivitis, the redness is maximal at the junction of bulbar and palpebral conjunctiva and the circumcorneal area is clear; whereas, the redness of uveitis and corneal disease often is painful and circumcorneal in location. If there is doubt about unilateral redness, ask the patient to close the affected eye and shine a light on the unaffected eye. If this causes pain in the affected eye, the problem is most likely uveitis (Au-Henkind test).

Flat-top papules on the tarsal conjunctiva may be seen in allergic children (vernal conjunctivitis). Redness of the bulbar conjunctiva with small vesicles that coalesce to form crescentic lesions along the corneal edge is seen in allergic children (limbal vernal conjunctivitis).

Bacterial thrombi may cause purpuric lesions of the conjunctiva (subacute bacterial endocarditis). Corkscrew vessels with thrombi may be seen in the fornices of patients with sickle cell disease.

Pallor, edema, and watery discharge together with follicles in the conjunctiva of lower lids may be seen in allergic conjunctivitis.

Chemosis is edema of the conjunctiva and is seen in severe allergies and angioneurotic edema. Pterygium is a membranous growth over the bulbar conjunctiva along the palpebral fissure medial to the cornea, often seen in allergic children. Follicles in the conjunctiva of upper lids occur in trachoma.

## Table 6-1. Differential Diagnosis of Red Eye

|  | **Conjunctivitis** | **Iritis** | **Corneal Injury/Ulcer** |
|---|---|---|---|
| Symptoms | Discomfort | Severe pain | Pain, variable |
| Discharge | Mucopurulent | Watery, slight | Watery, may be pronounced |
| Vision | Normal | Impaired | May or may not be |
| Hyperemia | Generalized | Circumcorneal | Circumcorneal |
| Cornea | Normal | Loss of luster | Surface reflection impaired; opacity |
| Pupil | Normal | Dilated; irregular | Small pupil |

Telangiectasis of the conjunctiva is seen in ataxia telangiectasia syndrome. Subconjunctival hemorrhage may indicate trauma, violent cough, or a bleeding disorder.

## Sclera

The normal *color* of the sclera is white. Yellow coloration of the sclera and conjunctiva indicates jaundice. White spots on the temporal side called "Bitot's spots" are seen in Vitamin A deficiency.

Injection of the sclera and overlying conjunctiva associated with mild pain and tendency to recur suggests episcleritis. Scleral redness, segmentally or of the entire surface with severe pain and bluish discoloration, suggests scleritis. Both of these are associated with rheumatic diseases.

Pigmented patches of the sclera and conjunctiva may be produced by melanocytes or by other causes. For example, blue sclera is seen in some normal people, iron deficiency anemia, osteogenesis imperfecta, and in Ehlers-Danlos syndrome. Metabolic conditions such as ochronosis and ingestion of a heavy metal such as silver also may cause pigmented sclera. Black patch on the sclera may be caused also by thinning of sclera, which allows the color of the choroid to show through.

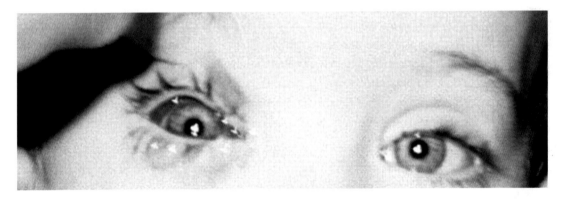

**Figure 6-6.** Conjunctivitis. Conjunctivitis with nonspecific conjunctival redness and watery discharge. Note that the circumcorneal area is relatively spared. (Courtesy of Sharon S. Lehman, MD, Chief Ophthalmology,Nemours Children's Clinic/Al duPont Hospital, Wilmington,DE and Robison D. Harley MD Endowed Chair in Pediatric Ophthalmology, Thomas Jefferson University-Jefferson medical Colege, Philadelphia,PA)

**Figure 6-7.** Iritis. Note the ciliary flush (corkscrew pattern of conjunctival vessels all the way to the rim of the cornea) (Courtesy of Sharon S. Lehman, MD, Chief Ophthalmology, Nemours Children's Clinic/Al duPont Hospital, Wilmington, DE and Robison D. Harley MD Endowed Chair in Pediatric Ophthalmology, Thomas Jefferson University-Jefferson medical Colege, Philadelphia,PA)

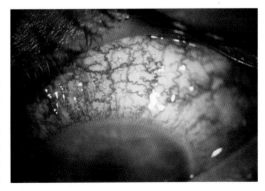

Flat patchy brown pigmentation of the conjunctiva (melanosis) around the limbus is benign and is seen in people with dark skin color. It is bilateral, stationary, and not associated with vascularity. When one sees pigmented conjunctiva together with pigmentation of the skin around the eye including the lids, it is the nevus of Ota. True nevus may be seen at birth or appear any time at the limbus or palpebral conjunctiva or the eyelid margin. They are flat and easily movable on the conjunctiva. If the nevus seems attached to the sclera, it suggests melanoma.

Asking the child to close the eyes and then palpating the eyeball over the closed eyelids with the index fingers may help estimate intraocular pressure. A hard (not just firm) feeling is a rough indication of increased pressure. Other clues to the presence of increased pressure are prominent eyeball, keratoconus, photophobia, excess tearing, and cloudy cornea. Causes of glaucoma include congenital glaucoma associated with syndromes such as Lowe oculocerebrorenal syndrome, Sturge-Weber syndrome, and STORCH complex.

To measure intraocular pressure accurately, tonometers are needed. This measurement should be performed by an ophthalmologist. A simple method to look at the depth of the anterior chamber is to use a penlight so that the beam falls at a right angle to the visual axis. Ask the patient to look straight ahead, hold the pen light at the side of the face just anterior to the ear, and shine the light so that the beam is directed at the bridge of the nose. If the iris is flat, there will be no shadow; if the iris is bulging, it will cause a shadow on the nasal side of the iris near the pupil.

Other points to note in the anterior chamber include blood (hyphema as in injury) and pus (hypopyon as in Behcet's disease).

## Cornea

The *size* of the cornea may be relatively large compared with the rest of the eye (megalocornea) in certain normal individuals and in newborns. The transverse diameter is 10 mm at birth and about 12 mm at age one year; this is about the size of an adult's cornea. A large cornea is seen as part of an enlarged globe of the eye in glaucoma. A small cornea (microcornea) is seen in many malformation syndromes.

Normal *shape* of the cornea is characterized by its roundness and slight anterior curvature. Increased anterior curvature (keratoconus) is seen in Down syndrome, osteogenesis imperfecta, and Ehlers-Danlos syndrome.

The *edge* of the cornea is usually clear. Occasionally, a patch of thickened conjunctiva (a pterygium) may grow over the edge of the cornea along the palpebral fissure. A phlycten is a small vesicle characteristically located on the corneal edge and is indicative of recent exposure to TB. Kayser-Fleischer ring is a greenish-gray ring along the outer margin of the cornea, seen in Wilson disease.

Circumcorneal injection is evidence of injury or infection of the cornea and uveitis. Corneal injury and infection are associated with foreign body sensation, pain, photophobia, tearing, and severe blepharospasm. Foreign body sensation, lid swelling, and photophobia due to irritation from a contact lens also may be seen.

Corneal *opacity* may be due to old injury, severe infection complicating a vitamin A deficiency, local inflammation (JRA or JIA), or also may be seen in certain syndromes (e.g., Hurler). Band keratopathy is a horizontal band of cloudiness of the cornea and may be visible to the naked eye. It is seen in JIA, sarcoid, and hypercalcemic states. Generalized haziness of the cornea is seen in glaucoma, certain metabolic syndromes (mucopolysaccharidosis), and early exposure keratitis. A salmon-pink patch of cornea is seen in acute interstitial keratitis.

The *continuity* of the cornea is disrupted by the presence of ulcers, which may be visible only as opacities or grayish infiltrates. If corneal injury, ulcer, or infection is suspected, a damp litmus paper impregnated with fluorescein or drops of fluorescein should be applied to the conjunctival side of an everted lid. Areas of injury will show up as green stained marks. Perforation of the cornea is seen following injury caused by sharp objects or following severe eye infection.

Corneal *deposits* are not easily visible to unaided eyes. Slit-lamp examination is essential to rule out corneal deposits (as seen in storage disease and chronic inflammation), and this is best done by an ophthalmologist.

## Iris

Complete absence of the iris is called "aniridia" and may be associated with Wilm's tumor. Loss of *continuity* of the iris is called "coloboma" (defect) and is seen as part of congenital malformation syndromes and after surgery for cataract. Coloboma of the iris has a high correlation with the presence of Wilm's tumor.

The *color* of a normal iris may vary (dark, dark brown, blue, and green). Young girls also may wear contact lenses which mask the normal color of the iris. The pale iris of albinism and the salt-and-pepper iris (Brushfield spots) of Down syndrome are easy to recognize.

The edge of the pupillary margin can be visualized using the +8 or +10 lens of the ophthalmoscope. The pupillary margin should be smooth. Irregularity with serrated edge suggests adhesions due to iritis. Nodular lesions along the edge of the iris may be seen in neurofibromatosis and in sarcoidosis (Koeppe nodules).

## Pupil

A dark pupil in the middle of a dark iris may be difficult to visualize. Shining the light obliquely or using a yellow light may facilitate visualization. The smaller circular light of the ophthalmoscope may help as well. Use the +8 or +10 lens of an ophthalmoscope to visualize the pupillary margin clearly.

The normal pupil is *round* and is *centrally* located, though it is occasionally oval. Coloboma of the iris makes the pupil irregular. The pupil may not be located in the center even in some normal children (eccentric pupil). Normally, the edge should be smooth. Look for irregularities and adhesions (synechiae).

*Size* may be normally small as in people with highly pigmented iris, or dilated as in those with light-colored iris. Pinpoint pupils give the person a beady-eyed, suspicious look; whereas, wide pupils are characteristic of children who elicit a pleasant response. Make sure that the same amount of ambient light falls on both eyes before making judgment on the equality of the size of the pupils. If a pupil is too large or too small, determine whether the abnormality is unilateral (asymmetric) or bilateral. If asymmetric, the next task is to identify the abnormal side.

Ulcers at the tip of the tongue usually indicate the presence of a severe cough from any cause (e.g., pertussis).

## Swelling

Isolated swelling of the tongue may be seen in angioneurotic edema or due to bleeding as in trauma and hemophilia resulting in a hematoma. Look for masses at the base of the tongue. Small masses at the base of the tongue in the midline may be due to lingual thyroid or thyroglossal duct cyst. Also look for ranula, which is a cystic mass under the tongue that does not extend to the floor of the mouth.

Ask the child to open the mouth and look for deviation of the tongue to one side or other. If it is deviated, observe jaw movements and exclude deviation of the jaw to one side that can give the appearance of deviation of the tongue. The other possible explanation for deviation of the tongue is paralysis of one half of the tongue (twelfth cranial nerve palsy), so that the normal side pushes the tongue to the weaker side.

## Movements

Some young children suck the tongue as a habit, instead of sucking the thumb. This causes movements the floor of the mouth as the child sucks the tip of the tongue held between the incisor teeth.

Some of the abnormal movements of the tongue are tremors (seen in thyrotoxicosis) and trombone tongue (seen in chorea). To elicit these findings, have the child stick his or her tongue out and keep it out as long as possible. In chorea, the tongue will involuntarily go in and out of the mouth giving the appearance of a trombone.

## Appearance of Papillae

The papillae may be *hypertrophic* as in strawberry tongue of scarlet fever, atrophic as in various anemias and pellagra, or absent as in familial dysautonomia in which fungiform papillae are absent. Black hairy tongue is characterized by the presence of a V-shaped brown to black area, anterior to the location of circumvallate papillae. This is due to hypertrophy of the filiform papillae and often is seen in hemophilia and purpura.

## Gums and Alveolar Ridges

The normal gum has three characteristics: 1) pinkish-bluish color, 2) a potential space between the marginal gingiva and the teeth, and 3) the area of gum that arches between the teeth does not extend through the entire height.

## Color

In gingivitis due to any cause (vitamin C deficiency or herpetic gingivostomatitis) and in periodontal disease, the gum is reddish and bleeds easily. In Dilantin (phenytoin)-induced hypertrophy, the gum is reddish, and there is true hypertrophy of gum overhanging the teeth. There is space between the gum and the crown of the teeth that can be demonstrated by passing the edge of a paper between the tooth and the gum. One can see the gum arching between the teeth, giving the appearance of a curtain on the stage.

Children with bruxism (grinding of teeth while awake or asleep) also show arching of the gum between the teeth since the teeth are ground down and there is relatively more gum than teeth. The gum is not red, however, and there is no space between the teeth and the overhanging gum.

A black line along the margin of the gum may be normal. It is also seen in heavy metal poisoning.

## Continuity (also see section on tongue)

Ulcers and vesicles on the gum are seen in herpetic gingivostomatitis. Vesicles and pustules along the alveolar ridges in a child with fever may be the only clue to pneumococcal septicemia. Hemorrhage in the gum is related to trauma, purpura, and leukemia.

## Alveolar Ridge

Hypertrophied alveolar ridges are seen in Hurler syndrome. A small swelling along the junction of the gum and tooth may be due to alveolar abscess, eosinophilic granuloma, or epulis. Epulis is a pearl-like tumor in the alveolar-buccal margin near the incisor teeth on the floor of the mouth, usually on one side only. An oral frenulum, attaching the upper lip to alveolar margin, is seen in Ellis-van Creveld syndrome.

## Mucous Membrane of the Cheek

Important clinical clues to be looked for on the mucous membrane of the mouth are:

- Small, thick, white plaques that are hard to remove and may leave bleeding points if removed (thrush/candidiasis).
- Whitish patch that is painful and friable because of healing areas of thermal burn, laceration, or abrasion.
- Vesicular lesions as in herpes simplex or Coxsackie virus infection.
- Bullous lesions as in erythema multiforme.
- Fewer numbers (less than three) of painful, round, shallow ulcers as in aphthous stomatitis.
- Large numbers of deep ulcers of varying sizes as in granulocytopenia.
- Pigmentation of the mucosa as in heavy metal poisoning or Addison disease.
- Severe gangrene of the buccal mucosa leading to perforating ulcer of the cheek (called "noma") as in severe malnutrition.
- Small bluish-white spots surrounded by a reddish zone opposite the molar teeth (Koplik spot) during the prodromal stages of measles.
- Reddish elevation around the orifice of parotid duct in mumps.

posterior surface of the pharynx are seen in chronic pharyngitis and in allergic individuals. Postnasal drip usually can be visualized when the pharynx is examined as described above.

A child with retropharyngeal abscess appears acutely ill with fever, dysphagia, drooling, and retracted neck. The abscess may be visible in the posterior pharyngeal wall. If such a mass is visible, *place the patient lying in lateral position, and be prepared to suction if the abscess should rupture.* As mentioned earlier, do not force the examination.

In chronic tonsillitis and adenoiditis, the child may have the following characteristics of "adenoid facies": an open mouth, "shiners" under the eyes, characteristic nasal voice or snoring at night, and inability to pronounce sounds which end with "ng" (e.g., "talking").

# TEETH

Describe the characteristics of (milk) primary teeth and permanent teeth under the following headings:

- Number
- Sequence and time of appearance
- Alignment within themselves and between upper and lower sets
- Color
- Texture
- Continuity
- Surface

## Normal Teeth

The milk teeth are 20 in number and should be present by 24 months of age. There are wide variations in the timing of eruption of teeth. Although this is not a good indicator of developmental milestones, lack of any primary teeth after two years is distinctly abnormal. Milk teeth are white in color and have a smooth edge in contrast to permanent teeth, which have an ivory (off-white) color and serrated edge. If the characteristic of the edge is not visible, gently palpating the edge with the index finger will help determine whether there are fine serrations.

Permanent teeth are 32 in number. The "sixth-year molar" is the first permanent tooth to erupt. Though the sequence of appearance of permanent teeth is definite, their timing is indefinite. The last molar may not erupt until adult life. The time of eruption and of budding of primary teeth is given in **Table 6-2**, and the time of eruption of permanent teeth is given in **Table 6-3**.

## Abnormality of Numbers of Eruptions

Complete absence of all teeth (anodontia) is seen in congenital ectodermal dysplasia. Complete absence of a few teeth is often related to normal cycle of loss and eruption and local conditions, such as cleft palate, impaction, and dentigenous cysts. Supernumerary teeth interfere with eruption of other teeth and therefore need attention.

*Premature* eruption of *deciduous* teeth may result in babies being born with teeth (natal teeth). They interfere with feeding and may be associated with early appearance of the corresponding permanent teeth. There is also the danger of aspiration.

*Premature* eruption of *permanent* teeth may be a clue to hyperpituitarism.

Delayed eruption of deciduous teeth (compare with normal values in **Table 6-2**) is seen in conditions such as hypopituitarism, hypothyroidism, cleidocranial dysotosis, and rickets. Delayed eruption of a single tooth occurs more commonly with permanent teeth and is due to factors such as retention of the primary tooth or hereditary traits.

## Size and Shape

Next, look at the size of the teeth. Microdontia and macrodontia are difficult to define. A localized form of microdontia often is seen in the maxillary lateral incisor and the third molar and is caused by genetic factors. Localized macrodontia of maxillary incisors, particularly in adolescents, leads to cosmetic problems.

**TABLE 6-2 : Chronology of PRIMARY DENTITION**

| Maxillary | Calcification starts | Eruption | Shedding |
|---|---|---|---|
| Central incisor | 3-4 mo in utero | 7 ½ mo | 7-8 yrs |
| Lateral incisor | 4½ mo in utero | 8 mo | 8-9 yrs |
| Canine | 5 ½ mo in utero | 16-20 mo | 11-12 yrs |
| First molar | 5 mo in utero | 12-16 mo | 10-11 yrs |
| Second molar | 6 mo in utero | 20-30 mo | 11-12 yrs |
| Mandibular | | | |
| Central incisor | 4½ mo in utero | 6/1/2 mo | 6-7 yrs |
| Lateral incisor | 4½ mo in utero | 7 mo | 7-8 yrs |
| Canine | 5 mo in utero | 16-20 mo | 8-11 yrs |
| First molar | 5 mo in utero | 12-16 mo | 10-12 yrs |
| Second molar | 6 mo in utero | 20-30 mo | 11-13 yrs |

*Modified from Table 304-1, Chapter 304, Section-2 The Oral cavity in Kliegman: Nelson Textbook of Pediatrics. Saunders/Elsvier. 18th ed. 2007. (copyright Elsevier 2007)*

## Color

Black teeth are seen in children taking oral iron preparations. Yellowish to yellowish-green discoloration is seen in children who were given tetracycline during infancy. In hypoplasia of enamel, the teeth look yellow to yellow-brown. Early lesions of caries appear brown, and established lesions are black and easy to identify. Other conditions that can be diagnosed from the color of the teeth are given in **Table 6-4**.

Look for mottling or pitting of enamel. This may be seen involving only a single tooth (trauma), or groups of teeth (severe febrile illness, malnutrition), or all teeth (amelogenesis imperfecta). Pitting and mottling of enamel also occur in fluorosis. Excess plaque formation over the teeth is due to poor oral hygiene.

**Table 6-3. Permanent Dentition.**

| Maxillary | Calcification starts | Eruption |
|---|---|---|
| Central incisor | 3-4 mo | 7-8 yr |
| Lateral incisor | 10 mo | 8-9 yr |
| Canine | 4-5 mo | 11-12 yr |
| First premolar | 1½-1¾yr | 10-11 yr |
| Second premolar | 2-2¼ yr | 10-12 yr |
| First molar | At birth | 6-7 yr |
| Second molar | 2½-3 yr | 12-13 yr |
| Third molar | 7-9 yr | 17-21 yr |
| **Mandibular** | | |
| Central incisor | 3-4 mo | 6-7 yr |
| Lateral incisor | 3-4 mo | 7-8 yr |
| Canine | 4-5 mo | 9-10 yr |
| First premolar | 1¾-2yr | 10-12 yr |
| Second premolar | 2¼-2½ yr | 11-12 yr |
| First molar | At birth | 6-7 yr |
| Second molar | 2½-3 yr | 11-13 yr |
| Third molar | 8-10 yr | 17-21 yr |

*Modified from Table 304-1, Chapter 304, Section-2 The Oral cavity in Kliegman: Nelson Textbook of Pediatrics. Saunders/Elsevier. 18th ed. 2007. (copyright Elsevier 2007)*

## Continuity and Surface

Broken front teeth are common in children and are characterized by a chipped cutting edge. A chipped tooth associated with hemorrhage from the gum line suggests fracture of the crown and of the root. If the tooth is also dislocated, it needs immediate attention.

Caries cause dark holes on the biting surfaces but also may occur on the medial borders of the central maxillary incisors particularly in babies who are constantly sucking bottles with sugar, whether from milk, juice, or sugar water (**Figure 6-11**). Some caries cannot be detected by clinical examination alone. Special lighting, instruments, and knowledge of tactile feel of small lesions are required to detect early lesions.

Normally, the edge of incisors is serrated and is usually broader than the root. However, the crown may be narrower than the root (peg-shaped) with a lobular occlusal surface in congenital syphilis. Hutchinson incisor teeth are characterized by rounded shape and notching along the biting edge. This is seen in congenital syphilis.

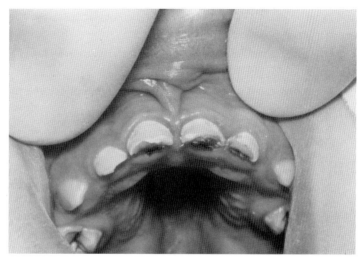

**Figure 6-11.** Bottle caries.
(Courtesy of RD Harshaw DMD)

### Table 6-4. Conditions Associated with Discolored Teeth

| Color | Diagnosis |
| --- | --- |
| Brown to black (portions of crown) | Caries |
| Yellow to yellow-brown to yellow-green | Enamel dysplasia |
| | Tetracycline therapy |
| | Excess fluoride |
| Dark gray to black | Oral iron therapy |
| | Pulp decay |
| Green | Erythroblastosis |
| Red | Porphyria |
| White | Poor enamel |

Dens invaginatus, which usually involves the maxillary lateral incisor is seen as a linear depression or defect in the continuity and is a common variation.

## Alignment

Have the child bite down on his or her teeth. Separate the lips and examine the bite. The occlusal surface of the teeth should appose with good alignment, with the posterior mandibular teeth interdigitating slightly ahead of the corresponding maxillary teeth. In malocclusion of class III variety, the posterior mandibular teeth are placed one or two teeth anterior to the corresponding maxillary teeth. A pronounced malocclusion of this type is called "prognathism" and is seen as a familial characteristic and in acromegaly. When the posterior mandibular teeth are aligned posterior to the corresponding maxillary teeth, it is a class II occlusion.

Hypognathia results in severe class II oral occlusion and may be a familial characteristic. It also may be seen in Pierre Robin syndrome and JIA.

Teeth may erupt in abnormal positions because of delayed shedding of deciduous teeth and result in crowding.

# BIBLIOGRAPHY

American Academy of Family Physicians, American Academy of Otolaryngology-Head and Neck Surgery; American Academy of Pediatrics Subcommittee on Otitis Media With Effusion. Otitis media with effusion. Pediatrics. 2004;113(5):1412-29.

Creighton PR. Common pediatric dental problems. Pediatr Clin North Am. 1998;45(6):1579-90.

Paradise JL. Testing for otitis media: diagnosis ex machina. N Engl J Med. 1977;296(8):445-8.

Smith's Recognizable patterns of human malformations. 6th ed. Jones K, editor. Philadephia: WB Saunders; 2005.

Smith DW, Gong BT. Scalp hair patterning as a clue to early fetal brain development. J Pediatr. 1973;83(3):374-80.

Wright JT. Normal formation and development defects of the human dentition. Pediatr Clin North Am. 2000;47(5):975-1000.

# Chapter 7

# CHEST (including heart and lungs)

## GENERAL EXAMINATION OF THE CHEST

The sequence of examination of the chest will vary depending on the cooperation of the child. In many situations, a cursory examination may be all that is possible. Auscultation of the chest for heart sounds and breath sounds is possible even with a crying child. If one waits for each inspiration during the cry, one can hear the adventitious sounds, except expiratory wheeze. Similarly, if one concentrates on the heart sounds during the expiratory phase of the cry, one can pick up important findings. Thorough examination of the heart, however, requires a quiet child and a quiet environment. Examination of the chest will be described under the traditional headings of inspection, palpation, percussion, and auscultation.

### Inspection

- Shape
- Visible abnormalities
- Movement with respiration
- Size (also see page 87)

The circumference of the chest is measured at mid-inspiration using a plastic or cloth tape at the level of the xiphisternum. Children up to age five years should be lying down during this measurement. After this age, the measurement is made with children standing. Chest circumference is 30 cm at birth (28.5 to 33.5 cm), 48 cm at one year of age (45 to 51 cm), and 52 cm at three years of age (50 to 56 cm). Chest circumference is smaller than that of the head in the first nine to 12 months of life. After one year of age, the chest circumference should be larger than the head circumference. Persistence of the infantile proportion suggests hydrocephalus. A small thoracic cage is seen in Ellis-van Creveld syndrome.

### Shape

In infancy, the transverse diameter and the anteroposterior diameter of the chest are equal, resulting in a chest that appears round. After two years, however, the transverse diameter increases so that the appearance is transversely oval. A round chest in an older child is due to chronic obstructive lung disease, such as asthma.

## Visible Abnormalities

Other abnormalities of the structure of the chest and thorax to be looked for include:

1. Absence of clavicle, as seen in cleiodocranial dysostosis.
2. Presternal edema, as seen in association with Henoch-Schönlein purpura and hemorrhagic edema of infancy.
3. Prominence of one side of the chest anteriorly, suggesting rib anomalies, scoliosis, or cardiac problems.
4. Hypoplastic nipples, as seen in Turner syndrome.
5. Supernumerary nipples (may be associated with renal anomaly).
6. Shield-shaped chest, as seen in Turner syndrome. (The distance between the nipples is normal in Turner syndrome.)
7. Depression of the sternum (pectus excavatum) seen as an isolated congenital anomaly and with chronic nasal obstruction due to adenoidal hypertrophy.
8. Protrusion of the sternum (pigeon breast) as seen in rickets, osteomalacia, and pectus carinatum.
9. Swelling of the costochondral junctions giving the appearance of rosary beads ("rachitic rosary") as seen in rickets.
10. A deep groove running along the sides of the chest parallel to the lower ribs as seen in some premature babies. This corresponds to the attachment of the diaphragm. Unless it is very pronounced, it has no clinical significance. Deep grooves (Harrison's sulci) are seen in rickets and in any chronic obstructive pulmonary disorder.
11. Absence of pectoralis muscle leading to flattened upper part of the chest on one side. This may be associated with absence of nipple, absence of breast development, and pleural herniation.
12. Location of one or both scapulae at a higher position with the lower angle turned toward the spine, as seen in Sprengel's deformity.

## Movement with Respiration

In newborns and young infants, respiration is mostly abdominal. A relatively flat abdomen with diminished abdominal excursions in a newborn suggests diaphragmatic abnormalities. Inflamed peritoneum also will shift the emphasis to movement of the intercostal muscles in this age group. After four to five years of age, most of the respiratory movements come from the intercostal muscles.

Normally, the chest moves evenly with each inspiration and expiration. Splinting of the chest with reduced total excursion during inspiration or cough suggests pleural irritation. A short grunt at the end of each expiration suggests a painful condition of the chest such as pneumonia or pleurisy (but children with pain anywhere may grunt). Remember that avoidance of deep inspiration and cough also may indicate irritation of the central nervous system and increased intracranial pressure.

Unequal movement of the chest suggests unilateral lung pathology. In children, the most important condition to remember is obstruction of the air passage due to a foreign body, and one should get a careful history of chewing on a foreign body or choking and coughing during a recent meal. Pleural effusion and empyema are associated with diminished excursion of the affected side of the chest as well.

During normal respiration, both the chest and abdomen move, and the abdominal movements are more easily visible than the thoracic movements, particularly in infants. During inspiration, the abdomen bulges (caused by the downward movement of the diaphragm), and the thoracic cage moves upward and outward (chest expansion). During expiration, the abdomen gets flatter, and the thoracic cage returns to the resting position. In diaphragmatic paralysis, the abdomen becomes prominent during expiration and flat during inspiration; this is called paradoxical respiration. Fluoroscopy is essential for actual demonstration of paradoxical respiration. Diaphragmatic paralysis (from whatever cause such as congenital poliomyelitis) and pneumothorax may be associated with paradoxical respiration.

*Accessory muscles of respiration* include the scalenii, the sternomastoids, the trapezii, the latissimus dorsi, and the abdominal muscles. In the presence of upper airway obstruction (as in croup, diphtheria) or in lower airway obstruction (asthma), accessory muscles of inspiration (scalenii, sternomastoids, and trapezii) come into play, resulting in supraclavicular and suprasternal retraction. In moderate lower airway obstruction, retraction of the lower intercostal spaces and epigastrium is seen as well. Accessory muscles of expiration (abdominal muscles and latissimus dorsi) are active in moderate to severe airway obstruction as in bronchial asthma. When patients with bronchial asthma sit up leaning forward slightly at the edge of the bed with the hands supporting them on either side, they fix the shoulder joint, so that the latissimi can act on the ribs and augment the expiratory effort.

The most standardized method for measuring chest expansion is one used by rheumatologists to evaluate restriction of chest expansion in ankylosing spondylitis. A conventional tape measure is used. Measurements are taken at the fourth intercostal space. Do not pull the tape too tightly. The difference between the circumference at the height of maximum inspiration and at the height of maximal expiration expressed in centimeters is the measurement of chest expansion.

# PALPATION

- Obvious swelling and tenderness
- Trachea
- Cardiac impulse
- Movements
- Vibrations (fremitus)

## Swelling and Tenderness

Palpate any obvious swelling for its texture, temperature, tension, and tenderness. In particular, note tenderness along the ribs, intercostal muscles, costochondral junctions, and manubrium. Sternal tenderness is noticed in leukemia. A prominent xiphoid process may cause a normal protrusion at the distal end of the sternum.

## Trachea

With the index finger and the ring finger on the sternal attachments of the sternomastoid, feel with the middle finger on the suprasternal notch for the position of the trachea. A shallow suprasternal notch with a trachea that is easily palpated may indicate anterior displacement of the trachea, as in mediastinitis; or the notch may be deep and the trachea not easily palpable, as in the presence of anterior mediastinal tumor. Very slight deviation of the trachea towards the right is normal. Marked deviation of the trachea to one or the other side may indicate either a pulling force on the lungs toward the side of the deviation of the trachea (e.g., collapse or fibrosis of the lung on the ipsilateral side) or a force pushing the trachea away from the affected side (e.g., pneumothorax or pleural effusion on the contralateral side). Take care to exclude scoliosis before interpreting tracheal deviation as secondary to lung disease (see pages 228 & 229). Look for pendular movement of the trachea, moving to one side during inspiration and to the opposite side during expiration. This can be appreciated with the same maneuver as for palpation of the trachea. Pendular movement of the trachea is seen in obstruction of a large bronchus or in a large pneumothorax. Also palpate for rhonchus or thud over the trachea. If present, it indicates tracheal or laryngeal obstruction.

## Cardiac Impulse

Next, locate the point of maximum cardiac impulse, which usually is located over the fifth left intercostal space on or just inside the midclavicular line. In the absence of obvious heart disease or scoliosis, a change in position of the apical impulse of the trachea suggests deviation of the mediastinum because of lung disease or, in infants, congenital defects in placement of the organs (dextrocardia or large diaphragmatic hernia).

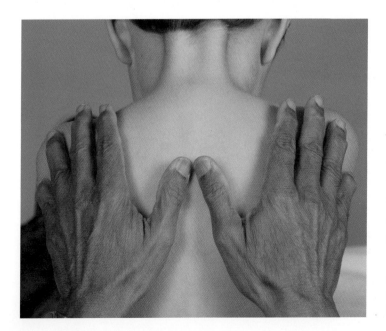

## Chest Excursion

The next step is to estimate the excursions of the two halves of the chest with respiration. Lay the palms of your hands on the posterior surface of the child's chest symmetrically with your thumbs touching each other in the midline (**Figure 7-1**). The fingers are spread over the sides of the chest. Steady your arms against the child's chest wall.

**Figure 7-1.** Method for estimating the equality of expansion of two halves of the chest.

Now, the excursions of the palm are noted with each inspiration. Normally, the palms move equally, as demonstrated by symmetrical movements of the thumbs going away from the midline with each inspiration and coming back together during expiration. When the two sides do not move symmetrically, the excursions are limited on one side and the thumb does not move away from the midline on the affected side, or the movements of thumbs are asymmetrical. This asymmetry suggests the presence of effusions or collapse or consolidation of the lung on the side with reduced excursions of the chest.

## Vocal Fremitus

Palpating for vocal fremitus also may help recognize changes in the conducting capacity of the lung. The child is asked to repeat the word "one" or "ninety-nine" while the examiner palpates all areas of the chest. The hand should detect distinct vibrations of equal intensity on corresponding areas of two sides of the chest. This is vocal fremitus. The intensity of the fremitus is diminished over areas where there is collapse of the lung (as in foreign-body obstruction of bronchus) or over pleural effusion. Vocal fremitus is increased over areas with consolidation or over a large cavity near the surface of the area being palpated. Occasionally, a to-and-fro *rub* may be palpable over an area of pleura which is inflamed. This is palpable pleural rub. A palpable thud over the chest usually indicates a foreign body in the trachea.

## Percussion

Observation made by percussion and auscultation of the chest should be described following the anatomic landmarks of the chest shown in **Figure 7-2**. The anterior aspect of the chest is divided into the presternal area and the right and left anterior portions. Each side is divided from above downward into supraclavicular (above the clavicle), infraclavicular (up to the level of the second rib), mammary (up to the fifth rib), and inframammary regions. On the lateral aspects, there are two areas: the axillary region (up to the level of the fourth rib) and the infraaxillary region. In the back, the regions are designated as suprascapular, interscapular, and infrascapular from above downwards. Description of physical findings using this anatomic surface landmark gives clinical precision. For example, a statement such as "stony dullness over right infrascapular area" is more precise than "dullness over right base." Why not be as precise about clinical descriptions as with the results of laboratory tests?

Auenbrugger, who was also a musician, got his idea for percussion of the chest from listening to the sounds when tapping barrels of beer to find out how full or empty they were. This is not a procedure relied on by present day clinicians, since more precise techniques are available. However, the following summary is given for the sake of completion.

One needs a cooperative patient to perform this procedure properly. It is preferable if the child is sitting or lying flat on his or her back so that observations on both sides of the chest can be compared. If there is scoliosis, percussion findings between the two sides cannot be truly compared.

The purpose of percussion is to make a comparison of the percussion note between corresponding areas of the two sides of the chest. Areas of altered resonance give clues to the presence of collapse of the lung, hyperaeration, cavitation or consolidation of the lung, and fluid in the pleural cavity. Direct percussion with one finger over the chest wall is done easily on smaller infants and gives valuable information. This requires experience.

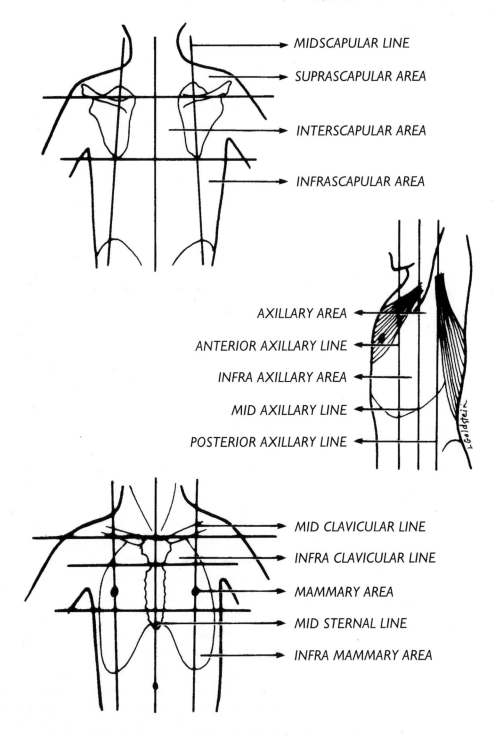

**Figure 7-2.** Surface anatomy of the chest used to describe location of abnormalities on percussion and auscultation.

The indirect, two-finger technique is the most commonly used method for percussion of the chest (**Figure 7-3**). The middle finger (pleximeter finger) of the left hand is placed on the chest wall so that it rests firmly, but not hard. The other fingers should not touch the chest wall since they may dampen the resonance. The middle phalanx of the middle finger (pleximeter finger) is then struck with the tip of the index or middle finger (plexor finger) of the right hand. The plexor finger should be bent in such a way that the strike lands perpendicularly—not at an angle. The striking finger should strike and spring back quickly so that it does not dampen the resonance. The movement of the striking finger should originate at the wrist and not at the elbow, which is likely to produce heavy percussion. Proper technique of percussion comes with experience, and experience comes from repeated practice.

It is best to start at the top (supraclavicular area) and proceed downward, systematically covering the front, sides, and back of the chest. Since the resonance is meaningful only in comparison to the opposite side, the percussion is done on the left infraclavicular area, right infraclavicular area, left mammary region, right mammary region, left inframammary region, right inframammary region, and so on. Remember to place the pleximeter finger parallel to the expected line of dullness. For example, to determine the upper edge of liver dullness, the finger is laid parallel to the ribs. But to percuss the right border of the heart, the finger is placed vertically on the chest, parallel to the right border of the sternum.

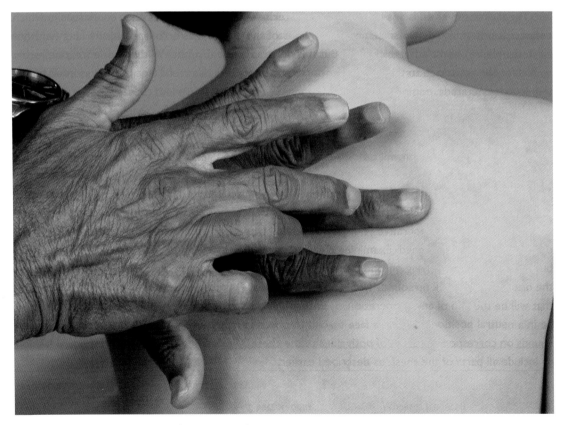

**Figure 7-3.** Two finger method of percussion of the chest.

# HEART

Examination of the heart should include arterial pulse, venous pulse, and blood pressure. These are discussed in Chapter 5, pages 95 & 96.

## Chest Landmarks

Before examining the precordium, learn the landmarks on the chest. The junction of the manubrium with the body of the sternum corresponds to the costochondral junction of the second rib and is called the "angle of Ludwig." Therefore, in defining the location of impulses or murmurs on the horizontal axis, feel for the angle of Ludwig (**Figure 7-5**). The space below this angle is the second intercostal space. From this definitive location, other landmarks can be identified easily. The xiphisternum starts at the level of connection of the sixth rib to the lower end of the sternum.

On the vertical axis, points of reference are midsternal line, lateral sternal line, and midclavicular line anteriorly. These are self-explanatory (**Figure 7-2**). Anterior-, mid-, and posterior-axillary lines on the lateral aspect of the chest and midscapular line over the posterior aspect of the chest are the other landmarks. In **Figure 7-5**, note that the anatomic location of the valves of the heart is different from the location at which sounds originating from that valve are best heard.

## Inspection

For proper examination of the chest, one has to undress the patient with due respect for privacy. There has to be a screen and it is best to have an observer, such as a nurse, particularly while examining

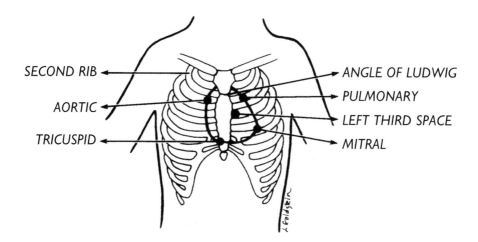

**Figure 7-5.** Surface anatomy of the chest to describe heart sounds and murmurs. Name of the location refers to the area at which sounds originating from the corresponding valves are heard best. Note that this area is located away from the anatomic location of the valve.

an adolescent. Observe for visible pulsation over various parts of the chest and in the epigastrium. If visible pulsations are seen on the right side, consider the possibility that the patient has dextrocardia, provided there is no scoliosis or pulmonary disease pushing or pulling the mediastinum. In coarctation of the aorta, collateral arterial circulation may develop, giving rise to visible pulsation of intercostal arteries of the chest wall. These are more visible over the posterior aspect of the chest wall.

Pulsations in the epigastrium normally can be seen in thin children or when children become excited. Occasionally, pulsations in the epigastrium are due to an enlarged right ventricle or pulsatile liver as in tricuspid regurgitation.

## Palpation

Apex beat corresponds to the lowermost and outermost point of the cardiac impulse. In normal older children, it is visible at or inside the midclavicular line on the fifth intercostal space. If it is not felt near this location, find out whether it is felt elsewhere over the anterior chest wall or is obscured. Apex beat is obscured in obesity, pericardial effusion, and emphysema. Apex beat may be displaced due to disease of the lung or scoliosis. If these causes are excluded, the common causes of displaced apex beat are cardiac enlargement, or rarely, dextrocardia. It is hyperdynamic in children during fever, in hyperthyroidism, in hypertension, and in impending heart failure.

Next, feel for the quality of the palpable *cardiac impulse*. A sensation of lifting of the palm on palpation of the precordium close to the sternum indicates right ventricular enlargement. The impulse hits the palm and stays with the palm. Left ventricular impulse is more forceful, stays only temporarily with the palpating palm, and is maximal farther to the left. In conditions of systolic overload (as in aortic stenosis), a forceful sustained heave is felt, but in diastolic overload (mitral regurgitation), the impulse is less forceful.

The pulmonary artery, if enlarged, can be palpated over the second left interspace at the lateral sternal line. An intense second pulmonary sound can be palpated as well.

Thrill is a "purring" sensation under the palm over the precordium in the presence of valvular diseases. If a thrill is felt, locate its point of maximum intensity and its relationship to the cardiac cycle. Use the diagram opposite (**Figure 7-5**) to recognize the location of the thrill. Time the thrill in relation to the maximum cardiac impulse.

Thrill over the pulmonary area may be systolic (pulmonary stenosis) or diastolic (pulmonary regurgitation). A to-and-fro thrill over the left infraclavicular area indicates a patent ductus. A systolic thrill over the left parasternal line may indicate pulmonary stenosis, ventricular septal defect, or auricular septal defect. A diastolic thrill along the left parasternal line is indicative of aortic regurgitation. A systolic thrill over the mitral area indicates regurgitation; whereas, a diastolic thrill over this area indicates mitral stenosis. Aortic stenosis is characterized by a systolic thrill over the aortic area and aortic regurgitation is characterized by a diastolic thrill best appreciated along the left parasternal line. A palpable thrill over blood vessels may indicate the presence of aneurysm or arteriovenous fistula.

Functional murmurs are almost never associated with a thrill except in children with a very thin chest wall.

Splitting of the first sound is difficult to detect. Even if detected, it is no indication of heart disease. Its importance is that it can be confused with systolic ejection click heard best near the apical impulse.

Listen to the heart in a quiet room and listen for the split during the peak of inspiration and at the end of expiration. Normally, the split is more marked and clearly recognized during the peak of inspiration. Ask the following questions while listening to the split:

- Is splitting present or absent? (If absent, consider aortic stenosis and extremely severe pulmonary stenosis.)
- If present, is it normally split?

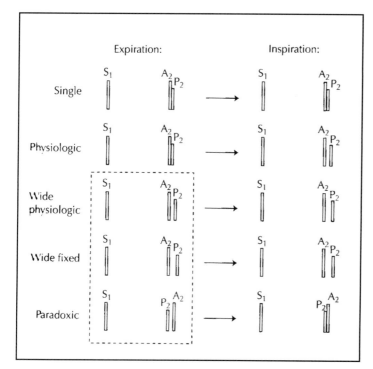

**Figure 7-6.** S2 Splitting. There are two normal patterns (single and physiologic) and three abnormal patterns (wide physiologic, wide fixed and paradoxic). All three abnormal forms of splitting are distinguished by audible expiratory splitting. Reproduced with permission from McGee S, Evidence-Based Physical Diagnosis. Philadelphia. 2001. W B Saunders Co. page 459. (Copyright Elsevier 2001)

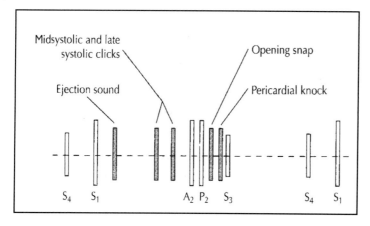

**Figure 7-7.** Miscellaneous Heart sounds. This figure shows the timing of miscellaneous systolic sounds (ejection sounds and mid- to late systolic clicks) and diastolic sounds (opening snap), in relation to the principle heart sounds (first, second, thord and fourth heart sounds) Reproduced with permission from McGee S, Evidence-Based Physical Diagnosis. Philadelphia. 2001. W B Saunders Co. page 483. (Copyright Elsevier 2001)

- If it is split widely with prolongation of the interval between the aortic and pulmonic component, does the wide split appear to be fixed (without any difference during inspiration and expiration)? If so, consider a large atrial septal defect.
- Is the split paradoxical (aortic component coming after pulmonary component)? If it is paradoxical, the split narrows during inspiration (instead of widening). This occurs in aortic stenosis, left bundle branch block, and patent ductus arteriosus (see **Figure 7-6**).

## Third heart sound (S3)

S3 is a low frequency sound normally heard during early diastole over the apex (mitral area) in many healthy children, including adolescents. It is caused by the rapid flow of blood to the ventricles early in diastole. Third heart sound is best heard with the bell of the stethoscope when the patient is in the left lateral position. It is loudest during expiration. Though the presence of third heart sound is not abnormal in the pediatric age group, increased intensity of this sound often is associated with a hyperdynamic heart, as in anemia or a large left-to-right shunt.

The third heart sound has to be differentiated from splitting of the first and second sounds, opening snap, and gallop rhythm. The differences between the third heart sound and normal splitting are listed in **Table 7-2** (also see Appendix 7-1).

## Opening Snap (**Figure 7-7 and Appendix 7-1**)

The opening snap is a high frequency sound heard in diastole almost immediately after the second sound and is indicative of a stenotic mitral valve with mobile anterior leaflet (sounds like "bu DUP" rather than just "DUP"). This occasionally may be mistaken for a widely split second heart sound. The differentiating points are 1) the opening snap is heard best over the precordium at the fourth intercostal space over the left lower sternal border, whereas the split second sound is heard over the pulmonary area, and 2) the opening snap is best heard in expiration or shows no variation with respiration, whereas the split is best heard in inspiration.

**Table 7-3. Characteristics of the Ejection Sound Heard Over the Aortic and Pulmonary Area**

|  | **Aortic** | **Pulmonary** |
|---|---|---|
| Location | Entire precordium | Upper left sterna border |
| Relation to heart sounds | Separated from first sound by a few milliseconds | Close to or on top of the first sound |
| Relation to respiration | No relationship to phase of respiration | Better heard during expiration, diminishes in intensity during inspiration |

Opening snap also has to be differentiated from the third heart sound which is heard over the apex, is low pitched, and muffled. Opening snap has a sharp quality and occurs earlier than S3 but later than split S2.

## Ejection Sounds and Clicks (Table 7-3)

Unlike opening snap, ejection sound (previously called ejection click) is heard during early systole very soon after SI (sounds like "bu *lub*"). It is a high pitched sound and is produced by an abnormal semilunar valve (pulmonary or aortic) or conditions leading to sudden dilatation of the pulmonary artery or the aorta. These sounds may be associated with a murmur.

The term *systolic click* is applied to sounds heard during mid or late systole. These sounds have a clicking quality and may or may not be associated with murmur. An apical midsystolic click is always abnormal and is indicative of a "prolapsed mitral valve." Occasionally clicks may be associated with a small pneumothorax. These clicks will be associated with respiratory movement.

## Triple Rhythm

Triple rhythm may be caused by a normal third heart sound or a gallop rhythm. Both are heard mainly over the mitral area. The differences are 1) the third component of gallop rhythm may be palpable, and 2) gallop rhythm appears in the presence of other serious heart disease.

## Gallop Rhythm

Gallop rhythm is the name given to heart sounds that resemble the sound of galloping horses rather than the "tick-tack," "lub-dup," to-and-fro characteristics of normal heart sounds. There is a third or fourth component with each cardiac cycle. A third sound gallop, also called "protodiastolic gallop," is located over the apex of the heart and is often a sign of heart failure. A fourth sound gallop is called a "presystolic gallop." A summation gallop is produced in the presence of tachycardia when these two components fuse. It is often difficult to differentiate between these subtypes of gallop rhythms.

## Fourth Heart Sound (S4)

The fourth heart sound is a low pitched sound heard just before systole. It is best heard over the apex of the heart with the patient in the left lateral position and with the bell of the stethoscope. It is accentuated during expiration. Fourth heart sound is said to be caused by atrial contraction and is heard just before SI. Many authorities consider the presence of S4 abnormal.

## Adventitious Sounds

Adventitious sounds are not heard in normal individuals (except the functional murmur) and are heard in addition to the heart sounds. These may be classified as murmurs, rubbing sounds, and cardiorespiratory sounds. The characteristics of the precordial murmur, if heard, should be discussed under the following headings: 1) location, 2) relationship to cardiac cycle, 3) intensity, 4) change in intensity in relation to respiration, 5) direction of spread, and 6) change in intensity in relation to posture.

## Murmurs (use Figure 7-7 and Appendix 7-1)

• (An internet search will lead one to several sites with audio recordings of heart sounds and murmurs. Also see references at the end of this chapter.)

## Location

Examples of murmurs in relation to the location of maximum intensity are listed in **Table 7-4**.

## Relationship to cardiac cycle

Heart murmurs are classified as *systolic* (when they occur with or immediately following the first heart sound and before the second sound), *diastolic* (when they occur after the second but before the first sound), or *continuous* (when they occur through systole and diastole).

**Table 7-4. Heart Murmurs: Location and Relationship to Cardiac Cycle**

| Location | Systolic | Diastolic |
|---|---|---|
| Mitral area | Functional murmur<br>Mitral regurgitation | Mitral stenosis |
| Pulmonary area | Functional murmur<br>Pulmonary stenosis<br>Atrial septal defect | Pulmonary hypertension<br>Pulmonary regurgitation |
| Lower left sternal border | Ventricular septal defect<br>Functional murmur<br>Aortic stenosis | Aortic regurgitation<br>Pulmonary regurgitation |
| Aortic area | Aortic stenosis<br>Coarctation of aorta | Aortic regurgitation |
| Tricuspid | Tricuspid regurgitation | Tricuspid stenosis |
| Left second intercostal space | Patent ductus arteriosus | Patent ductus arteriosus |
| Neck | Venous hum<br>Aortic stenosis<br>Pulmonary stenosis | |
| Back | Usually a valvular stenosis | |

The following steps may help recognize this relationship. While listening to the heart, concentrate on the first sound for five or six cardiac cycles while saying "one" as the first sound is heard. Then try to locate the relationship of the murmur to the first sound. Repeat the same steps now with attention on the second sound, to recognize the characteristics of the diastolic murmur.

If systolic murmur is heard over any area, try to determine whether it is heard very early in systole, in midsystole, or throughout systole. Systolic murmur may be:

- Holosystolic—occurring throughout systole, beginning with the first heart sound and ending with the second sound. Murmurs of ventricular septal defect and mitral regurgitation are holosystolic.

- Early systolic murmur—occurring very early, beginning with the first sound and ending in midsystole. These also are called "ejection murmurs." These murmurs are usually short and soft. Murmurs of aortic stenosis and functional murmurs belong to this class. The location, mild intensity, lack of spread, and absence of thrill will help differentiate the functional murmur.

- Midsystolic—starting a few milliseconds into the systole (not at the very beginning), peaking in midsystole, and ending before the second heart sound. These also are called "flow murmurs." Examples of this type of murmur are functional murmurs, murmurs of mild aortic and pulmonary stenosis, and murmurs of atrial septal defect. A beginner may find it hard to recognize these characteristics. During the training sessions, listening to sound recordings of heart sounds and murmurs should help.

- Diastolic murmurs are always pathologic. They may be early diastolic, as in pulmonary and aortic regurgitation, or mid-diastolic as in early mitral stenosis. Continuous murmurs are heard in patent ductus arteriosus and in arteriovenous fistula.

## Intensity

The intensity of the murmur is not necessarily related to the seriousness of the disease. For example, the small ventricular septal defect can produce a very rough harsh murmur, whereas the diastolic murmur of aortic regurgitation may be hardly audible. Murmurs due to obstruction of flow through a narrowed valve are rough, whereas murmurs due to leakage of blood through incompetent valves are soft and blowing in character.

The murmurs are usually graded from 1 to 4 with Grade 1 being the softest and Grade 4 being the loudest (Levine grading system).

Grade 1.    Soft, not heard immediately on auscultation; have to focus on systole
            for a few beats.
Grade 2.    Soft, heard immediately on auscultation but not loud.
Grade 3.    Loud and heard easily, no thrill.
Grade 4.    Loud, associated with a thrill.

Some include Grades 5 and 6 for loud murmurs heard even without the stethoscope touching the chest wall.

## Intensity in relation to respiration

Murmurs originating on the right side of the heart increase in intensity during inspiration caused by an increase in stroke output of the right side. Conversely, murmurs arising on the left side are accentuated during expiration. This is the reason for listening to the parasternal area during expiration to listen for aortic diastolic murmur. The Still's type of functional murmur also may vary in intensity with the respiratory cycle.

Ask the patient to hold his or her breath for a few seconds and listen to the intensity of the murmur. After the patient starts breathing normally, keep listening to the intensity of the murmur for 10 to 12 more cardiac cycles. Murmurs originating on the right side of the heart (atrial septal defect, pulmonary stenosis) tend to return to the basic level of intensity very quickly, whereas murmurs originating on the left side of the heart (ventricular septal defect) return to control intensities slowly.

## Direction of spread

The murmur is said to radiate if it is heard with equal intensity some distance away from the point of maximum intensity. Presence of a thrill and radiation of murmur away from the point of origin indicate that the heart murmur is a pathological murmur. Innocent murmurs are not associated with thrill and do not radiate to the back. The innocent murmur of the pulmonary ejection type may radiate down along the parasternal line to the fourth intercostal space.

A list of heart lesions with their characteristic murmur and the direction of the spread of the murmur are given in **Table 7-5**.

## Relationship to posture

Next, determine the effect of posture on the murmur. For example, if a murmur is heard over the root of the neck on the right side with the patient sitting, listen to the same area with the patient supine. If the murmur disappears, it is probably cervical venous hum. On the other hand, the ejection type of functional murmur heard over the pulmonary area is heard best in the supine position. The murmur of aortic regurgitation is heard better when the patient is sitting up and leaning forward (and is holding the breath in expiration).

Murmurs of mitral regurgitation and aortic stenosis decrease in intensity when the patient goes from a recumbent to a sitting position.

Ask the patient to sit up from a lying down position repeatedly 10 to 15 times, then lie down on the left side and auscultate over the apex of the heart. This may accentuate the soft systolic murmur of acute rheumatic fever, which may not be heard in a patient resting in bed.

Repeatedly going from a standing to squatting position may accentuate the systolic murmur of mitral valve prolapse.

## Innocent Murmurs (Functional Murmurs, Physiologic Murmurs)

During his favorite routine of listening to murmurs over various areas of the body, Dr. Donald Cassels (1957) of the University of Chicago mentions seven locations where *functional murmurs* can be heard. These locations are 1) a systolic murmur over the head of young children particularly before the closure of the fontanel, heard symmetrically above both ears and over the parietal areas; 2) a murmur near the tip of the mastoid close to where the vessels enter the base of the skull, also symmetrical; 3) a cervical venous hum (continuous murmur) over the right side of the neck; 4) a murmur at the root of the neck but only in systole; 5) murmurs originating at sites above the clavicle (items 3 and 4) but radiating below the clavicle; 6) basal systolic functional murmur; and 7) Still's murmur.

Innocent or *physiologic murmurs* are so common in the pediatric age group that they deserve some explanation. The most common of these are 1) the "twanging-string" murmur of Still, 2) basal ejection murmur, and 3) the venous hum (items 3, 6, and 7 of the preceding paragraph).

### Table 7-5. Characteristics of Radiation (Spreading) of Heart Murmur

| Lesion | Murmur | Radiation to |
|---|---|---|
| Mitral regurgitation | Mitral stenosis | Lateral and posterior aspect of the chest |
| Mitral stenosis | Mitral diastolic | Lateral and posterior aspect of the chest |
| Pulmonary stenosis | Pulmonary systolic | Left side of neck, left infraclavicular area and the back |
| Pulmonary regurgitation | Pulmonary diastolic | Left parasternal line |
| Aortic stenosis | Aortic systolic | To the neck along carotids; may transmit to apex |
| Aortic regurgitation | Aortic diastolic | Along the left lateral sternal border |
| Patent ductus arteriosus | To-and-fro over left infraclavicular area | Second and third left intercostal spaces, parasternally |
| Atrial septal defect | Second and third left intercostal spaces, parasternal line | Poor transmission |
| Ventricular septal defect | Third to fifth left intercostal spaces, parasternal line | To the right of the sternum, to entire precordium |

The "twanging-string" murmur of Still has a musical quality and is best heard over the mid-precordium to the left of the lower sternum. It is heard in the first one-third of systole and has crescendo-decrescendo characteristics. It is best heard when the patient is supine. The intensity is variable and may increase with exercise.

Basal systolic murmur is heard over the left second interspace in the first one-third of systole with the patient supine. The intensity diminishes on sitting. It has a harsher quality, and therefore may be mistaken for the murmur of pulmonic stenosis. Absence of thrill and absence of transmission to posterior chest wall differentiate this from an organic murmur.

Venous hum is a low pitched continuous murmur (systole and diastole) heard best at the base of the neck. Cervical venous hum is heard commonly on the right side of the neck, may be accompanied by a thrill, and often is transmitted to the second right intercostal space. It is accentuated when the patient is sitting. It disappears when the patient lies down and is obliterated by the Valsalva maneuver. The Valsalva maneuver is performed by straining (as done during difficult bowel movements) in which the patient attempts forced expiration with the mouth and nose closed.

Cervical venous hum is physiologic but is more common in the presence of high output states, such as anemia. Venous hum is obliterated in the presence of constrictive pericarditis or superior vena cava obstruction.

## Rubs

A pericardial rub is a to-and-fro leathery, scratching sound heard with systole and diastole. It often is heard for only a short duration of time, disappears, and reappears again. If there is effusion, the rub disappears. Pericardial rub is best heard with the patient sitting up and the chest piece of the stethoscope held over the left second and third intercostal space immediately to the left of the sternum.

*Cardiorespiratory murmurs usually* are heard at the apex or over areas where the heart and lung are close together. They are heard as if they originate close to the chest piece of the stethoscope, vary with respiration, are mid or late systolic, and have a high pitch. They often are heard in pericarditis and in emphysema.

**Special maneuvers** to increase the intensity of murmurs include deep inspiration, Valsalva, squatting from a standing position, and sustained abdominal pressure. To appreciate the increased intensity, auscultate at the edge of the murmur's radiation. Inspiration and abdominal pressure increase the venous return to the heart and increase the intensity of right heart murmurs. Both venous return and arterial resistance are increased when the patient squats from a standing position or on passive elevation of the leg. These maneuvers increase the intensity of murmurs of hypertrophic cardiomyopathy and mitral valve prolapse. The Valsalva maneuver decreases the venous return, increases systemic arterial resistance, and decreases the intensity of aortic stenotic murmur and the venous hum.

*Evidence based examination: When cardiologists and trainees in cardiology examined adult patients in a clinical setting, the reliability of detecting systolic murmurs was fair (0.30 to 0.48). If a cardiologist assessed a murmur as "normal," the likelihood of finding a cardiac abnormality was low. Conversely, if a cardiologist assessed a murmur as significant, the likelihood of finding a cardiac abnormality was high. The presence of any one of the following increased the likelihood of aortic stenosis as the final diagnosis: effort syncope, slow rate of rise in carotid artery, late timing of peak murmur intensity, and decreased intensity of the second heart sound. Absence of a mitral murmur or a late systolic or holosystolic murmur (as documented by a cardiologist) reduced the likelihood of finding mitral regurgitation. A systolic click with or without systolic murmur is strong evidence for mitral valve prolapse.*

*One study in pediatrics, based on examination by pediatric cardiologists, showed the following significant features for predicting cardiac abnormality: 1) murmur of harsh quality, pansystolic in timing, intensity of Grade 3 or more, and located over the left upper sternal border; 2) presence of a click; and 3) abnormal second heart sound.*

## Sounds Produced By Prosthetic Valves

The opening and closing sounds are louder with a clicking or metallic quality and may even be heard without a stethoscope. Whether the sound is loud during opening of the valve or the closure depends on the type of the valve. The aortic valve is associated with a midsystolic murmur heard on either side of the upper part of the sternum. The murmur of prosthetic mitral valve is also midsystolic and heard over the left sternal border. *Any diastolic murmur with these prosthetic valves suggests a leak.*

## Some Physical Principles of Auscultation

Immediate or direct auscultation by applying the ears to the chest was practiced by Hippocrates, Harvey, and Corvisart long before Laennec's description of the stethoscope.[2] Laennec was forced to think up a method for indirect auscultation when he encountered a 16-year-old obese girl with heart disease. Laennec described his two-part, 12-inch-long cylinder of wood with one funnel-shaped end in 1819. This was obviously monoaural. C. J. B. Williams described the first binaural stethoscope in 1843. In this device, a rigid lead tube connected the chest piece and the earpiece. The prototype of the modern stethoscope with a flexible tube was described by Dr. George Cammann in 1855. All of these stethoscopes had a bell-type chest piece. The first diaphragm-type chest piece with a flexible membrane was invented by Dr. Marsh of Cincinnati in 1851. After many modifications, the modern bakelite chest piece was patented by Dr. R.C.M. Bowles of Brookline, Massachusetts, in 1901 and his name has since been used almost synonymously with the diaphragm-type chest piece.

During auscultation, vibrations set up inside the chest and transmitted through the chest wall are picked up by the chest piece of the stethoscope, transmitted through the column of air in the tubing, and reach the ear. The ear is only the recording mechanism. The brain has to interpret these sounds. It is logical to conclude that the final interpretation of the sounds originating in the chest is subject to the following variables:

***Variables Related to the Source of Sound***
- Origin of sound (heart or lung)
- The frequency of vibrations
- The sound pressure (energy) of the sounds
- The conducting medium of the chest

[2] *The word stethoscope means "to measure the chest" (scope meaning measure; stethos meaning chest).*

### Variables Related to the Stethoscope
- Type of chest piece
- Tubing
- Earpiece

### Variables Related to the Interpreter of the Sound
- Age and experience of the physician
- The characteristics of the human ear and brain

The following is a summary of the characteristics of these variables. The normal heart sounds originate from the closure and opening of atrioventricular valves and the closure and opening of the semilunar valves. The normal breath sounds are due to the passage of air to and from the alveoli through bronchi of varying sizes. The contents of the chest have an attenuating effect on the sound waves. Therefore, the sounds originating in the major four valves are heard best over that area of the chest wall which is reached via a path of minimum attenuation. This is the reason why the sound originating in the mitral valve is heard best over the apex of the heart though the valve itself is located more medially.

The frequency cycles of the heart and lung sounds range from 120 to 1000 cycles per second (cps). Most of these are below the 660 cps range. It is obvious therefore that an efficient transmitting mechanism is required to hear these sounds, though an occasional click or pericardial rub can be heard by the patient or observer without any aid. As a general rule, breath sounds have a higher pitch than heart sounds. The frequencies of various heart and lung sounds are listed in **Table 7-6**.

During auscultation, we hear sounds of varying pitch and intensity. The human ear is a good detector of change in frequency cycles, if the change is gradual. But it is not adequate for detecting changes in intensity at the very low energy levels characteristic of the heart and lung sounds. Presence of sounds of varying pitch introduces the problem of masking. As the intensity increases, the low-pitched tones become more prominent, since the high-pitched tones are masked or attenuated. Obesity has a definite effect on the quality of the heart sounds. Another type of masking is seen when

### Table 7-6. Frequency Cycle of Various Heart and Lung Sounds

|  | Sounds | Frequencies (cycle per sec) |
|---|---|---|
| Heart | Low pitched heart murmurs | 400 |
|  | High pitched heart murmurs | 660 |
|  | Systolic and diastolic murmurs | 120 to 650 (up to 1000) |
|  | Presystolic murmurs | 140 |
|  | Pericardial rub | 140 to 660 |
| Lungs | Rales | 120 to 1000 |
|  | Amphonic breathing | 240 to 660 |
|  | Bronchial | 240 to 1000 |

There are various techniques to relax the abdominal wall. The central theme is distraction. Some children distract easily if you engage them in a conversation. Others will relax with laughing, and some standard jokes are in order. Some children have to be examined when they are sitting up or lying prone. Flexing the hips and asking the child to take a deep breath will relax the abdominal wall in most children. In some, asking the child to take deep breaths and palpating quickly during expiration will work. The same is accomplished in a crying child. Wait until the child relaxes the tension on the abdominal wall at the end of the expiratory phase of crying and, when the child takes a deep breath, press your fingers as the abdomen relaxes. In ticklish children, place your hand on top of the child's hand, but with the index finger somewhat overlapping. Palpate the abdomen with the child's own hand, except your index finger can dip in a little just over the edge of the child's hand (**Figure 8-1**).

Before palpating the abdomen, ask the child to point to where it hurts and palpate this area last. Normally, abdominal palpation should cause no pain. If there is an area of tenderness, note its location and point of maximum intensity. Also, try to elicit rebound tenderness. Press firmly over one area of the abdomen. If there is no pain, suddenly release and remove the fingers from the abdominal wall. Tenderness on withdrawal of the fingers ("rebound tenderness") indicates peritoneal irritation.

Tenderness along the edge of the liver is seen in hepatitis. Tenderness over the right upper quadrant to the right of the midline is seen in duodenal ulcer. Tenderness of the right lower quadrant is seen in appendiceal infection. Left upper quadrant tenderness may be indicative of splenic rupture or infarct. Tenderness along the left upper and lower quadrants along the flanks is seen in ulcerative colitis and amebiasis. Loin tenderness is seen in perinephric abscess. Diffuse tenderness of the abdomen indicates peritonitis. Pain due to spasm of the intestines may be relieved by pressure and squeezing, whereas pain due to intraabdominal inflammatory conditions is aggravated by pressure.

Note whether the tone of the abdominal wall is soft, firm, or tense. A hard tense feeling usually indicates serious intraabdominal pathology. Board-like rigidity indicates peritonitis. Diffuse firmness may indicate chest disease or muscle spasm, as in tetanus. Localized firmness indicates a mass (e.g., a midline firm mass may be a full bladder). Very soft texture of the abdominal wall is seen in prune-belly syndrome. A palpable mass in the right lower quadrant may be the cecum or the appendix. A mass in the right upper quadrant usually is related to the liver; in the left upper quadrant, it is related to the stomach or the spleen. Flank masses usually are related to the kidneys.

## Pyloric Stenosis

Examine the infant after the stomach has been emptied to palpate the pyloric mass in congenital pyloric stenosis. Ask the mother to hold the baby in a relaxed position. It will be helpful to give the baby some sugar-water to drink just before palpating for the mass. Sometimes it is necessary to feed clear liquids until the baby vomits and palpate the abdomen soon after the vomiting. Gently flex the hip with one hand to relax the anterior abdominal wall, and palpate the abdomen with the other hand at a point midway between the umbilicus and the costal margin along the lateral border of the right rectus muscle. The fingertips should be used with a kneading up-and-down motion to feel for a firm olive-like swelling of the pyloric mass.

**Table 8-1. Expected Liver Span of Infants and Children (in cm)**

| | Males | | | Females | |
| --- | --- | --- | --- | --- | --- |
| Age/yr | Mean Estimated Liver Span | SEM | Age/yr | Mean Estimated Liver Span | SEM |
| 6 months | 2.4 | 2.5 | 6 months | 2.6 | 2.6 |
| 1 | 2.8 | 2.0 | 1 | 3.1 | 2.1 |
| 2 | 3.5 | 1.6 | 2 | 3.6 | 1.7 |
| 3 | 4.0 | 1.6 | 3 | 4.0 | 1.7 |
| 4 | 4.4 | 1.6 | 4 | 4.3 | 1.6 |
| 5 | 4.8 | 1.5 | 5 | 4.5 | 1.6 |
| 6 | 5.1 | 1.5 | 6 | 4.8 | 1.6 |
| 8 | 5.6 | 1.5 | 8 | 5.1 | 1.6 |
| 10 | 6.1 | 1.6 | 10 | 5.4 | 1.7 |
| 12 | 6.5 | 1.8 | 12 | 5.6 | 1.8 |
| 14 | 6.8 | 2.0 | 14 | 5.8 | 2.1 |
| 16 | 7.1 | 2.2 | 16 | 6.0 | 2.3 |
| 18 | 7.4 | 2.5 | 18 | 6.1 | 2.6 |
| 20 | 7.7 | 2.8 | 20 | 6.3 | 2.9 |

SEM: standard of error of the mean.

Reprinted from: Lawson EE, Grand RK, Neff RK, Cohen LF. Clinical estimation of liver span in infants and children. Am J Dis Child. 1978;132: 474-6. (Copyright 1978, American Medical Association. All rights reserved)

# Appendicitis

Appendicitis starts in children with a history of persistent but vague and diffuse abdominal pain, often in the periumbilical area. Soon it localizes to the right lower quadrant. The appendix may not be in its classical location in the right lower quadrant; therefore, symptoms and signs may vary depending on the location. Flank pain may be seen with location of the appendix along the paracolic gutter. There also may be loss of appetite, lowgrade fever, and change in bowel habits. Constipation is the usual manifestation though diarrhea may occur with retrocecal or pelvic appendix.

The classical finding on examination is focal point tenderness over the inflamed appendix. This may be located on the McBurney's point, which is midway between the right anterior superior iliac spine and the umbilicus. If the appendix is located along the paracolic gutter, the tenderness may be over the flank of the abdomen or felt only on deep palpation. If the appendix is in the retrocecal or pelvic position, tenderness is elicited on a deep rectal examination. Cough also may aggravate the pain and cause the child to wince.

If the appendix has perforated, the findings will be those of peritonitis. The child will appear toxic and pale, lying still with grunting respiration. The abdomen will feel rigid on palpation with generalized guarding, and the bowel sounds will be absent. A mass may be palpable in the right lower quadrant, either on examination of the abdomen or on rectal examination.

## Liver

The liver is normally located on the right side and its size varies with the age and size of the child. In addition, size of the liver as determined by palpation will be different from the size determined by percussion. Neither of these is as accurate as the size determined by imaging techniques. Normal data for total height of the liver and for the size of the liver palpable below the costal margin are available (**Table 8-1**).

With the child lying supine without a pillow, stand on the right side of the child (if right-handed) and palpate starting from the lower right quadrant gradually moving up. If the liver edge is palpated, measure the size below the costal margin at the mid-clavicular line using a ruler or tape measure. Normal values are 3.0 to 3.5 cm below the costal margin up to six months of age, 0 to 3 cm in children between six months to four years of age, less than 2 cm in children between four and 10 years of age, and less than 1 cm in children over 10 years of age.

To measure the total height of the liver, percuss along the midclavicular line anteriorly with the pleximeter finger held parallel to the ribs using heavy percussion. A mark is made at the intercostal space when dullness is first noted. To determine the lower border of the liver, percussion is started at the right lower quadrant and gradually moved towards the costal margin. Light percussion is used. The point at which the tone changes to dullness is marked, and this denotes the lower edge of the liver. The vertical height between the two points is now measured. Normal values for vertical height of the liver (liver span) at various ages are given in **Table 8-1**.

Be sure to palpate the left lobe of the liver at the epigastrium. This is particularly important in the tropics, where amebic abscess of the liver and portal hypertension are common. In both of these conditions, the left lobe of the liver is more prominent than the right lobe. It is good to auscultate over the liver, since a hepatic rub can be heard in the presence of perihepatitis, liver abscess, and leukemic infiltration of the liver.

*Evidence based examination: The conclusion of a study on the size of the liver in adults is as follows: "a palpable liver is not necessarily enlarged or diseased, but does increase the likelihood of hepatomegaly." Since half of all palpable livers are not enlarged, measurement of vertical liver span is required.*

## Spleen

The spleen is normally located on the left side. It usually is not palpable unless it is enlarged at least three times its size. Remember to start palpating over the right lower quadrant and proceed diagonally toward the left upper quadrant. Recognizing an enlarged spleen depends on feeling the edge of the organ. A very large spleen may cross the midline with the palpable edge on the right side, and the edge can be missed if palpation is done only on the left side.

If the spleen is not palpable with the patient in the supine position, examine the patient in the right lateral position. With the patient lying on the right side, place your left hand over the left lower ribs on the midscapular line pushing the spleen gently, and use your right hand to palpate the spleen. This is called "Short's maneuver."

Castell described a percussion sign for determining an enlarged spleen. (*Caution: Do not percuss if there is suspicion of a ruptured spleen.*) With the patient in the supine position, percussion of the lower intercostal spaces on the anterior axillary line produces a resonant note both in inspiration and expiration. If the spleen is enlarged, the percussion over the lower intercostal spaces is resonant during expiration and dull during inspiration. Another method is to show dullness over the Traub's space (an area delineated by the sixth rib superiorly, midaxillary line laterally, and the left costal margin inferiorly). Also remember to listen over the spleen with the stethoscope since a splenic rub may be heard in perisplenitis.

*Evidence based examination: In one study on adults, no one method was found to be superior to others for palpation of the spleen. Splenic percussion had high sensitivity but poor specificity.*

## Other Intraabdominal Organs and Masses

Masses over the right lower quadrant usually are related to the appendix but may be due to cecal mass or to ovarian masses in the female. In intussusception, an ill-defined sausage-shaped mass is felt over the right upper quadrant. Associated with this, the right lower quadrant is found to be empty.

Palpation of the kidneys may be difficult in obese children. In normal children, one uses deep bimanual palpation to feel for the kidneys. With the patient supine and the abdomen relaxed, place the palm of one hand posteriorly at the flank, pushing the kidneys forward. Place the other hand anteriorly, over the anterior abdominal wall below the costal margin, and feel for the kidney during deep inspiration.

After feeling for the liver, spleen, and urinary bladder feel for any other intraabdominal masses. If any mass is felt in the abdomen, describe its characteristics by answering the following questions:

- Where is it located?
- Where are the upper and lower borders?
- Does it cross midline or is it in midline?
- Is it attached to abdominal wall?
- Is it firm, hard, soft, or cystic?
- Does it move with respiration?
- Is it movable?
- Is there bruit or murmur? Is it pulsatile?

## Percussion (for Fluid)

Normally, the abdomen sounds tympanic on percussion except when percussed over solid organs such as the liver or a full bladder. A highly tympanic note is heard in intestinal obstruction or paralytic ileus. If the abdomen is enlarged due to free fluid in the abdominal cavity, obesity, or a mass, the percussion note will be dull.

The following methods may be used to detect free fluid in the abdomen:

1.  Bulging flanks may indicate free fluid or obesity.

2.  If the flanks are full, percussion starting from the umbilicus and moving towards the flank and listening for transition from resonant to a dull note may indicate the presence of fluid. However, if the patient is obese, the dullness on percussion may not necessarily indicate fluid.

3.  Further evidence for free fluid may be obtained by eliciting *shifting dullness*. With the patient in the supine position, place a finger on the flank parallel to the midline. Percuss over an area of dullness. Now ask the patient to roll over and lie on the opposite side to the percussed dullness, while keeping the pleximeter finger in place. After the fluid has time to settle at the dependent position, percuss again. Percussion now will give a tympanic note over the same area where it was dull when the patient was supine.

4.  The following method is used to elicit *fluid wave*. With the patient supine, have another observer place the edge of his or her hand vertically on the midline of the abdominal wall (**Figure 8-2**). Now place the palm of your hand on one side and tap with the fingers on the opposite flank. If free fluid is present, you can feel a fluid wave created by the tap.

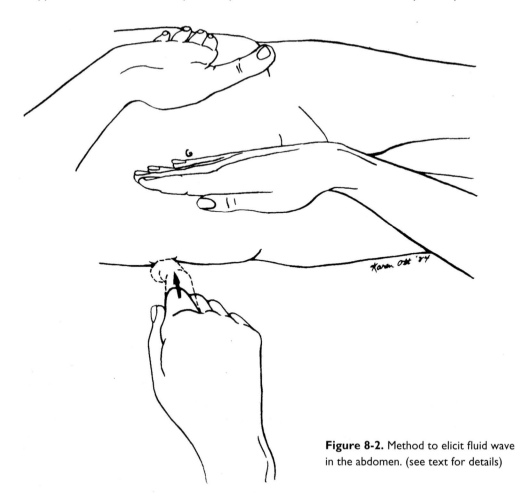

**Figure 8-2.** Method to elicit fluid wave in the abdomen. (see text for details)

5. To detect very small amounts of fluid, place the patient in a knee-chest position and percuss over the periumbilical area. Normally this produces a resonant sound. A dull note on percussion suggests free fluid in the abdomen. This is called the "puddle sign."

*Evidence based examination: The most useful findings for diagnosing ascites are fluid wave, shifting dullness, and peripheral edema. No single sign is both sensitive and specific. Puddle sign and auscultatory percussion have low sensitivity and are not recommended.*

## Bowel Sounds (Auscultation)

Listen to the bowel sounds before starting palpation. Normally, the bowel sounds are best heard along a diagonal line six inches long, starting one inch to the left and above the umbilicus and running toward the right lower quadrant. The sounds have a gurgling quality. These sounds are increased and have a higher pitch in the presence of gastroenteritis. The sounds have a metallic quality during early stages of intestinal obstruction. These sounds are absent in paralytic ileus and in late obstruction. In the presence of ascites and peritonitis, the sound may be distant.

In addition, listen to murmurs over the abdomen, particularly over the flank, since renal artery stenosis can produce a systolic murmur. Bruit may be heard even in normal individuals, over the anterior abdominal wall between the xiphisternum and the umbilicus, particularly in thin individuals. These are usually systolic sounds, which rarely spread to the flanks. Loud murmurs heard over other areas are most likely pathologic.

# INGUINAL REGIONS

Hernia, hydrocele, undescended testicle, and lymph nodes are common causes of swelling in the inguinal region. If a swelling is present in this area, describe the characteristics as outlined earlier (page 6, **Table 1-1**). In addition, describe whenever there are fluctuations in size, either spontaneously or related to coughing or crying.

## Hernia

Indirect inguinal hernia is the most common variety (direct inguinal and femoral hernia are rare). It occurs more often in boys. Classically, there is a bulge in the inguinal region extending into the scrotum. This enlarges and becomes tense when the child cries. Usually the swelling becomes smaller in size when the child is not straining, or when reduced by external manipulation.

Another way to locate subtle evidences of inguinal hernia is as follows: palpate the spermatic cord and compare its texture with the opposite side and with that of normal children. A thickened cord is evidence of indirect inguinal hernia. Also, palpate the cord gently and roll it along its longitudinal axis under the fingers. A silky texture to the cord may suggest an indirect inguinal hernia. This is a very subjective sign, and surgical hernia repair should not be initiated on the basis of the "silky cord" sign alone.

level than the right, but one side is not larger than the other. If one side appears larger than the other, determine if the larger side is abnormal (due to swelling of the testes or swelling around the testes) or the smaller side is abnormal (due to absence of the testis in its usual location). Palpation of the testicle and the soft tissues of the scrotum should help decide this question. In addition, look at the wrinkles over the scrotum. If the distance between the wrinkles is narrower on the small side compared with the larger side, the testis most likely has not descended into that scrotum.

The scrotum may be small if the testis has not descended. If the scrotum is empty, palpate along the inguinal canal between the anterior superior iliac spine and pubic tubercle for the testis. The testes may appear to be in a higher position when the child is lying supine. When he sits up or stands, however, the testes descend into the scrotum. If on palpation a testicular mass is felt along the inguinal canal, gently push it into the scrotum with the thumb and index finger of the other hand. If this can be done, the testis is descended, even if it goes back up quickly. This is called a "retractile testis." If the mass is felt along the inguinal canal, but cannot be pushed down into the scrotum by the above technique, it is an undescended testis. If the testis is not felt anywhere, the testis is probably inside the abdomen (provided it is a male). The presence of penis without any testis, suggests the possibility of ambiguous genitalia.

Another useful technique to palpate the testis along the inguinal canal suggested by C. Everett Koop is as follows: moisten the fingertips with liquid soap and rub the fingers gently but firmly along the inguinal canal from above downward. If the testis is present, it will "plop" under your finger.

A large scrotum may indicate one of the following: 1) thickened skin (as in elephantiasis of the scrotum), 2) fluid in the sac (hydrocele), 3) intestines in the scrotum (hernia), 4) large testis, and 5) large epididymis. A large scrotum that becomes small when the child is lying down or when the child is relaxed but gets large from a cough or straining, is probably a hernia. Masses that cannot be reduced may be normal structures within the scrotum, such as the testis, or they may be testicular tumors. Hydrocele cannot be reduced completely, although it may become smaller with pressure.

Tenderness of the scrotum may be due to orchitis, epididymitis, or torsion of the testis or of the appendix of the epididymis. Ultrasound examination of the testis is indicated since torsion of the testis requires urgent correction.

The normal color of the scrotum is darker than the rest of the body. Red color with tenderness indicates inflammation (orchitis) or torsion of the testis. Blue lines along the scrotal sac indicate varicocele. Normally the scrotum is not tender to palpation, although the testis has a peculiar characteristic sensation. Tender scrotum may indicate inflammation of any of the tissues, torsion of the testis, or a strangulated or incarcerated hernia.

In older children and adolescents, determine the state of sexual development by examining the size of the penis, scrotum, testicular size, and pubic hair. Normal stages of sexual development are given in Chapter 12B, page 323.

## Female Genitalia

Examination of the genitalia may be a traumatic experience for children of any age. Therefore, proper preparation and good explanations are essential. One should be sensitive to the child's feelings and shyness. The examination should not be abrupt or threatening. When examining adolescent girls, make sure a female nurse or the mother is present. Examine under good light. Proper positioning is essential for a good examination of the genitalia. In young infants and children who cannot cooperate, examine the child sitting on her mother's lap in a semirecumbent position. Support the child's feet on your knees and ask the child to place the soles of her feet together. This diverts the child's attention and also fully abducts the thighs. Now, grasp the labia majora between the thumb and index finger and draw outwards, thus exposing the labia minora, urethral meatus, and vagina. Most of the findings can be observed easily on inspection alone.

In the newborn, the genitalia are highly pigmented and edematous, particularly in breech delivery.

In older prepubertal children, the labia minora may have receded in size compared with the remainder of the external genitalia. The glans clitoris is no longer than 3 mm and is 2 mm wide. The hymen is seen just interior to the introitus. The vaginal mucosa is red and appears thin. If the older child is placed in the knee-chest position, the introitus will be easier to visualize, allowing a view of the vagina and cervix; foreign bodies may be seen in this position.

Points to be looked for on examination of the female genitalia (other than in newborns) are:

1.  Normal secondary sexual development: look for the appearance and distribution of pubic hair. Tanner's classification of various stages of sexual development are given in Chapter 12B, page 326.
2.  Look at the general hygiene, smell, and staining of pants; don't forget to look for lice if pubic hair is present.
3.  Urethral discharge is uncommon at any age. If present, it may indicate mechanical irritation (tight panties, foreign body, masturbation), physiological (for two to three years before menstruation starts), or inflammation anywhere along the tract.
4.  Look for cyst, caruncle, or prolapse around the urethral orifice.
5.  Look for foreign bodies by separating the labia. A foreign body in the vagina is a common cause for vaginal discharge and bleeding. (Occasionally, careful bimanual palpation with one finger in the rectum and one in the vagina may be needed to palpate a foreign body. The finger should not be forced into the fornix which is very short.)
6.  Look for discharge and the characteristics of the vaginal discharge. Bloody vaginal discharge seen in the newborn period often is due to estrogen withdrawal and is physiologic. In older infants, a foreign body is a common cause for vaginal discharge, which is intermittent, blood stained, and foul smelling. In adolescent girls, bloody vaginal discharge usually is due to normal menstruation. A rare cause is sarcoma botryoides. Watery discharge may be caused by local irritation or local infections. Purulent discharge, particularly in adolescent girls, suggests gonococcal infection. Whitish cheesy discharge is associated with Candida infection, whereas watery or gray discharge may be associated with trichomonas infection.
7.  Examine the clitoris. A large clitoris may be a normal variation or may indicate precocious puberty. In gonadal dysgenesis and hypopituitarism, the clitoris is small. If there is no tissue surrounding the superior aspect of what appears to be the clitoris, it is probably not a clitoris.

8. In prepubertal girls, synechiae may fuse the two sides of the labiae. Normally these can be separated easily, and they will always separate spontaneously in association with the vaginal pH change in puberty.

9. Next examine the labia majora. They may be fused in congenital adrenal hyperplasia, giving the appearance of a scrotum. Labia majora are hypoplastic and the clitoris appears large in Trisomy-18 syndrome.

10. Look for an imperforate hymen, particularly in the presence of what appears to be an enlarged uterus in an adolescent girl.

11. Also, examine the child for physical evidences of sexual abuse (page 351).

## Ambiguous Genitalia

Ambiguity is suggested by the presence of:

1. Large clitoris
2. Small penis
3. Hypospadias
4. Undescended testis
5. Fused labia majora
6. Inguinal hernia with a mass in a "female" infant

If ambiguous genitalia are suspected in the newborn period, investigation is required prior to sex assignment.

When there is a discrepancy between the morphology of the gonads and of the external genitalia, it is intersexuality. If in an XX female with ovaries the external genitalia are virilized, the child is a female pseudohermaphrodite. If, in an XY male with testes, the external genitalia are ambiguous or female, the child is a male pseudohermaphrodite.

# ANUS AND RECTUM

Proper preparation and gentle methods are crucial for a good examination and future cooperation. It is best to examine these areas with the child lying on his or her left side (left lateral position).

On inspection, look at the location of the anus. In certain congenital malformations of the rectum, the opening may be too far forward, close to the genitalia. There may be no opening at all, the opening of the rectum may be through a small fistula, or into the vagina (female) or urethra (male). Passage of meconium through the vagina or urethra suggests that rectourethral or rectovaginal communication exists.

Next, look for pinworm or segments of tapeworm close to the anal opening. Presence of cracks and fissures in the mucocutaneous junction is called "fissure-in-ano." This may be related to a variety of causes, such as pinworms, constipation, eczema, or other mechanical irritation. Painful fissure may cause constipation and blood streaks in the stools.

Conditions that cause nodular lesions in and around the anus are 1) rectal tag, 2) polyps, 3) hemorrhoids, 4) prolapse of the rectum, and 5) anorectal abscess. Small rectal tags are of no clinical significance. If there are rectal polyps, remember to look for oral mucous-membrane pigmentation (Peutz-Jegher syndrome). Polyps are pedunculated and reddish in color. Hemorrhoids are uncommon in children and are characterized by solid dark protrusions. If they occur, look for some underlying cause such as venacaval or mesenteric obstruction. A true prolapse of the rectum is seen in chronic diarrhea, amebic dysentery, cystic fibrosis, severe cough (pertussis), or severe worm infestations. Also look for anorectal abscess, which will be tender, warm, indurated, or fluctuant.

Fistulae are uncommon in children except in the presence of a congenital anomaly, in which case they open into the vagina or urethra. Acquired fistulae are due to abscesses and open into the perianal skin. This is particularly common in Crohn's disease. A probe, used gently, can help establish the presence of a fistula.

*Rectal examination* is done with the child in the left lateral position. In most children, particularly the small ones, it is better to use your little finger. In older children one may use the gloved index finger. The glove over the finger should be greased properly. As the finger enters the rectum, feel for the sphincter tone. If the anal opening is tight, it may denote anal stenosis or an anxious child, but if the examining finger cannot be moved in at all, think of agenesis of the rectum or imperforate anus. Do not force. In conditions associated with spinal cord lesions (such as myelomeningocele and traumatic paralysis), the sphincter does not grip the finger since the sphincter tone is poor or absent. Exquisite tenderness on entering the rectum may indicate anorectal abscess or acute prostatitis. Usually, fecal masses can be felt in the rectum. An empty rectum may suggest intestinal obstruction or megacolon. In megacolon, a sudden widening of the ampulla proximal to the line of agenesis of ganglia may be felt. If any mass (other than feces) is felt, determine whether it is part of the gut, a polyp, or a mass in the pelvis. Bimanual palpation with one finger in the rectum and the fingers of the other hand over the anterior abdominal wall will help determine the nature of the pelvic mass.

On bimanual palpation, the uterus (in girls) and the bladder (both sexes) usually may be felt on the midline. Foreign bodies in the vagina and rectum may be felt during this procedure.

**Remember to**: 1) look at the face of the child for evidences of pain and tenderness, such as wincing, during the rectal examination, and 2) examine the stool obtained by rectal examination for ova, parasites, and blood.

# BIBLIOGRAPHY

Barkun AN, Camus M, Green L, Meagher T, Coupal L, De Stempel J, Grover SA. The bedside assessment of splenic enlargement. Am J Med. 1991;91(5):512-18.

Deligeorgis D, Yannakos D, Panayotou P, Doxiadis S. The normal borders of liver in infancy and childhood: Clinical and x-ray study. Arch Dis Child. 1970;45(243):702-4.

Jean Emans SJH, Laufer MR, Goldstein DP. Pediatric and Adolescent Gynecology. 5th ed. Baltimore: Lippincott Williams & Wilkins; 2004.

Koop CE. Visible and Palpable Lesions in Children. New York: Grune & Stratton; 1976.

Naylor CD. The rational clinical examination. Physical examination of the liver. JAMA. 1994;271(23):1859-65

Cyanosis is blue color of the skin. Determine whether it affects only the distal parts of the body (peripheral) or affects the lips and tongue also (central).

Jaundice is yellowish discoloration of the skin and conjunctiva. The intensity of staining may vary from the minimal yellow of Gilbert's disease to the intense green-yellow of biliary atresia. Presence of associated itching and dark stool suggests biliary obstruction.

Next, look at the normal pigmentation of the skin, which varies among different ethnic groups. Even within each group there are variations. If there is hypo- or depigmentation, find out whether it is localized or generalized. Also inquire about the time of onset. Congenital generalized absence of melanin pigment is seen in albinism, in which the scalp hair and eyebrows are also pale. A congenital form of localized hypopigmentation is partial albinism (piebaldism), in which the forehead, anterior scalp (white forelock), elbows, and knees are involved.

Hypopigmented lesions along the lines of Blaschko from early childhood may be indicative of hypomelanotic nevi of Ito. Often, these hypopigmented lesions are in swirls.

Vitiligo is an acquired disorder causing localized areas of hypopigmentation. Areas commonly affected are the face (around the eyes and mouth), hands, feet, elbows, and knees. This may be associated with autoimmune conditions.

Other causes of patches of hypopigmentation include tinea versicolor, poikiloderma, xeroderma pigmentosum, and tuberous sclerosis.

Skins lesions are seen in over 90% of patients with tuberous sclerosis. Hypopigmented macules (formerly called "ash leaf spots") are seen in infancy. These lesions are visible to the naked eye but may need examination under a Wood lamp. Other skin lesions associated with tuberous sclerosis are shagreen patches, facial angiofibroma, also known as adenoma sebaceum, and periungual fibroma.

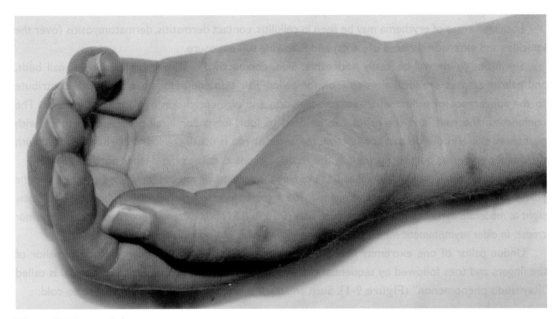

**Figure 9-1.**Raynaud phenomenon

*Excess pigmentation* may be due to racial characteristics or exposure to the sun. Determine whether it is generalized or localized in distribution.

A generalized slate color is seen in Addison's disease and in congenital adrenal hyperplasia. This pigmentation of Addison's disease also involves the buccal mucosa. Some drugs (Quinacrine) and heavy metals (silver, arsenic) may cause generalized hyperpigmentation.

Examples of localized hyperpigmentation include overproduction of melanin (freckles and moles), chronic inflammation (as in eczema), or cafe-au-lait spots (**Figure 9-2**). Swirls of hyperpigmentation may be seen in incontinentia pigmenti. Other examples of localized hyperpigmentation include acanthosis nigricans (axilla, nape of the neck), ochronosis (over the cartilage portion of the external ear), and porphyria (sun exposed areas).

Alternate areas of depigmentation and excess pigmentation may be seen in scleroderma and vitiligo.

## NATURE OF LESIONS

Describe lesions of the skin (rashes) under the following headings: primary lesion, secondary lesion, and distribution/configuration.

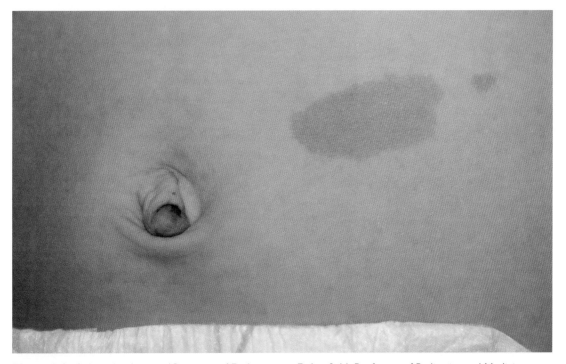

**Figure 9-2.** Café au lait lesions (Courtesy of Dr.Lawrence Eichenfield, Professor of Pediatrics and Medicine (Dermatology), University of California at San Diego,and Chief, Pediatric and Adolescent Dermatology, Rady Children's Hospital and Health Center, San Diego, CA)

The *primary* lesions are:

1. *Macules*: flat lesions flush with the surface of the skin. These may be erythematous (**Figure 5-6**) or pigmented (**Figure 9-2**). Erythematous macules blanch when pressure is applied (petechiae do not).

2. *Papules*: thickened, elevated lesions and small in size (up to 1 cm). *Papules, nodules, and tumors* are different gradations of morphologically similar lesions except for variation in size and depth of involvement. Papular lesions may coalesce to form *plaques* that are larger than 1 cm, slightly elevated, and circumscribed (**Figures 9-3, 9-4,** and **9-5**).

3. *Vesicles*: fluid-filled lesions projecting above the surface of the skin (herpes zoster, **Figure 9-6**). Small lesions are called "vesicles" and larger ones are called "bullae" or "blebs."

4. Pustules: similar to vesicles but containing pus (**Figure 9-7**). Deeper lesions with pus are called "abscesses."

5. *Wheals*: slightly elevated lesions of the skin with the central portion paler than the periphery.

6. *Petechiae* and *purpura*: bloodcolored spots in the skin. They do not blanch on pressure. Petechiae are smaller (less than 0.2 cm), and purpura are larger (up to 1.0 cm). Lesions larger than this are called "ecchymosis" (**Figure 9-8**).

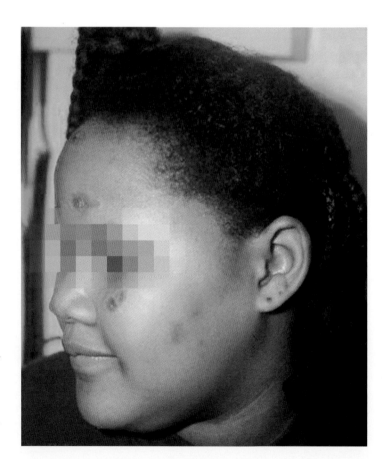

**Figure 9-3**. Discoid lesion of Systemic Lupus Erythematosus (Reproduced with permission from 1972-2004 American College of Rheumatology Slide Collection)

The secondary lesions are:

1. *Excoriations*: caused by scratching, leaving nail marks. Lichenification is hyperpigmented dry plaques with accentuated skin markings (atopic dermatitis, **Figure 9-9**).
2. *Crust*: formation due to dried fluid (serum, blood, or pus), if the primary lesion is a vesicle or pustule (as in impetigo, **Figure 9-7**).
3. *Desquamation*: a scaling of the primary lesion with desiccated plates of cornified epithelial cells.
4. Increased or decreased *pigmentation* around the primary lesion.
5. *Ulceration*: a depressed lesion due to loss of both epidermis and part of the dermis.
6. *Scar* formation: caused by replacement of dermis and subcutaneous tissue with fibrous tissue following injury (no normal markings of the skin, no hair follicles, no sweat pores, and no melanin).
7. *Atrophy*: characterized by an "ironed-out" appearance and increased translucency so that veins are prominent.

## DISTRIBUTION OF LESIONS

In the differential diagnosis, combine the characteristics of the primary and secondary lesions with the areas of distribution. When describing the lesion, remember to answer the following questions:

1. Is it a primary lesion?
2. Is it a secondary lesion?
3. What is the distribution?
4. If elevated, is it rounded or pointed?
5. If vesicle, is it umbilicated?
6. Is there redness around it?
7. Is there pigmentation around it?
8. Does it "feel" more than it "looks"?
9. Is it superficial or deep?
10. If it is an ulcer, describe the base and the edge of the ulcer. Also look for induration under or around the ulcer.

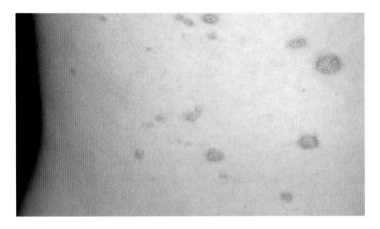

**Figure 9-4.** Plaque lesion of Psoriasis ((Courtesy of Dr.Lawrence Eichenfield, Professor of Pediatrics and Medicine (Dermatology),University of California at San Diego,and Chief, Pediatric and Adolescent Dermatology, Rady Children's Hospital and Health Center, San Diego, CA)

The pattern of distribution of skin lesions gives valuable clues to diagnosis. For example, red pointed papules and pustules over the face and on the back of the upper part of the trunk in an adolescent most likely are caused by acne. The classic facial rash of systemic lupus erythamatosis is seen over the sun-exposed malar area (**Figure 5-6**). Lesions of pityriasis rosea are seen mostly on the trunk. Lesions of scabies (grayish linear lesions with a vesicle or pustule at one end) are seen over the palms, creases of the wrist, axilla, perineal area, and dorsum of the penis. In infants, lesions may be seen on the face and neck as well. Grouped vesicles along dermatome distribution are seen in herpes zoster. Gottron's papules and plaques of dermatomyositis are seen over the extensor surface of small and large joints (**Figure 9-10**).

Rash in the diaper area involving the groin folds is the result of retention of moisture. Rash in the same area sparing the folds but involving the convexities probably is due to contact dermatitis. Rash in the diaper area with satellite lesions indicates secondary infection, most often fungal (candida).

## PALPATION OF LESIONS

### Texture

Normal skin has a smooth, soft, moist feeling. Rough skin may be due to a simple cause, such as excess bathing and dryness or a serious condition, such as congenital icthyosis (collodion baby is the extreme variant). A rough coarse skin commonly is seen in various allergies and hypothyroidism.

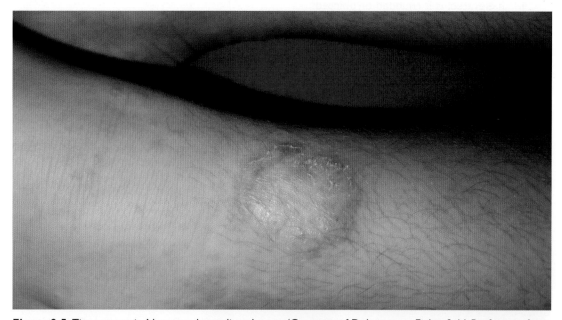

**Figure 9-5.** Tinea corporis. Note annular, scaling plaques. (Courtesy of Dr.Lawrence Eichenfield, Professor of Pediatrics and Medicine (Dermatology),University of California at San Diego,and Chief, Pediatric and Adolescent Dermatology, Rady Children's Hospital and Health Center, San Diego, CA)

# Edema

Pitting on pressure signals the presence of edema. Edema may be acute or chronic, pitting or non-pitting. An area of skin may appear edematous in the presence of subcutaneous emphysema. Palpation or auscultation over an area of subcutaneous emphysema will elicit crepitus.

Dependent edema is seen over the pretibial region. In bedridden patients, edema will be over the sacrum. The usual causes of edema are hypoalbuminemia, increased central venous pressure, and capillary leak. One has to think of several conditions under each of these three major categories. Periorbital edema more often is indicative of nephrosis and hypoalbuminemia rather than of congestive heart failure. Scrotal edema is seen in any condition with massive edema, such as in nephrosis and cirrhosis. Local causes of scrotal edema include epididymitis and torsion of testis.

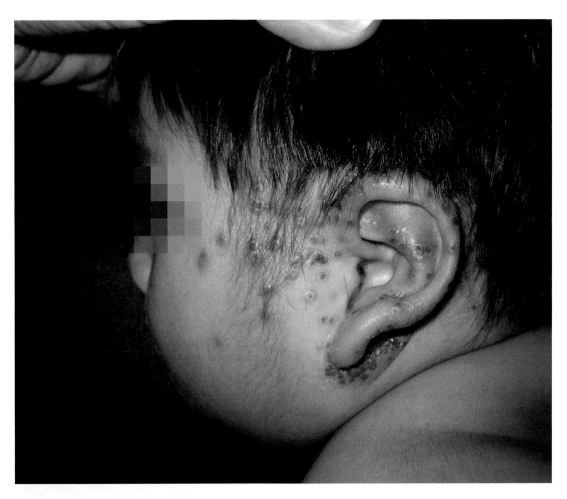

**Figure 9-6.** Vesicles in Herpes zoster. Note blistering and erythema. (Courtesy of Dr. Lawrence Eichenfield, Professor of Pediatrics and Medicine (Dermatology), University of California at San Diego, and Chief, Pediatric and Adolescent Dermatolgy, Rady Children's Hospital and Health Center, San Diego, CA)

Occasionally a child may be born with very large pigmented lesions often elevated above the surface and with an angular margin. These lesions are seen over the upper back, shoulders, and thighs, often in a dermatome distribution. These are called "giant congenital pigmented nevi" with descriptive names such as "bathing trunk," "coat-sleeve," and "stocking nevi." Some of these lesions are associated with coarse brown hair. These giant hairy nevi may be associated with neurological problems.

*Nevus of Ota* is a bluish-gray lesion usually present at birth over the trigeminal area (face). These individuals also may have bluish discoloration of the sclera on the affected side.

*Freckles* are light or dark brown lesions usually seen over sun-exposed parts of the body such as the face. These lesions are not present at birth. In contrast, *lentigines* are also dark brown lesions but they can affect any part of the body and are present from birth.

*Café-au-lait* spots (**Figure 9-2**) are hyperpigmented light tan macules of varying sizes present at birth or developing during childhood. Normal children may have a few *café-au-lait* spots (fewer than three), but six or more lesions with a diameter of 0.5 cm or greater are considered to be characteristic of neurofibromatosis. Usually the border is regular, but large unilateral café-au-lait spots with an uneven border are considered characteristic of McCune-Albright syndrome (polyostotic fibrous dysplasia). Other conditions associated with *café-au-lait* spots are Bloom syndrome and tuberous sclerosis.

Classic descriptions of a few skin diseases are given in **Table 9-1**. Morphological descriptions of skin lesions and some examples are given in **Table 9-2.** Distribution of skin lesions as a clue to diagnosis is given in **Table 9-3**. Classic configurations are described in **Table 9-4.**

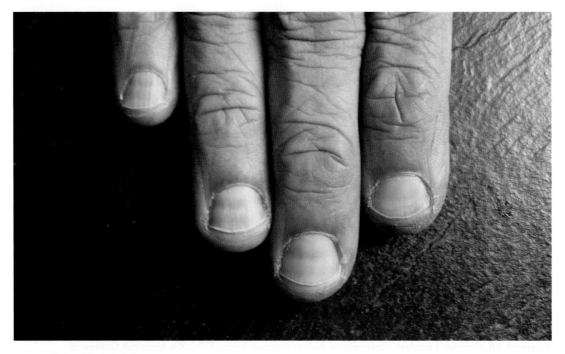

**Figure 9-11.** Muehrke's lines

# NAILS

Examination of the nails can give many diagnostic clues. The changes in the nails can be grouped under two classes: quantitative and qualitative.

| | |
|---|---|
| Quantitative: | Area of nail—increased/decreased |
| | Thickness of nail—increased/decreased nail bed |
| | changes—increased thickness |
| Qualitative: | Color |
| | Surface consistency adherence to nail bed |

## Table 9-1. Classic Description

| | |
|---|---|
| Allergic urticaria | Wheals that are raised (edema), smooth, pink or red, surrounded by bright flare. If the center clears, the lesion may look annular. Clears within 24 hours at any one site. Associated with itching. May involve any part of the body. |
| Vasculitic urticaria | Wheals are similar to the allergic variety; however, they stay longer than a day at the same site. Less itching but more burning and tingling. Most often trunk and limbs. |
| Pityriasis rosea | Pink, oval, scaly plaques along the stretch lines of the skin giving the "Christmas tree" appearance. May be preceded by a single herald patch over the trunk. |
| Erythema multiforme | Abrupt onset of fixed red papules within a day, which evolve within a period of 2 to 3 days and may become annular. Lesions often have an outer red zone, middle dusky zone, and a central blister giving the bull's eye lesion (as opposed to urticaria which keeps appearing over several days, migrate to areas not involved initially, and have central clearing). May be seen over any part of the body; bull's eye lesions often on the palms. |
| Tinea capitis | Some lesions may look like dandruff with scales, erythema, alopecia, and with broken shafts of hair (gives appearance of black dots in the center of the lesion). In severe inflammation (kerion), the lesions are larger with evidence of vesicles, inflammation, and alopecia. (**Figure 9-13**) |
| Tinea corporis | Erythematous plaque with a clear elevated margin and cluster of vesicles. The center may appear clear. (**Figure 9-5**) |
| Acne | Face, upper trunk, and upper arms are involved the most. The lesions are vesiculonodular with dark follicular plug (comedo). Other lesions are "whiteheads," pustules, and cysts. |

## Quantitative Changes

In acromegaly the total area of the nail is increased. In hyperparathyroidism the nails are large in surface area, broad and rounded, and not clubbed.

A thickened nail plate characteristically is seen in chronic fungal infections. A thickened nail bed is seen in chronic inflammatory conditions or in the presence of fibrous tumors.

A decreased amount of nail is seen following accidental removal of nail, in nervous nail biters, and in epidermolysis.

## Qualitative Changes—Color

The nail beds will be blue in both central and peripheral cyanosis. A red or blue area under the nail most commonly is caused by an injury resulting in subungual hematoma. The other important lesion to recognize is the subungual hemorrhage of subacute bacterial endocarditis. This is usually a narrow red band parallel to the long axis of the finger, and also may be seen in other conditions. Various other color changes have been noticed in chemical poisoning, kala-azar, and Addison's disease. Fungal infections of the nail are associated with color changes (white flecks to yellow patches). One should not forget the nail polish, particularly in young girls.

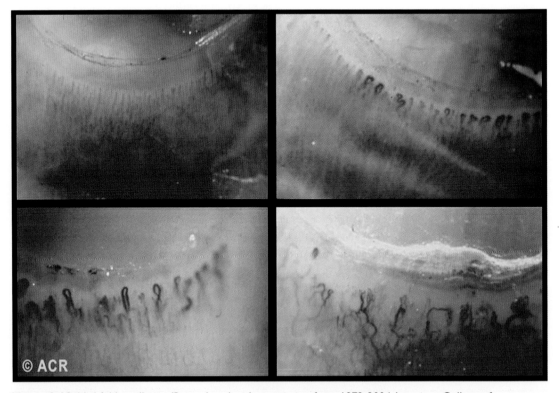

**Figure 9-12.** Nail fold capillaries (Reproduced with permission from 1972-2004 American College of Rheumatology Slide Collection)

# Surface

Normally the surface is smooth with slight convexity. Concave nails (koilonychia) are classically associated with iron-deficiency anemia though one sees such changes very rarely. Increased convexity of the nail surface is seen in many normal adults, but not so much in children.

Loss of continuity of the surface with pits classically is seen in psoriasis and in eczema. Longitudinal and transverse ridges and bands are more common in adults than in children. Malnutrition and severe chronic inflammatory conditions such as eczematous dermatitis are the usual associated conditions.

Transverse opaque bands that run across the width of the nail are known as "Muehrcke's lines" (**Figure 9-11**). They may be associated with any metabolic stress such as infection or malignancy. Reil's line (often following a major febrile illness) and Beau's lines (seen after any major catabolic event) are non-pigmented indented transverse bands. These are palpable, unlike the Muehrcke's lines.

## Table 9-2. Morphological Descriptions and Associated Conditions

| Morphology | Associated Conditions |
| --- | --- |
| Macular | exanthematous diseases |
| Macular pigmentary | vitiligo, postinfectious, freckles, lentigenes |
| Maculopapular | drug eruptions and exanthems |
| Papulonodular | localized or generalized<br>causes of localized nodules are granuloma, erythema nodosum, foreign body |
| Generalized nodules | rheumatic fever, rheumatoid nodulosis, sarcoid, panniculitis |
| Papulosquamous | psoriasis, seborrhea, pityriasis rosea |
| Annular | systemic lupus erythematosus, granuloma annulare, erythema multiforme, erythema annulare centrifugum |
| Eczematous | atopic, contact dermatitis |
| Vesiculobullous | herpes zoster, erythema multiforme, pemphigus |
| Pustular | acne, impetigo, pyoderma |
| Ulcer | stasis, vasculitic, ischemic, infections |
| Urticaria | drug eruption, cold urticaria, vasculitic urticaria |

*SLE=systemic lupus erythematosus*

## Consistency

The nail may be excessively soft, as in chemical injury or malnutrition. This is seen particularly after excess use of nail polish and polish removers. A very friable nail is seen in fungal infections and psoriasis.

## Adherence

Partial separation of the nail from the nail bed is seen commonly after trauma. It also is seen after severe dermatitis or exanthem, such as in erythema multiforme exudativum or exfoliative dermatitis. Look for redness and swelling around the edge of the nail as well.

Nail-fold infection is called "paronychia," if acute. Though it often is caused by staphylococci, paronychia also may result from *Candida* and rarely from herpes simplex.

Pterygium is a layer of cuticle that grows over the proximal portion of the nail and is seen in dermatomyositis. Periungual erythema also is seen in dermatomyositis.

Periungual telangiectasia is seen in scleroderma and is part of a series of changes seen in the nail-fold capillaries. Ideally, examine the capillary bed at the base of the nail in children with Raynaud's phenomenon and scleroderma using a stereomicroscope under oil-immersion, at 25X to 40X magnification. In a routine clinic setting, use the +40 magnification of an ophthalmoscope. In normal children, capillary loops of uniform size and distribution will be seen. Dilated capillary loops, areas of avascularity, and excess branching raise suspicion of juvenile scleroderma or dermatomyositis (**Figure 9-12**).

**Table 9-3. Characteristic Distribution of Skin Lesions**

| Condition | Distribution |
| --- | --- |
| Acne | face, upper chest, upper back |
| Seborrhea | scalp, behind the ears |
| Atopic dermatitis/eczema | flexor surfaces of joints |
| Psoriasis | hair margin, peri-umbilical, around the anus |
| Pityriasis rosaea | upper chest and back |
| Pityriasis alba | face (blotchy, improves in winter) |
| Scabies | palmar creases, between fingers, behind the ear |
| Acral | rocky-mountain spotted fever |
| Sun-sensitive areas | drug induced, photosensitivity |
| Diaper area | diaper rash, intertrigo, candida, acrodermatitis, Kawasaki |

# HAIR *(also see Chapter 6, pages 110-112)*

The characteristics of the hair to be observed are:

Quantitative:    Increase:    generalized
                                  localized
                  Decrease:    generalized
                                  localized

Qualitative:    Color
                  Texture

Surface characteristics (straight, curled, or beaded)
                  Strength (brittle)

Some of these items have been described under scalp hair. The *quantity* of hair may be increased all over the body in Cushing's syndrome, steroid therapy, de Lange syndrome, diphenyl hydantoin (Dilantin) therapy, and porphyria. Children with chronic illness also tend to show hirsutism. A localized area of hypertrichosis may be seen in association with a nevus (nevus pilosus). Areas of the body placed in a cast show hypertrichosis soon after removal of the cast.

Generalized *hypotrichosis* is seen in conditions such as hypothyroidism, congenital ectodermal defect, and drug toxicity (thallium, cytotoxic drugs, and vitamin A). If the loss of hair is localized, consider alopecia areata (smooth skin with no inflammation and a band pattern), local infections (tinea capitis **Figure 9-13**), and psychological hair pulling with unilateral patches having an odd shape (trichotillomania). Telogen effluvium occurs after major illness or stress with diffuse loss of hair.

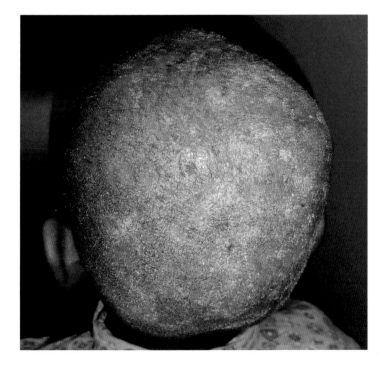

**Figure 9-13.** Tinea capitis (Courtesy of Dr. Lawrence Eichenfield, Professor of Pediatrics and Medicine (Dermatology), University of California at San Diego, and Chief, Pediatric and Adolescent Dermatology, Rady Children's Hospital and Health Center, San Diego, CA)

The *color* of hair is better appreciated in the scalp hair. If the color of body hair is abnormally pale, consider albinism.

Changes in *texture* have been described already in the section on scalp hair. Dry coarse hair is common in hypothyroidism, whereas fine thin hair is seen in conditions such as homocystinuria.

*Surface characteristics* such as a beaded appearance of the hair (monilethrix) and nodular swellings (*trichorrhexis nodosa*) also are appreciated better with scalp hair. Lice and their nits have to be looked for in pubic hair of adolescent boys and girls. The hair is fragile in many congenital syndromes and in areas of fungal infections.

## SPECIAL SIGNS TO ELICIT

### Dermatographism

Simple stroking of the skin results in a wheal and flare reaction so that if an alphabet is written on the skin, a raised alphabet appears at the site of the stroke. This may be associated with atopic skin or systemic onset-JIA, but often is not indicative of any disease.

### Flaying

When the hand is rubbed rapidly over an area on the arms or legs with sufficient pressure, small nodular lesions, not visible on inspection, may be appreciated.

### Koebner Phenomenon

On stroking the skin of an unaffected area, lesions present in other areas seem to jump to the site of pressure, as seen in JIA.

### Table 9-4. Configurations of Lesions that May Be Helpful

| | |
|---|---|
| Grouped vesicles | Herpes |
| Dermatome | herpes zoster |
| Blaschko lines | Hypomelanosis |
| Annular | erythema migrans, subacute lupus |
| Linear | Self-inflicted, poison ivy |
| Sun exposed areas | photosensitive eruptions, both congenital (porphyria) and acquired (SLE) |

*SLE=systemic lupus erythematosus*

# BIBLIOGRAPHY

Fitzpatrick TB, Walker SA. Dermatological differential diagnosis. Chicago: Year Book Medical Publishers; 1962.

Goodheart HP. Goodheart's Photoguide of Common Skin Disorders: Diagnosis and Management. 2nd ed. Baltimore: Lippincott Williams & Wilkins; 2003.

Paller AS, Mancini AJ. Hurwitz Clinical Pediatric Dermatology: A Textbook of Skin Disorders of Childhood and Adolescence. 3rd ed. Philadelphia: Elsevier Saunders; 2005.

# Chapter 10

# MUSCULOSKELETAL SYSTEM

Limb pain, joint pain, muscle pain, limp, sprains and strains, fractures, and swollen joints are some of the most common reasons children are brought to the physician. It is therefore important for every physician to be proficient in the examination of muscles, bones, and joints. A screening history and physical examination developed in the UK called the GALS (Gait, Arms, Legs, and Spine) is a general functional assessment of the musculoskeletal system in adults.

A modified assessment tool for children (pGALS) is also available. (The details of an examination using the pGALS system are given in **Table 10-1**. A DVD is available from Arc Trading, James Nicholson Link, Clifton Moor, York YO30 4XX, UK). The system consists of three basic questions and a physical examination. The questions are: 1) Does the child have any pain or stiffness of muscles, joints, or back? 2) Can the child dress and feed self completely without any difficulty (at an age-appropriate level)? 3) Can the child walk up and down stairs without difficulty? (This question also may include walking, running, playing, and gait abnormalities.) A positive answer to any one of these questions merits a more thorough questioning and examination.

## MUSCLES

In the perinatal period, the following points in the history give important clues to the presence of muscle disease: 1) reduced intrauterine movements, 2) neonatal respiratory distress, 3) poor suck, and 4) reduced activity of limbs.

In older infants and children, the following points in the history may indicate the presence of a muscle disease: 1) floppy baby, 2) delayed milestones, 3) trouble walking or running, 4) frequent tripping and falling, 5) easily tired (fatigue), 6) double vision at the end of the day, 7) trouble climbing stairs and getting up from a sitting position, 8) muscle pain (spontaneous or after exercise), 9) swallowing difficulty, and 10) trouble letting go of objects.

Family history is extremely important. The differential diagnosis of various muscle diseases is made easier when there is a family history of similar illness.

Physical examination includes 1) inspection, palpation, and percussion of the muscle(s); 2) evaluation of the strength of individual or groups of muscles; 3) exclusion of nervous system disorders with associated myopathy; 4) exclusion of joint diseases associated with disuse atrophy; 5) observation of gait; and 6) assessment of activities of daily living (ADL). Also remember to examine all the other systems, looking for clues to systemic diseases.

### Table 10-1. Modified Pediatric GALS System

Three questions:

Any pain and/or stiffness in joints or muscles or back?

Can dress or feed self without difficulty? (if appropriate for age)

Can go up and down stairs without difficulty? (if appropriate for age)

**GAIT:**

Observe child walking, running and making a quick turn

Symmetry

Smooth movements

Heel strike/toe off

Stance–swing through

Observe child walk on tip of toes and on heels

Also look for in-toeing and out-toeing (not part of GALS or pGALS)

**ARMS:**

Ask the child to put the hands in front

Ask the child to turn the hands over and make a fist

Ask the child to touch the tips of the fingers with the thumb

Squeeze the metacarpophalangeal joints

Place the hands in the Indian Greeting position

Place the hands so the dorsum of the hands appose

Ask the child to reach up and "touch the sky"

Ask the child to put the hands behind the occiput

Ask the child to put the hands behind the back below the scapula (not part of GALS or pGALS)

**LEGS:**

| | |
|---|---|
| Standing: | Look for quad wasting, symmetry, valgus, varus |
| | Look for swelling of the knee and feel for effusion |
| | Look at the plantar arches |
| | Look at the arch when the child stands on tips of toes |
| Lying supine: | |
| | Flex hips and knees |
| | Feel for crepitus |
| | Rotate each hip |
| | Squeeze metatarsus |
| | Look at the sole of the feet |

(In infants, ask the parent to put the child over his/her shoulder. The examiner then will be standing behind the child and can then bend the knee, extend the knee, and rotate the hips gently.)

**SPINE:**

Look from in front, side, and behind

Look for scoliosis, kyphosis, and gibbus

Ask the child to bend over and touch the toes or the floor if possible; observe the prominence of scoliosis and increased flexibility (not part of GALS or pGALS)

Ask the child to look up at the ceiling

Ask the child to touch the shoulder with the ear (lateral flexion of cervical spine)

Ask the child to open the mouth as wide as possible (must be able to accommodate three of the child's own fingers)

*Modified from: Doherty M, Dacre J, Dieppe P, Snaith M. The 'GALS' Locomotor Screen. Ann Rheum Dis.1992;51:1165-69; and Foster HE, Kay LJ, Friswell M, Coady D, Myers A. Musculoskeletal Screening Examination (pGALS) for school-age children based on the adults GALS screen. Arthritis Rheum (Arthritis Care Res). 2006;55(5):709-16. (Reprinted with permission from John Wiley & Sons Inc)*

# Inspection

Look into the following characteristics of muscle:

- Size
- Shape
- Symmetry

Size can be small or large. Shape depends on the normality of each muscle. Symmetry refers to muscles with bilateral distribution.

Congenital absence of certain muscles is easily recognizable. This may be present as an isolated abnormality (e.g., pectoralis major) or associated with a syndrome (e.g., depressor labii oris with congenital heart disease, pectoralis muscle with leukemia, or temporalis with myotonia).

Certain muscles may be small due to wasting (best example, quadriceps wasting following injury to or inflammation of the knee or after casting). Wasting may be due to disuse, primary muscle degeneration, or secondary to anterior horn cell or peripheral nerve disease. Wasting of individual muscle is identified best in relation to the opposite side. If there is wasting, determine whether it is generalized or localized. Generalized wasting is easily recognizable in anyone with a chronic disease. It often is correlated with loss of weight. If the wasting is localized, determine whether it is related to one muscle, one group of muscles, one limb, or one half of the body. In long-standing hemiplegia, one side may be atrophic compared with the other. In peripheral nerve paralysis, only one group of muscles is involved.

If hypertrophic muscle is found, determine whether it is normal and healthy, as in an adolescent or an athlete, or is suggestive of disease. Also make sure that the hypertrophic side is the one that is abnormal. Determine whether the muscle hypertrophy is localized or generalized. For example, congenital hemihypertrophy involves one half of the body and should always alert the physician to serious disease. Hypertrophy of an isolated muscle classically is seen in Duchenne muscular dystrophy in which calf muscles are unusually large. Generalized hypertrophy of muscles is seen in congenital adrenal hyperplasia. *Appearance of hypertrophy* of muscles may be seen in lipodystrophy and hypothyroidism.

Fasciculation of muscle bundles is seen in conditions associated with irritation of the anterior horn cells (e.g., poliomyelitis or Werdnig-Hoffmann disease).

# Palpation

A feeling of induration over the muscles is seen in fasciitis, dermatomyositis, infectious myositis, and in pyomyositis. Tenderness of muscles is seen in any myositis, particularly pyomyositis and dermatomyositis. When testing muscles with very little strength, palpating along the tendon when the patient is attempting a particular movement may help recognize muscle movements not otherwise demonstrable.

# Percussion

Contraction of percussed muscle with delay in relaxation typically is seen in myotonia congenita. This may best be tested on the biceps. This can be demonstrated in the tongue muscles as well.

## Muscle Strength

The following screening tests will help recognize significant muscle weakness:

1. Ask the patient to lift the neck off a pillow from a supine position. (tests anterior neck flexors, if weak, the patient cannot perform this task.)
2. Ask the patient to shrug the shoulders (to test trapezius).
3. Ask the patient to elevate the arms over the head (to test weakness of deltoids).
4. Ask the patient to flex the elbow with palm facing upward (tests the biceps).
5. With the patient sitting at the edge of the table and with the popliteal space flush with the edge, ask him or her to extend the knee (tests the quadriceps).
6. With the patient lying on the right lateral side, have him or her flex the knee (to reduce the effects of the iliotibial) and abduct the hip on the left side (tests the left gluteus medius). Repeat the test with the patient lying on the left side to test the right gluteus medius.
7. With the patient lying prone and the knees flexed (to eliminate the hamstrings), ask him or her to lift the hip off the table (tests the gluteus maximus).
8. Ask the patient to push down on your palm with the sole of the foot while sitting and to walk on the toes ( tests gastrocnemius and soleus).

When examining for strength of various muscles, the usual method is to ask the patient to move in one direction and apply resistance to that muscle. A better method is for the patient to move the joint with the muscle being tested to the maximum possible range, and then you apply force to bring it back to neutral. For example, while testing for biceps, let the patient flex the elbow. Then ask the patient to resist when you extend his or her elbow.

If a more detailed evaluation of strength of various muscles, for active and passive ranges of movements, with and without gravity, with and without resistance is needed and for proper grading of muscle strength (**Table 10-2**), use the help of a physical therapist or a physiatrist

If there is weakness of muscles, note the pattern of distribution. Proximal muscle weakness is seen in dermatomyositis; distal extremity weakness alone is seen in peripheral neuritis; one-sided weakness is seen in unilateral cerebral insult; unequal lower limb weakness is seen in myelomeningocele; and equal complete lower limb weakness is seen in paraplegia.

### Table 10-2. Grading of Muscle Strength

| | |
|---|---|
| 0 | No movement of muscle |
| Trace (1) | Palpable contraction No movement of joint |
| Poor (2) | Full range, gravity eliminated |
| Fair (3) | Full range, against gravity |
| Good (4) | Full range against gravity and moderate resistance |
| Normal (5) | Full range against gravity and normal resistance |

# Activities of Daily Living (ADL)

Evaluation of ADLs is important for helping children with physical handicaps due to neuromuscular or musculoskeletal diseases. An ADL evaluation also is used for functional classification of severely handicapped children. The functional categories are given in **Table 10-3**.

Certain simple functional tests are very useful in following the degree of muscle weakness in dermatomyositis. They are as follows:

1. elevation of neck from supine lying,
2. elevation of extended lower limb (in seconds),
3. ability to get up from lying down without help,
4. ability to get up from sitting with arms folded in front.

These may be useful to follow children with generalized muscle weakness. However, specially designed evaluation tools must be used for proper follow-up of patients with dermatomyositis, muscular dystrophy, etc.

Involvement of other systems in the presence of muscle weakness should suggest specific diagnoses. They are listed in **Table 10-4**.

## Table 10-3. Functional Category

I.  Fully independent

II. Mostly independent—minimal help required

III. Wheelchair-bound—but can take care of certain items

IV. Totally dependent on others

## Table 10-4. Helpful Associated Clues in Diagnosing Diseases of Muscle

| Presence of | Suggests |
| --- | --- |
| 1.  Myotonia | Mental retardation |
| 2.  Exaggerated reflexes | Diseases of central nervous system |
| 3.  Fasciculations | Anterior horn cell disease |
| 4.  Rashes | Collagen vascular disorders |
| 5.  Sensory changes | Peripheral nerve disease |
| 6.  Dark urine | Myoglobinuria |

## Gait

The importance and details of analysis of gait have been summarized already (Chapter 5, page 67). Certain characteristic gaits associated with weakness of specific muscle groups include:

- waddling—proximal weakness around hip, specifically gluteus medius, called "Trendelenburg gait,"
- toe walking—Duchenne/tight heel cord,
- slapping gait—peripheral neuropathy,
- high-stepping gait—lesions of the posterior column.

Ask the child to walk and to run. Also make the child walk on the toes (tests plantar flexors) and heels (tests dorsiflexors). Also test the child for the ability to stand on one leg (tests gluteus medius, Trendelenburg sign).

## JOINTS AND BONES

- History
- Inspection
- Palpation
- Auscultation
- Testing for range of movement
- Functional evaluation (including gait)
- Examination of bone, tendon, and periarticular tissues
- Examination of other systems

## History

Pain, swelling, inability to move a joint, excessive movement, or dislocations and contractures are some of the symptoms related to joint disease. There may be symptoms involving other systems, such as characteristic rash or pleuritic pain, which point to a systemic diagnosis; therefore, complete a careful review of systems.

Pain in the joint is a common symptom. Children fall and get hurt so often that history of trauma may not help in the diagnosis. However, this is an important piece of history and should be sought in all cases of joint pain.

Pain in a joint (arthralgia) is not synonymous with arthritis. If there is joint swelling in addition to pain, it is more likely to be arthritis. Arthritis is defined as "swelling, effusion, or presence of two or more of the following signs: limited range of motion, tenderness or pain on motion, and increased heat over the joint."

Acute onset of pain suggests trauma or inflammatory disease. Pain that comes on slowly is more suggestive of a rheumatic disorder. Pain in one joint likely is due to trauma or inflammation, whereas polyarticular pain suggests a generalized disorder. Pain in a joint for one or two days most often is due to trauma, but also may indicate infection. Pain in a joint for a few days or months may be due to one of the rheumatic diseases.

Intense, acute pain is seen in trauma, acute rheumatic fever, or septic arthritis. Extreme grades of pain are associated with vasomotor disease. Moderate pain is seen in JIA. Arthritis with no pain suggests a neuropathic joint.

True migrating pain is characterized by pain in one joint in the morning, moving away to another joint by evening. This is called "flitting, fleeting pain." Such pain is seen in acute rheumatic fever and in gonococcemia. Non-migrating polyarticular pain is seen in other rheumatic disorders.

Relief of limb pain with aspirin is characteristic of osteoid osteoma. Relief of joint pain with one of the nonsteroidal anti-inflammatory drugs also may indicate acute rheumatic fever or JIA.

The relationship of pain to activity and sleep is another important point. Pain worse on activity is indicative of mechanical or degenerative joint disease, such as acute cartilaginous necrosis; whereas, pain and stiffness early in the morning are indicative of rheumatic disorders such as JIA.

Pain so severe that it interferes with sleep often is seen in vasomotor problems and bleeding into the joint. A child who goes to sleep but wakes up in the middle of the night complaining of pain probably has "growing pains" but such a history also makes one think of septic arthritis, osteomyelitis, osteoid osteoma, or periosteal reaction due to various causes. Pain that does not interfere with sleep but gets worse in the morning is seen in JIA.

Pain in one location may indicate a problem elsewhere (referred pain). For example, pain due to hip disease may be referred to other sites, such as the outer aspect of the ilium over the gluteus medius, to the inguinal triangle, or to an area over the anterior aspect of the thigh just above the patella. Pain in the sacroiliac joint is referred to deep in the buttocks. Cervical spine involvement may give rise to pain over the occiput. Pain arising from intervertebral disc inflammation may be felt around the chest wall.

## Inspection

Look for the presence or absence of swelling and its relation to the joint. Periarticular swelling and cellulitis easily can be mistaken for arthritis. Periarticular swelling usually involves only one side of the joint. Cellulitis usually extends well above and below the joint. Swelling of a joint with poorly defined edges merging into the surrounding area usually suggests effusion into the joint, whereas swelling of the joint with clearly defined edges suggests synovial thickening.

Look for symmetry in the length of the extremities, size of the joint, muscle bulk around the joints, and range of motion (of bilateral joints).

Sternoclavicular swelling can be recognized easily if present. Consider JIA if swelling is chronic and gonococcemia if it is acute. Swelling of the elbow is characterized by obliteration of the dimples on either side of the olecranon. Swelling of the carpal joints of the wrist is seen on the dorsal aspect, is diffuse without a clear edge, and is associated with limitation of wrist extension. Swelling of the extensor tendon sheath of the wrist is characterized by a clear, distal, oblique transverse edge. Diffuse swelling of the entire dorsum of the hand may suggest periosteal reaction of the metacarpals as in sickle cell disease or leukemia, tenosynovitis of flexor tendons with lymphedema, or serum sickness.

Flexed fingers and edema of the dorsum of the hand characterize flexor tenosynovitis of the hand.

Swelling of the knee joint can be appreciated easily. The bony landmarks, such as those of the patella, may become indistinct and there may be a fullness of the suprapatellar space. There may be a bulge above and lateral to the patella. Slight limitation in the final few degrees of extension suggests effusion.

If the joint is not visibly swollen and fluid collection is suspected, look for the "bulge sign." To elicit a bulge sign, keep the knee in extension and push the fluid by rubbing vertically along the medial border of the patella. This gets the fluid into the suprapatellar pouch laterally. Now, one gentle stroke with one or two fingers along the lateral edge of the patella should produce a bulge just medial to the medial border of the patella. Make sure patellar movement is not mistaken for the fluid wave.

Another method to elicit evidence of effusion in the knee is patellar ballotment. Squeeze all the fluid from the suprapatellar space into the joint. Now gently press on the patella. Normally, in the absence of fluid, there should be no movement. If there is fluid, the patella will strike the deeper structures and bounce back.

While examining the knee, also look in the back for fullness over the posteromedial corner of the popliteal space. This is the location of Baker's cyst. In the presence of a large effusion, this sac may swell and rupture into the calf. The fluid collection in the calf may be large enough to compress the popliteal vein and cause the syndrome of pseudothrombophlebitis. This may be difficult to differentiate from true thrombosis of the popliteal vein. The history is often helpful. If there is doubt, an ultrasound examination of the calf is indicated.

Two signs associated with ruptured popliteal cysts are 1) a crescent-shaped ecchymotic area around the malleoli, and 2) Homan's sign, which is discomfort in the popliteal area on forced dorsiflexion of the foot. (This sign is used as an indicator of deep vein thrombosis. However, this test is unreliable, associated with high false positivity, and has been "disowned" by Dr. Homan himself.)

Swelling of the ankle joint is characterized by swelling on either side of the tendoachilles posteriorly. If it is only on one side of the tendoachilles, it is probably a tenosynovitis. Swelling of the anterior aspect of the ankle is seen in edema. Swelling of the plantar aspect of the foot with tenderness is seen in plantar fasciitis associated with spondyloarthropathy syndromes. Swelling of sole and dorsum of the feet without tenderness is seen in serum sickness.

## Palpation

Mild *temperature* differences over the skin of the joints can be appreciated easily. Heat over a joint is one of the primary requirements for the diagnosis of inflammatory arthritis. This is particularly easy to appreciate over the knee joint. It is best to compare the temperature of the skin over the anterior aspect of the patella with that of the skin over the upper end of the tibia. The patellar area is cooler than the pretibial area in normal children (Fries' sign).

*Tenderness* over joints is another important clue to the diagnosis of inflammatory arthritis. Place one finger into the external auditory meatus and feel forward (anteriorly) to test the temporomandibular joint. The cartilage will be palpable directly under the finger, and tenderness can be elicited easily. Test the tenderness of the small joints of the fingers by gently squeezing each small joint individually.

Percussion along the flexor tendon produces exquisite tenderness in flexor tenosynovitis, whereas tingling sensation along the outer three fingers when tapping the flexor aspect of the wrist suggests carpal tunnel syndrome.

There is no direct way of testing for tenderness of the hip. However, pain so severe that the hip cannot be moved even five to ten degrees in any direction suggests septic arthritis, unless proven otherwise.

Palpate along the joint line of the knee between the femur and the tibia both on the medial and the lateral sides to locate tenderness over the collateral ligaments and the menisci. The details of this examination are given in a following section on Sports Injuries. If the knee is kept straight (extended) and the patella is pressed down against the femoral condyle and gently rubbed, pain is elicited in chondromalacia of the patella. (This condition also is called "patellafemoral syndrome." In an athletic girl, pain in the knee with frequent buckling of the knee suggests this diagnosis.)

Subtalar tenderness is elicited by gripping the ankle firmly and moving the foot into inversion and eversion. Test the small joints of the foot individually as described earlier for the fingers.

The other most important point in testing for tenderness is to *exclude* tenderness of the periarticular structures. Bony tenderness close to a joint may appear as if the pain or tenderness is coming from the joint. Careful examination will differentiate bony tenderness from joint tenderness. For example, during examination of a child with pain in the knee, remember to feel for tenderness over the tibial tubercle, as the child may have osteochondritis dissecans (Osgood-Schlatter disease). Always feel for tenderness of the bone proximal and distal to the joint because pain at the metaphysis due to osteomyelitis may mimic joint pain. Bone pain of leukemia may mimic the joint pain of arthritis. Tenderness along the tendon attachment may mimic arthritis. This is important to recognize, since enthesitis of tendoachilles is seen in ankylosing spondylids and polytendonitis in hyperlipidemia.

The sacroiliac joint does not require examination routinely in children. Local tenderness is useful if present. If not, elicit tenderness of this joint by performing the "Pretzel Test." Hold and cross one *lower limb* over the other lower limb (**Figure 10-1**) while crossing the *opposite upper limb* across the trunk. In this semi-twisted position, hold the shoulder (of the upper limb being crossed over) and knee (of the lower limb being crossed over) and give a gentle spring-like stretching. This may elicit pain and wincing in the presence of sacroiliac joint disease, though no one clinical test is good enough to define and localize sacroiliac disease. Another method is to place the hands on the patient's pelvis so that the palms are over the iliac crests and the thumbs over the anterior superior iliac spines. Gentle compression of the pelvis towards the midline may elicit pain over the sacroiliac joints.

Minimal synovial thickening over any joint can be appreciated after a few years of practice. Always compare the feeling over a joint with the corresponding joint on the opposite side and with a normal joint. Feel for the amount of tissue between your finger and the underlying bone. Also feel for its texture. Gentle palpation is necessary to appreciate synovial thickening because the synovium collapses on firm pressure. A "cashmere velvet" feeling is the best description of hypertrophic synovium.

During palpation, also feel for nodules along the flexor tendons and periarticular tissues.

*Percussion* along the flexor tendon produces severe pain in tenosynovitis. Percussion on the flexor aspect of the forearm just above the wrist causes pain along the outer three fingers in carpal tunnel syndrome.

Abduction and adduction are tested with the patient in the supine position. Now lift each lower limb with the knee in extended position and move it away from mid-line and towards mid-line. (Remember to keep fingers on the pelvis so that if the whole pelvis is rocking, it is recognized.)

To test for *rotation* at the hip, the best position is with the child lying prone. Actually, four different observations may be made in this prone position (**Figure 10-4**).

1. Have the child lie prone and flex the knees as far as they will go. Normally, both heels should touch the buttocks. Also, both knees should be capable of the same range of movement. Thus, limitation of range of movement of the knee is demonstrated.

2. If the hip rises off the table when the knee joints are flexed fully, suspect hip flexion contracture.

3. With the knees in 90 degrees of flexion, rotate the femurs. When the heels cross over, external rotation at the hip is tested and when the heels go apart, internal rotation at the hip is tested (**Figures 10-5 and 10-6**).

4. With the knee flexed, lift the thigh off the table. Ask the child to hold the flexed limb in the air. This tests the gluteus maximus in isolation.

Significant limitation of internal rotation is seen in many intraarticular diseases of the hip including chronic arthritis, slipped epiphysis, and Legg-Perthes disease. Up to 18 months of age, excessive external rotation is a common normal finding. The external rotation may remain excessively greater, with limitation of internal rotation, particularly in hypotonic infants who lie supine all the time.

Another well-known test for examining restricted range of movement of the hip is the FABER (Flexion, ABduction, External Rotation) test. With the patient in the supine position, ask him or her to

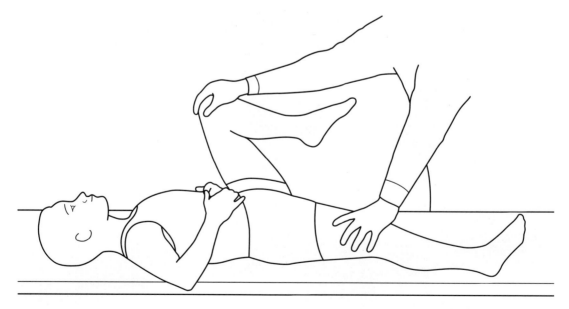

**Figure 10-3.** Testing for hip flexion contracture. The left hip is flexed fully to prevent the lumbar spine from compensating and the right hip is extended as far as possible. Normally, the posterior part of the right thigh should touch the examining table.

place the foot of the affected limb over the opposite knee. This puts the hip into abduction and external rotation and a little pressure over the knee also will stretch the hip into mild extension. If there is hip disease, the patient may not be able to accomplish this task or will have pain over the inguinal area.

The *knee* should extend to a straight line. In girls, and in a standing position, it may even reach 5 to 10 degrees of hyperextension. Loss of full extension is seen in various arthritides. Pain below the knee causing limitation of full flexion is seen in Osgood-Schlatter disease. Limitation of flexion of the knee may be due to fracture or infection of the patella and quadriceps contracture.

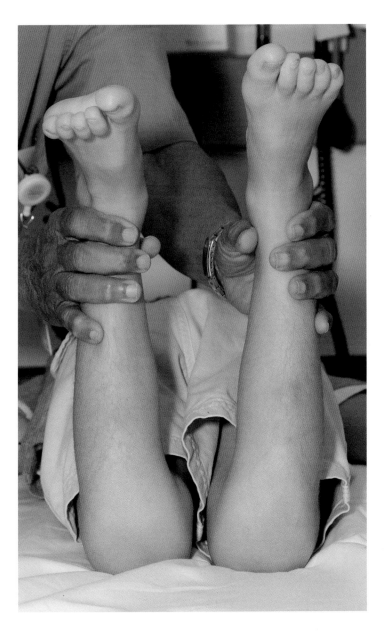

**Figure 10-4.** Patient prone with knee joints in flexion. This is a good position to test the ankle, knee and hip joints.

The *ankle* has normal dorsiflexion and plantar flexion of about 30 degrees. Have the child sit at the edge of a table with the legs hanging freely. Ask him or her to dorsiflex and plantar flex with and without resistance. Test the range both in active motion and passively. Subtalar motion is usually 10 to 15 degrees and is tested by fixing the ankle, holding the foot by the calcaneum, and inverting and everting the foot.

*In-toeing* and *out-toeing* gaits are common complaints during the growing years. The etiological causes of these gait abnormalities are given in **Table 10-5**.

During evaluation of a child for in-toeing and out-toeing, obtain a history on the following points: 1) When was it noticed? Pronounced metatarsus adductus will be visible even at birth, whereas a flat foot is appreciated only when the child starts walking. 2) What is the rate of progression? Most of these problems correct themselves by the age of seven or eight years. Continuing observation is essential. If there is rapid progression, it may be necessary to treat the condition. 3) Obtain a family history of similar problems in other members.

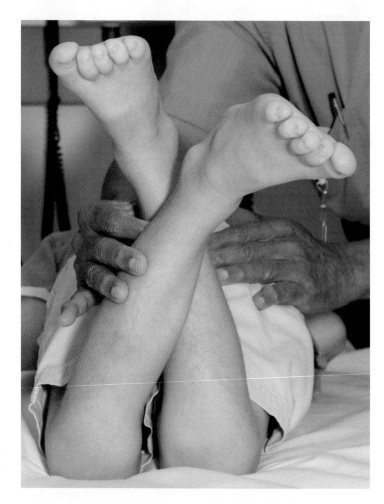

**Figure 10-5.** Testing for external rotation of the hip with patient in prone position.

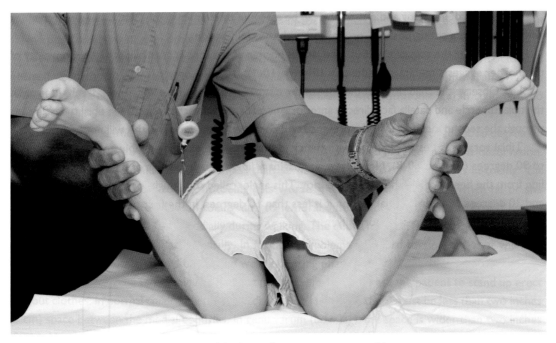

**Figure 10-6.** Testing for internal rotation of the hip with patient in prone position.

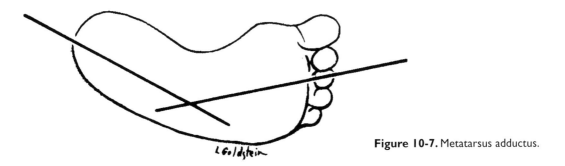

**Figure 10-7.** Metatarsus adductus.

## Table 10-5. Torsional Deformities of the Lower Limb

|  | In-toeing | Out-toeing |
| --- | --- | --- |
| Hip | Femoral anteversion | Physiologic (infancy) |
| Tibia | Internal torsion | External torsion |
| Foot | Metatarsus adductus | Flat foot or curved foot |

*Modified from: Staheli LT. Torsional deformity. Pediatr Clin North Am. 1977; 24(4):801. (Copyright Elsevier 1977)*

# SPINE

## Inspection

Examine the child from the front, side, and back. Presence of a short neck or elevated shoulder and scoliosis in a young child indicates the possibility of hemivertebrae. If a child walks extremely carefully as if to avoid pain, suspect the possibility of intervertebral disc inflammation or caries of the spine. A bunch of hair over the lower end of the spine suggests the presence of lipomeningocele, particularly if associated with paraparesis, tight heel cord, or urinary problems. A dimple at the lower end of the spine may be a sacrococcygeal dimple or pilonidal sinus. The points in favor of pilonidal sinus are its location (higher), color (tan, blue), and surrounding hair.

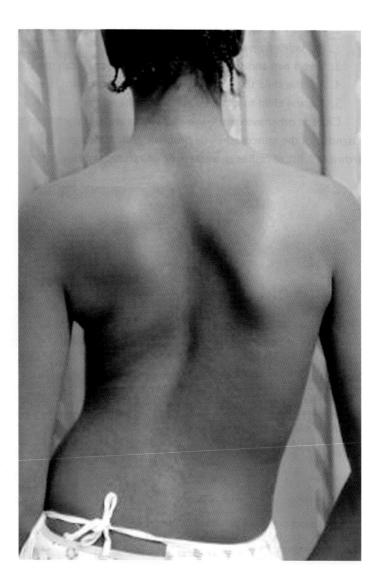

**Figure 10-14.** Scoliosis with the patient erect, viewed from behind the patient. Note the asymmetry in the positions of the shoulders, and the space between the side of the torso and the inside of the arms. (Photo courtesy of Sukhen Shah M.D. Department of Orthopedics, A I DuPont Hospital for Children, Wilmington, DE)

Normally, when the child is looked at from the side, the cervical spine and lumbar spine show concave curves, and the thorax shows a convex curve. Loss of C-curve in the cervical spine suggests either JIA or tuberculosis of the spine. Prominent thoracic curvature may indicate kyphosis, as in Scheuermann disease or Morquio disease. If there is a distinct angle at the apex of the kyphosis of the thorax, it is called "gibbus" and indicates the possibility of fracture or collapse of a vertebra, as in tuberculosis.

Loss of lumbar lordosis is seen in ankylosing spondylitis. Prominent lumbar lordosis may be familial, developmental (up to seven or eight years), secondary to severe hypotonia, or due to hip flexion contracture.

Points that suggest *scoliosis* (even before removing the clothing) are elevated shoulder on one side, family history of scoliosis, prominent scapula, apparent leg-length discrepancy, and complaint about unequal bra cup size in girls.

Scoliosis is easily visible on examining the spine from the back (**Figure 10-14**), and is described traditionally as "scoliosis with convexity to the right (or left)." Since scoliosis can be primary or secondary, make sure that there is no neuromuscular disease or leg-length discrepancy.

To measure for leg-length discrepancy, lay the patient down in the supine position. With the lower limbs in equal degrees of abduction from midline, measure the distance from the anterior superior iliac spine to the medial malleolus. Run the measuring tape across the thigh, over the medial surface or the front of the knee, and along the medial aspect of the tibia. This is the true leg length.

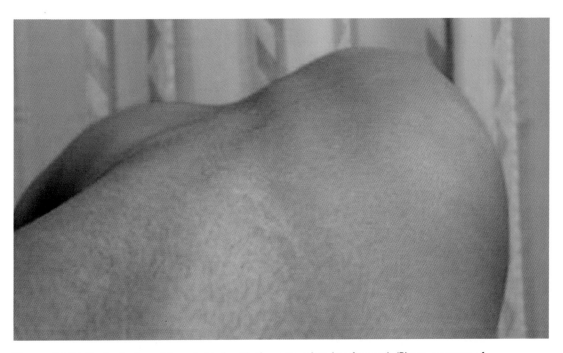

**Figure 10-15.** Scoliosis viewed from behind, with the patient bending forward. (Photo courtesy of Sukhen Shah M.D. Department of Orthopedics, A I DuPont Hospital for Children, Wilmington, DE)

Apparent leg length is measured from the umbilicus to the medial malleolus with the legs lying parallel. This may be abnormal, even if the legs are of equal length, in the presence of hip flexion contracture and asymmetry of the pelvis.

Since the scoliosis may be a fixed lesion, test for this by asking the child to lean forward as if to touch the feet with the hands (**Figure 10-15**). A curve that corrects during this procedure obviously is not fixed. In a small child, lift the child by the arms and hands vertically. A nonfixed curve will disappear. True scoliosis will become prominent during flexion.

Test for *mobility of the lumbar spine* using a modified Schober's method. Place a horizontal line across the back in the midline at the level of the sacral dimples with the patient standing erect. Place another mark on the skin in the midline over the spine at a point 10 cm above the first point. Place a third mark 5 cm below the first point. Now ask the patient to bend over to touch the feet. Measure the distance between the upper and lower marks. Normally, the back should stretch to at least 5 cm between the two points during this maneuver. A more simple clinical method is to place two fingers on the adjacent spinous processes and estimate the separation of fingers when the patient bends forward.

## Palpation

Palpate the spine for local tenderness, particularly if osteomyelitis or a vertebral tumor is suspected. Tenderness between the vertebrae may be elicited in disc inflammation.

## HAND

The hand gives clues to the diagnosis of many systemic diseases. The subheadings under which hands should be observed are:

- General clues: handedness, involuntary movements, neurologic
- Size of the hand and of the phalanges
- Shape
- Hand position
- Trophic changes
- Color of the palm and of the fingers
- Rash (palm, fingers, and nail)
- Nodules (palm, tendons, and fingers)
- Fingers: size, numbers, alignment, thumb
- Dermatoglyphics

## General Clues

The general examination starts with observation of handedness while receiving a toy or an object. Since definite handedness may not be established until two and a half to three years of age, a consistent approach with one hand at a very early age arouses suspicion of weakness on one side. A child with no dominant handedness at seven to eight years of age also arouses suspicion of neurological problem.

One can recognize the *handedness* of the child by looking for certain clues. Clinical clues are significant only in relation to a cluster of other findings. One cannot, therefore, swear by any of the following findings. 1) The dominant hand will have a wider base at the proximal end of the nail of the thumb compared with the non-dominant side. The corner of the nail on the dominant side is also more squared than rounded. 2) If the web-space between the thumb and the index finger is spread, the angle is more obtuse on the dominant side. 3) If the child is asked to put his or her hands behind the back and raise the hands as far as possible between the shoulder blades, the dominant hand will reach higher.

*Tremors* (also see pages 54 & 279) may be observed on even a casual scrutiny of the hands. Tremor at rest is seen in essential tremor and Wilson disease. Tremor seen in sustained posture suggests anxiety and fatigue and, rarely, disease states such as thyrotoxicosis and cerebellar disease. Intention tremor (tremor which comes on with an activity such as in the finger-nose test) is seen in cerebellar disease or in stress.

Athetosis is characterized by writhing movements of the distal parts of the body and is observed most commonly in the hands. Carpopedal spasm also may resemble athetosis but is elicited by occlusion of vessels with a sphygmomanometer cuff. Asterixis (liver flap) is a flopping movement of the outstretched hand and is seen in hepatic failure (e.g., Reye syndrome).

One can feel the *power of grasp* during a handshake. Though a weak grasp by itself may not indicate disease, look for neurologic and joint diseases (juvenile idiopathic arthritis) which interfere with grasp. On sustained grasp, alternate squeezing and relaxing by the patient (inability to sustain the grasp) is seen in chorea and is called "milk-maid's hand." During the hand grasp, a sweaty palm may suggest an anxious child. Also look for clues of nail biting and thumb sucking.

The easiest way to test for the motor components of all *three major nerves* of the upper extremity is by testing the mobility of the thumb. Abduction and extension of the thumb are lost in radial nerve paralysis, adduction of the thumb is lost in ulnar nerve paralysis, and apposition of the thumb is lost in median nerve paralysis. The sensory portions of these three nerves are evaluated by testing sensation over the ulnar aspect of the little finger (ulnar nerve), the tip of the index finger (median nerve), and the dorsal aspect of the web between the thumb and index finger (radial nerve).

# Size

The size of the hand and of the fingers may be small (feet also small) as in achondroplasia, Down syndrome, and de Lange syndrome. The fingers are also small. Large hands are seen in gigantism, and long hands with spidery fingers are seen in arachnodactyly and homocystinuria. Hypoplasia of the radial aspect of hand is seen in Holt-Oram syndrome and Fanconi syndrome.

# Shape

The shape of the hand in athetosis has been described above. "Mitten hand" with fused fingers is seen in Apert syndrome. Bifid claw-like hand is seen in Thalidomide syndrome.

Clinodactyly is the shortening of the radial aspect of the middle phalanx, resulting in radial deflection of the terminal phalanx. It is common in females and is seen in 0.3% of the normal population (**Figure 10-17**).

Hypoplasia of the metacarpal bones of all fingers is seen in syndromes such as Coffin-Siris and *cri-du-chat*. Look at the knuckles when the patient makes a fist. Instead of a row of knuckles at the same level, if a dimple is seen at the head of the fourth metacarpal, it suggests hypoplastic fourth metacarpal, as in pseudohypoparathyroidism.

The appearance of the *thumb* can give clues to many diagnoses. **Table 10-7** lists various abnormalities of the thumb and associated syndromes. The thumb sign of Marfan syndrome is elicited by asking the patient to clench the fist with the thumb held inside the palm. The tip of the thumb protrudes past the ulnar border of the palm and the metacarpophalangeal joint of the thumb is also protruding at the radial side in Marfan syndrome (thumb sign) (**Figure 10-18**). The sign is absent in homocystinuria, a condition in which other morphologic features are very similar to those of Marfan syndrome. A short thumb is seen in several syndromes. When the thumb is placed along the side of the palm parallel to the other fingers, the tip normally should be between the proximal and the middle crease of the index finger.

## Dermatoglyphics

The epidermal ridges and creases of the palms of the hand are unique for each individual. The thumbprint has been used as an equivalent to a signature in India and China for many centuries. Sir Francis Galton established the study of fingerprints (derma-skin; glyphic-curve), though Purkinje recognized the characteristics of finger patterns. The three components of the dermatoglyphic patterns are:

1. Flexion creases
2. Ridge arrangement of palms
3. Finger patterns

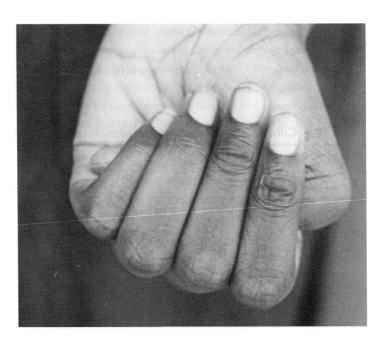

**Figure 10-18.** Thumb sign in Marfan syndrome.

## Flexion Creases

Usually there are three palmar creases. When the two distal creases are fused and run as a single crease across the entire palm reaching the ulnar border of the palm, it is called the "simian crease" (**Figure 10-19**). This is classically seen in Down syndrome. When there are two transverse creases and the proximal one runs across the entire palm, it is called "Sydney line," and is seen in congenital rubella syndrome.

Look for a crease on the palmar surface of the fingers corresponding to the interphalangeal joints. Normally, there are two or three creases over the proximal interphalangeal joints but only one over the distal interphalangeal joints. Two creases over the palmar aspect of the distal interphalangeal joints are seen in patients with sickle cell disease. Usually the second crease is located just beyond the distal interphalangeal flexion crease.

## Ridge Arrangement of Palms

The ridges of the palm run in different directions. In areas where three ridge systems meet, there are triradiate structures, aptly called "triradii" (**Figure 10-20**). There is one proximal (axial) triradius on the palm close to the wrist. This is designated as t. There are four other triradii (digital) situated one each under the index, middle, ring, and little fingers. They are designated A, B, C, D. The angle between the triradii located on A, t, and D is called the "AtD" angle and usually measures 40 degrees. If, however, the axial triradius is located distally in the center of the palm, the AtD angle becomes obtuse (75 to 80 degrees). Such a situation occurs in Down syndrome, Turner syndrome, and congenital rubella syndrome.

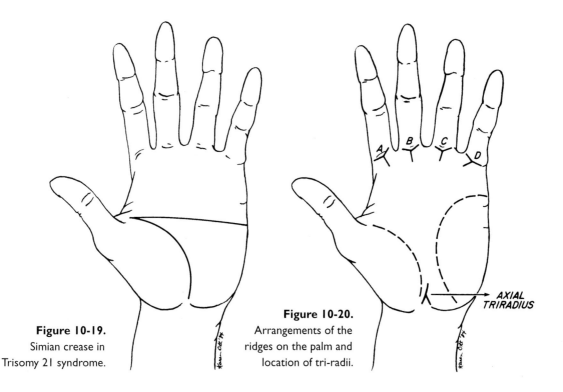

**Figure 10-19.**
Simian crease in
Trisomy 21 syndrome.

**Figure 10-20.**
Arrangements of the
ridges on the palm and
location of tri-radii.

AXIAL
TRIRADIUS

### Finger Patterns

There are three characteristic patterns on the fingertips: loop, whorl, and arch (**Figure 10-21**). The loop has only one triradius, whereas the whorl has two. The loops may be ulnar loops (opening toward the ulnar side) or radial loops (opening toward the radial side). The usual pattern is ulnar loop of the little finger, radial loop of the index finger, and whorl or arch of the middle finger. One occasionally may have the same pattern in all fingers. This is rare in normal children and is seen more often in congenital rubella syndrome (more whorls), Trisomy-18 (more arches), and Down syndrome (ulnar loop in all fingers). In Trisomy-18, there may be no patterns at all on the fingertips.

The number of ridges cutting across a line joining the center of a loop or whorl to the nearest triradius may be counted in each of the 10 fingers (**Figures 10-21** and **10-22**) and added together to get the ridge count. The average value is 145 for males and 127 for females. The ridge count is increased in Turner syndrome and congenital rubella syndrome, since they have more whorls (average is 169) and decreased in Klinefelter syndrome (average is 27).

## SPORTS INJURIES OF KNEES AND ANKLES

Trauma to soft tissues is common in sports-related injuries. It could be a strain (injury to muscle-tendon unit) or a sprain (injury to ligaments).

In children, when there is a stress on a joint, fracture is more common than ligamental tears. However, ligamental injury can occur in sports, particularly in adolescents. The knee and ankle joints are the most commonly injured joints.

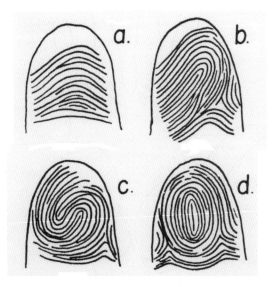

**Figure 10-21.** Deramatoglyphic patterns on fingers. A. arch; B. loop; C. double loop. D. whorl.

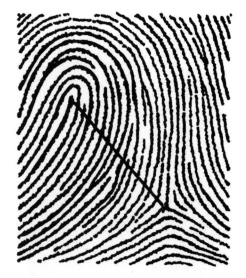

**Figure 10-22.** Ridge count. See text for description.

The patella may be completely displaced from the intercondylar notch due to an acute violent force pushing the patella laterally. This can occur particularly in those with hyperextensible joints. There is pain and swelling on the medial aspect of the patella and your attempts to move the patella laterally produces great anxiety in the child (apprehension test).

The lateral collateral ligament of the knee is tested as follows. Holding the lower end of the leg with one hand, place the palm of the other hand just below the knee on the medial aspect of the upper part of the leg. The knee should be in just a few degrees of flexion, so that it is not locked in extension. Give gentle outward pressure on the upper part of the tibia and inward pressure on the lower part of the leg. This should stretch the lateral collateral ligament and cause pain if it is injured.

To test the medial collateral ligament, use the same procedure but apply inward pressure over the upper part of the tibia with the palm held on the outer aspect and apply outward pressure on the lower leg. There should be less than 5 degrees of motion and no pain. Damage to the medial collateral ligament is associated with greater than 5 degrees of motion and a palpable gap in the medial joint line. Pain inside the joint suggests damaged articular cartilage.

Presence of gliding movement of the tibia on the femur suggests loss of integrity of the cruciate ligaments. To test the cruciate ligament of the knee, ask the patient to lie supine with the knee in flexion and the sole of the foot touching the examining table. Gently maintain the position of the foot flat on the table and grasp the upper end of the tibia with both hands. Now rock the tibia gently forward. If the anterior cruciate ligament is intact, the forward motion of the tibia will stop abruptly at a specific point. If it is damaged, the tibia can be moved forward without an abrupt stop. This is the *anterior drawer* sign. To look for posterior cruciate ligament damage, place the patient in the same position as above. If the tibia appears to be sagging behind the femur, a slight push from behind will correct the subluxation.

Look for meniscal injury using the McMurray's test with the patient in the supine position. Stand on the same side as the injured knee. Holding the heel on one hand and the knee on the other, slowly extend the flexed knee to full extension while applying a medial rotation force on the knee. If there is pain along the joint line during extension, if the knee cannot extend fully, or if there is a popping sensation, suspect medial semilunar cartilage damage. Repeat the same test but while rotating the tibia externally to test for lateral semilunar cartilage injury.

The severity of sprains of the ligaments around the ankle joints may be graded as I (minimal swelling and pain-no disability), II (moderate swelling, severe pain, and some disability), or III (complete rupture of the ligament resulting in a snapping noise, severe pain, and disability). Type III sprain is associated with instability of the joint which may be tested as follows: 1) Stabilize the lower leg with one hand, grasp the heel firmly with the other hand and try to move it anteriorly to look for excess anterior movement of the talus in the ankle mortise as compared with the opposite side. This tests the talofibular ligament. 2) To test for the calcaneofibular ligament, grasp the heel as described in the first step, and look for excess inversion of the foot (as compared with the opposite side).

# BIBLIOGRAPHY

Beetham WP, Polley HF, Slocumb CH, Weaver WF. Physical examination of the joints. Philadelphia: WB Saunders; 1965.

Care of the young athlete. Andy J, Sullivan MD, Anderson SJ, editors. Elk Grove (IL): American Academy of Pediatrics; 2000.

Foster HE, Kay LJ, Friswell M, Coady D, Myers A. Musculoskeletal screening examination (pGALS) for school-age children based on the adults GALS screen. Arthritis Rheum (Arthritis Care Res). 2006;55(5):709-16.

Homans J. Venous thrombosis and pulmonary embolism. N Engl J Med. 1947; 236:196-201.

Holt SB. The significance of dermatoglyphics in medicine. A short survey and summary. Clin Pediatr. 1973;12(8):471-84.

Metzl JD. Sports Medicine in the Pediatric Office: A Multi-media Case-based Text with Video. 1st ed. American Academy of Pediatrics. 2007.

Rang M. The Easter Seal Guide to Children's Orthopedics. Ontario, Canada: Easter Seal Society; 1982.

Staheli LT. Fundamentals of Pediatric Orthopedics. 4th ed. Philadelphia: Lippincott-Williams & Wilkins Publishers; 2007.

# Chapter 11

# CENTRAL NERVOUS SYSTEM

Some common complaints associated with diseases of the central nervous system are: loss of consciousness, seizures, developmental delay, developmental regression, weakness of parts of the body, unsteady gait, limping, clumsiness, involuntary movements, floppiness, and headaches. Loss of vision, loss of hearing, and vertigo as presenting symptoms are less common in children.

*Weakness, reduced selective motor control, ataxia*, and *apraxia* were recently defined and classified as negative motor signs.

*Weakness* is defined as "inability to generate normal involuntary force in a muscle or normal voluntary torque about a joint."

*Reduced selective motor control* is defined as "impaired ability to isolate the activation of muscles in a selected pattern in response to demands of a voluntary posture or movement." This is different from weakness and may be manifested as abnormal postures or unusual movement patterns (e.g., synergic movements).

*Ataxia* is defined as "inability to generate a normal or expected voluntary movement trajectory that cannot be attributed to weakness or involuntary muscle activity about the affected joints." Specific deficits that may be seen as components of ataxia include dysmetria (inaccurate motion to a target either undershooting [hypometria] or overshooting [hypermetria], dyssynergia (decomposition of multi-joint movement), and dysdiachokinesis (excessive difficulty performing repetitive movements).

*Apraxia* is defined as "impairment in the ability to accomplish previously learned and performed complex motor actions that cannot be explained by ataxia, reduced selective motor control, weakness, or involuntary motor activity." Developmental apraxia is defined as "failure to have ever acquired the ability to perform age-appropriate complex motor actions that is not explained by the presence of inadequate demonstration or practice, ataxia, reduced selective motor control, weakness, or involuntary movements."

***Quick and easy neurological examination***: In a practical essay on neurological examination, John Freeman describes how to perform a screening neurological examination of a child in an office setting. (*For details read Freeman JM. The three-cent neurological examination and other tools for an era of managed care. Contemp Pediatr. 1997;14:153-64.*) The first step is a good history. At the end of taking a history, one should know whether there is a neurological problem, if so what kind of a problem it is, and whether it is possible to localize it to one of the components of the central nervous system. History also should establish whether the problem is acute and progressive (needs immediate referral), chronic, or episodic. If it is chronic, determine whether it is static, progressive, or improving.

The three-penny examination, which is a playful, nonthreatening screening neurological examination, follows. By dropping a shining penny on the floor behind the child (on a surface that is not carpeted so the coin will make noise) and observing, one can find out whether the child hears ordinary sounds and is able to localize. Now ask the child to pick up the penny and give it to the mother or to the doctor and observe how the child performs this task (intact hearing, understanding of the request, and ability to follow commands are being tested). If there is no response to voice command, gesturing may be needed. Watching the child pick up the coin from the floor may demonstrate problems with balance, coordination, developmental delay, weakness, handedness, posturing, muscle weakness, and associated movements. Using two more coins, test the field of vision, extraocular movements, and nystagmus (described in page 270). Then place two coins on the child's outstretched hands and make him or her walk (tests weakness, involuntary movements, ataxia).

# EXAMPLES OF HISTORY TAKING

Before describing the methods of physical examination, loss of consciousness and seizure will be discussed in detail with emphasis on history taking and classification.

*Loss of consciousness (coma)*: There are different levels of diminished consciousness that include *confusion and delirium* in which the patient is unable to maintain a coherent stream of thought, *drowsiness* in which a patient appears to be asleep but easily arousable with verbal or light stimuli, *stupor* in which the patient appears to be asleep and does not respond to light or verbal stimuli but responds to noxious stimuli, and coma in which the patient does not respond to noxious stimuli either.

When dealing with a child in a coma, the following points in the history are relevant. Was the onset sudden or gradual? Is there a history of trauma (intracranial bleeding)? If there was trauma, did the patient lose consciousness at once (severe intracranial bleeding, cerebral contusion) or after a period of lucid interval (middle meningeal bleeding)? Is there a history of headache and vomiting preceding the onset of coma (encephalitis, tumor)? Did the patient have fever before onset of coma (encephalitis, meningitis)? Is there a history of ingestion of drugs or toxins? Are there any members of the family taking medications (possibility of ingestion of drugs)? Is there a history of preceding illness such as diabetes, SLE, or sickle cell disease? If so, has the patient been taking any drugs for this illness? Also look for history of substance abuse.

*Concussion* is defined as "a state of momentary loss of consciousness or a state of confusion or amnesia following head trauma." Head trauma is a common problem for which medical care is sought particularly after automobile accidents, sports injuries, and child abuse. Some of the factors that lead to further investigations in a child with concussion are headache and vomiting, retrograde amnesia, evidence of skull fracture, and seizure.

*Seizure* is defined as "a momentary or transient alteration in consciousness, behavior, motor activity, sensation or autonomic function caused by excessive rate and hypersynchrony of discharges from a group of cerebral neurons."

In the current classification of epilepsy, old terminologies such as petit mal, grand mal, and psychomotor seizure are included under the more generalized classification of "focal" (partial) and "generalized" seizures. Focal includes motor and sensory seizures. Generalized includes tonic, clonic, and absence seizures (**Table 11-1**).

*Seizures:* Some of the important points in the history to be obtained in any patient with seizures include the following questions. What is the nature of involuntary movement? Are they tonic-clonic? Are they sudden, single, or repetitive muscular contractions (myoclonic)? Are they complex, seemingly purposeful acts (focal motor with automatism, formerly known as psychomotor attacks)? Are they confined to one extremity or to one side of the body? Does the attack start in one area of the body and "march" in a definite sequence, or does it come all at once? How long does the attack last? (Tonic-clonic attacks and complex partial seizures last longer than a minute or two. Absence seizure and syncope last for less than a minute.) Does the patient lose consciousness? (Patients with tonic-clonic, absence, and complex partial seizures lose consciousness). Does the patient fall down? (In generalized tonic-clonic and akinetic seizure, the patient collapses to the floor. In tonic-clonic seizure, the tone is increased; this is not so in the akinetic type.) Does the patient lose control of the bladder and bowel? (This occurs in generalized tonic-clonic seizure, and loss of control of bladder and bowel at night may suggest a seizure that no one witnessed). What happens after the attack? (In generalized tonic-clonic type, the patient may sleep for a few hours and appear dazed; in absence type, the patient may appear momentarily confused, or have lip-smacking and chewing movements; some patients with focal seizures may show associated behavioral motor activity such as lip-smacking or chewing movements and be amnesic to events that happened during the seizure.) How many attacks are there per day? (This establishes the severity and seriousness of the problem.) Are there any precipitating events? (Examples are light stimulation or a startle response.)

## Table 11-1. Seizures in Children

Generalized: Due to involvement of both hemispheres. May be with motor activity (convulsive) or without. May be associated with loss of consciousness.

    Tonic-clonic (grand mal)

    Tonic

    Clonic

    Myoclonic

    Atonic-akinetic (drop attack)

    Absence (petit mal)

Partial:

    Simple without loss of consciousness

    Complex with altered mental status (temporal lobe seizures)

Lennox-Gastaut: intractable mixed seizures

Benign Rolandic epilepsy: nighttime seizures during sleep

Juvenile myoclonic epilepsy

Infantile spasm (old salaam epilepsy with hypsarrhythmia)

# PHYSICAL EXAMINATION OF THE GENERAL NEUROLOGICAL STATUS

## Appearance

Normal components of appearance include:

- Awareness
- Position and spontaneous movements of the body
- Responsiveness to touch and handling
- Activity
- Orientation

### Awareness

A normal child is alert and responsive. A comatose child is unresponsive and not aware of his or her surroundings. The vacant looks of a retarded child or a blind child are easy to recognize after some experience. Certain children may be aware of their surroundings, but not able to verbalize, as seen after head injury and meningitis.

### Table 11-2. Glasgow Coma Scale

| | |
|---|---|
| Eye opening | |
| Spontaneous | 4 |
| Reaction to speech | 3 |
| Reaction to pain | 2 |
| No response | 1 |
| Best motor response | |
| Spontaneous | 6 |
| Localizes pain | 5 |
| Withdraws in response to pain | 4 |
| Abnormal flexion in response to pain | 3 |
| (decorticate posture) | |
| Abnormal extension in response to pain | 2 |
| (decerebrate posture) | |
| No response | 1 |
| Best verbal response | |
| Oriented | 5 |
| Confused/disordered | 4 |
| Inappropriate words | 3 |
| Incomprehensible sounds | 2 |
| No response | 1 |

During the management of a patient with coma, a standardized examination can be administered quickly to assess the integrity of important neurologic functions and the severity of coma. The most commonly used clinical scoring system for the assessment of severity of coma is the Glasgow Coma Scale. In this system (**Table 11-2**), the patient is assessed for eye opening, the best motor response, and the best verbal response. The highest score is 15 with an intact and normal level of consciousness. The lower the score, the deeper is the level of coma. However, this scale is not useful for children under three years of age, since the subscale for the best verbal response is not applicable. Therefore, a modified Glasgow Scale called the "Children's Coma Scale" has been developed (**Table 11-3**). A score of 13-15 is defined as mild, 9-12 as moderate, and less than 8 as severe.

**Table 11-4** is a more comprehensive list of all important items in the history and physical examination of a child in a coma. Routine neurologic examination is discussed later in this chapter. The following comments refer to the neurologic profile and the Coma Scale.

## Table 11-3. Childhood Coma Scale

| | |
|---|---|
| Eye opening | 4 |
| Spontaneous | 3 |
| Reaction to speech | 2 |
| Reaction to pain | 1 |
| No response | |
| Best motor response | 6 |
| Spontaneous | 5 |
| Localizes pain | 4 |
| Withdraws in response to pain | 3 |
| Abnormal flexion in response to pain | |
| (decorticate posture) | 2 |
| Abnormal extension in response to pain | |
| (decerebrate posture) | 1 |
| No response | |
| Best verbal response | 5 |
| Smiles, oriented to sound, follows objects, interacts | 4 |
| Crying, consolable, inappropriate interactions | 3 |
| Inconsistently consolable, moaning | 2 |
| Inconsolable cry, irritable and restless | 1 |
| No response | |

*With kind permission from Springer Science & Business Media. Hahn YS, Chyung C, Barthel MJ, Bailes J, Flannery AM, McLone DG. Head injuries in children under 36 months of age: demography and outcome. Childs Nerv Syst. 1988; 4:34-40.*

## Table 11-4. Examination of the Comatose Patient

History (from parents and friends)

    Onset of coma (abrupt, gradual)

    Recent complaints (headache, depression, focal weakness, vertigo)

    Recent injury

    Previous medical illnesses (diabetes, uremia, heart disease)

    Previous psychiatric history

    Access to drugs (sedatives, psychotropic drugs)

General Physical Examination

    Vital signs

    Evidence of trauma

    Evidence of acute or chronic systemic illness

    Evidence of drug ingestion (needle marks, alcohol on breath)

    Nuchal rigidity (examine with care)

Neurologic Profile

    Verbal responses

        Oriented speech

        Confused conversation

        Inappropriate speech

        No speech

    Eye opening

        Spontaneous

        Response to verbal stimuli

        Response to noxious stimuli

        None

    Pupillary reactions

        Present

        Absent

    Spontaneous eye movements

        Orienting

        Roving conjugate

        Roving dysconjugate

        Miscellaneous abnormal movements

        None

    Oculocephalic responses

        Normal

        Full

        Minimal

        None

**Table 11-4. (Continued)**

Oculovestibular responses
>    Normal
>    Tonic conjugate
>    Minimal or dysconjugate
>    None

Corneal responses
>    Present
>    Absent

Respiratory pattern
>    Regular
>    Periodic
>    Ataxic

Motor responses
>    Obeying commands
>    Localizing
>    Withdrawal
>    Abnormal flexion

>    ## Abnormal extension
>    None

Deep tendon reflexes
>    Normal
>    Increased
>    Absent

Skeletal muscle tone
>    Normal
>    Paratonic
>    Flexor
>    Extensor
>    Flaccid

*From: Plum F and Posner JB. The Diagnosis of Stupor and Coma. 3rd ed. Philadelphia: FA Davis Co; 1980. Reprinted with permission from Oxford University Press.*

For each category, enter the best level of function on admission and periodically thereafter. A flow sheet with these data will be of great help in the management of patients in a coma. The best verbal response is oriented speech and gets the highest score; whereas, no speech obviously indicates a deeper state of coma. Patients with spontaneous eye opening and movements get the best score and are obviously not comatose, though many may not be aware of their surroundings. Those with

or in the doctor's office. One may have to rely on the history and careful observation of whatever communication is available. If there are sufficient reasons, refer the child to a speech pathologist for a thorough examination. Certain points, however, are within the reach of all interested clinicians and can be evaluated with most children. These normal milestones in speech and pre-speech developments are given in **Table 11-5**.

### Table 11-5. Sequence of 29 Linguistic and Auditory Milestones

| Sequential Milestone Item | Months of Age |
|---|---|
| Alerting* | 1 |
| Social smile* | 1-1 ½ |
| Cooing | 3 |
| Orient to voice* | 4 |
| Orient to bell (1)* | 5 |
| "Ah-goo" | 5 |
| Razzing | 5 |
| Babbling | 6 ½ |
| Orient to bell (11)* | 7 |
| Gesture | 7 ½ |
| "Dada/mama" (inappropriate) | 8 |
| Orient to bell (111)* | 9 ½ |
| "Dada/mama" (appropriate) | 10 |
| One word | 11 |
| One-step command (w/gesture)* | 12 |
| Two words | 12 |
| Three words | 14 |
| One-step command (w/o gesture)* | 15 |
| Four to six words | 15 |
| Immature jargoning | 15 |
| Seven to twenty words | 18 |
| Mature jargoning | 18 |
| One body part* | 18 |
| Three body parts* | 21 |
| Two-word combinations (N+N) | 21 |
| Five body parts* | 23 |
| Fifty words | 24 |
| Two-word sentences (S+P) | 24 |
| Pronouns (I, me, you; inappropriate) | 24 |

*Age levels are approximate and still need to be standardized on different normal populations. The sequence of development for items at different age levels demonstrates much less variability, especially in delayed subjects. Attempts should be made to directly observe asterisked items; when a child is uncooperative during a particular evaluation, parental observation may be recorded.*

*From Capute AJ, Accardo PJ. Linguistic and auditory milestones during the first two years of life: a language inventory for the practitioner. Clin Pediatr. 1978;17: 847-53. (Reprinted by permission of SAGE publications)*

## Quality

In testing for quality of speech, find out whether the patient can produce an adequate *volume* of air. Patients with intercostal muscle paralysis (as in myopathies, poliomyelitis) may not be able to speak long sentences without frequent pauses. They may have no voice or a breathy voice. A simple way to test for this is to make the child take a deep breath and count as many numbers as possible in one breath. Another simple method is to have the child blow out a match held at a distance of two to five inches.

Vocal cords are essential for *phonation*. The patient may have normal respiration and strong respiratory muscles, but if vocal cords do not move normally, one may have aphonia (no voice). The vibration of air by vocal cords gives rise to pitch and intensity of the sound. Listen, therefore, to the pitch. Monotonous speech without inflections is seen in deafness. A deaf child also may have a very high-pitched voice if the deafness is central. Some normal children may have a high-pitched voice, particularly in the prepubertal period.

Coordinated movement of the tongue, palate, and lips are required for *articulation*. A simple test for articulation is to make a child say "ka, pa, ti, ka" repeatedly and quickly. Because the sound "ka" comes from the back of the throat, the word "pa" produced by the lips, and "ti" produced by the tongue and the palate, these three sounds test the major components of articulation effectively. Problems of coordination also will be evident when the child tries to say these words fast. Test words such as "methodist, episcopal," or "round the rugged rock the ragged rascal ran" can be used in older children and adolescents to assess intelligibility and coordination.

The *content* of the speech as to appropriateness and orientation and irregularity of *rhythm* (stuttering) are easily discerned just by listening to the child's conversation.

Nasal resonance during phonation is seen in cleft palate, chronic adenoiditis, or palatal paralysis. If this is suspected, ask the child to say words that end with "ng" (e.g., coming, walking). The child will say "comig," walkig," etc.

# CRANIAL NERVES

## Olfactory Nerve (First Nerve)

Testing the sense of smell is difficult, even in adults. In children it is even more so. Present common items such as toothpaste, oranges, and chewing gum to each nostril with the other side closed. The child should have his or her eyes closed and should guess the item from the smell. In infants, change of facial expression may be the only clue.

## Optic Nerve (Second Nerve) (Figure 11-1)

- Presence or absence of vision
- Acuity
- Fields
- Fundus

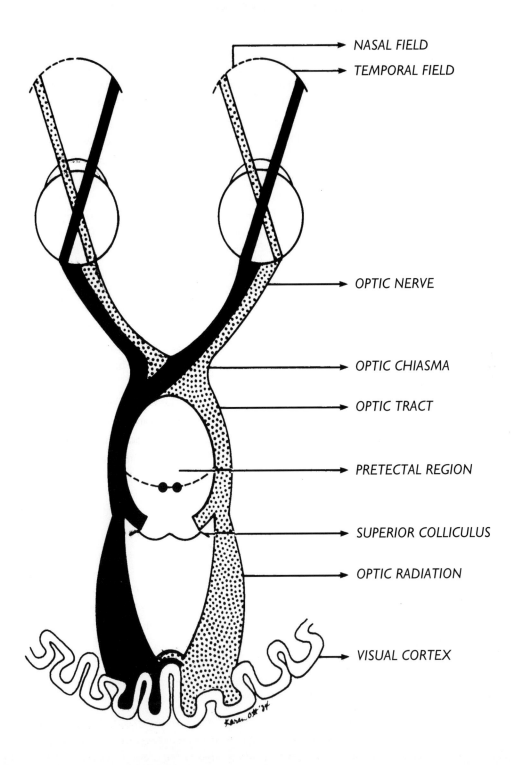

NASAL FIELD

TEMPORAL FIELD

OPTIC NERVE

OPTIC CHIASMA

OPTIC TRACT

PRETECTAL REGION

SUPERIOR COLLICULUS

OPTIC RADIATION

VISUAL CORTEX

**Figure 11-1.** Diagram of visual pathway

*Vision Screening.* Vision screening of infants and children is an essential part of well-child care and is summarized in **Table 11-6** and **Appendix 11-1**. For a detailed discussion of this topic, the reader is referred to the Recommendations of the American Academy of Pediatrics Section on Ophthalmology, in cooperation with the American Association for Pediatric Ophthalmology and Strabismus, and the American Academy of Ophthalmology Committee published in Pediatrics [2003;111(4):902-7].

In infants, a pen light or an attractive toy may be used to test for the presence of vision. An infant with intact vision should be able to fix on a target and track by the third month of age. A threat response to a rapidly approaching object such as a menacing hand gesture may help to detect intactness of vision. A threat stimulus coming from different directions may help test the field of vision. Unilateral cover test (explained below) may be used to determine the intactness of vision in each eye. Infants and children with poor vision may not like the normal eye being covered or may not follow an object with one eye.

Current screening methods used in preschool children have not been validated. However, monocular acuity of vision can be tested using one of the standard vision charts such as HOTV, Lea, and Tumbling E. This is done with both eyes open at first and then with one eye covered. Tendency for amblyopia is tested using the Random Dot E stereogram.

Older children should be tested using standard visual charts (**Table 11-6**).

## Table 11-6. General Guidelines for Examination of Eyes in Infants and Children

1. Use methods appropriate to age and developmental level.
2. All newborns should be examined within the first two months to evaluate fixation, ocular alignment, and red reflex.
3. Special screening is recommended to look for amblyogenic factors in infants and children with developmental disabilities.
4. Formal vision screening should start at three years of age using standard guidelines.
5. Physical examination of the eye should include: external structures, visual acuity, ocular alignment and motility, and an ophthalmoscopic examination.
6. Children wearing eye glasses should be tested initially with the glasses on. Vision testing should be performed in a well-lit area.
7. Most vision screening charts require the subject to be seated at a distance of 10 feet (3 meters).
8. For younger children, picture charts (e.g., Allen) are appropriate. For older children, use one of the standard charts (e.g., Snellen, E, HOTV).
9. Proper occlusion of the untested eye requires properly fitting patches.
10. Most children have a visual acuity of 20/50 by three years of age.

*Source: American Academy of Pediatrics, Section on Ophthalmology. Red reflex examination in Neonates, Infants and Children. Pediatrics. 2008;122(6):1401-4.*

*And* **Committee on Practice and Ambulatory Medicine, Section on Ophthalmology, American Association of Certified Orthoptists, American Association for Pediatric Ophthalmology and Strabismus and American Academy of Ophthalmology.** *Eye examination in Infants, Children, and Young Adults by Pediatricians. Pediatrics. 2003;111(4) 902-7.*

## Presence of Vision

If a child follows a moving light or object, intact cortical vision is confirmed. A simple test to document intact cortical vision is to make a menacing gesture, as if to poke the eye. A consistent blink response indicates cortical vision. However, this response is not present routinely before 10 months of age. Inconsistent response indicates that the vision is intact, but the interpretation of vision is impaired, as in parietal lobe lesions of children recovering from head injury or coma and in the presence of retardation.

## Acuity

Testing for visual acuity has been described previously under vision screening. Place screening charts at a distance of 10 feet. Test each eye separately and then both together. At least 50% or more of the letters in each line should be recognized correctly by the child to get a "pass" for that line. Physiologically, children are farsighted until six to seven years of age. Myopia is common in older school-aged children. Children in the first three grades of school should be able to read 20/20 or better with each eye. A compact eye testing machine which projects the charts in front of the child's visual field is easier to administer and takes very little space in an office, but is not accurate.

## Field of Vision

The field of vision is tested by a confrontation method until the child is old enough to cooperate with perimetry. Some simple methods are 1) use a colorful toy or finger puppet and approach the eye from each side sequentially. If the child turns to the object when approached from one side but not the other, suspect hemianopsia. 2) If the child tilts the head to read, hemianopsia or muscle imbalance is suspected. 3) Ask the child to look at a measuring tape when it is being pulled out of its container. Ask the child to fix the eye on the opening in the container from which the tape comes out. Do it first with the tape coming out from right to left and then from left to right. Normally, the eye will follow the tape for a short distance as it comes out and return back to the opening of the tape container. This is called "opticokinetic nystagmus." If there is hemianopsia, this reflex will be absent in the direction opposite of the hemianopsia. 4) Ask the child to sit and look at your eyes, which you are holding level with his or her eyes. Now dangle two objects on threads behind the child's head and slowly bring them forward. As soon as the peripheral field of the eye catches the object, the child will move the eye. If this occurs consistently in one direction but not the other, it indicates a field defect. 5) In older children, use the static or the kinetic confrontation method. In the static method, ask the child to look into your eyes (fixation), which are placed at the same level as his or her eyes. Now take your hands to the periphery of the visual field (**Figure 11-2**), with your index fingers extended and at diagonally opposite positions. Quickly flex one of these fingers and ask the child to show which finger moved. This is repeated at the other two quadrants of the field. This method is more helpful in adults with parietal lobe lesions. In the kinetic method, the physician tests one quadrant at a time by slowly moving an object from the extreme periphery to the center of the field.

When the defective visual field crosses the vertical meridian, the lesion is most likely in the retina or the optic nerve. If the defects are strictly confined to one half, the lesions are most likely in the chiasma, optic radiation, or the occipital cortex.

Beware of false positive findings. Cooperation is needed for these tests, and staring at a child's eyes can frighten him or her.

## *Fundus*

The optic fundus is examined with an ophthalmoscope. The following is a brief description of the parts of the ophthalmoscope and their use.

The *ophthalmoscope* consists of a handle, batteries, and the ophthalmoscope head. Most models operate on batteries (3 volts). Some models (particularly those used by ophthalmologists) can be connected to electric outlets through a transformer (12 volts). Always use fresh batteries to obtain maximum light and good visualization.

The head of the ophthalmoscope has a rubber guard to prevent scratches to the examiner's glasses if he or she wishes to use the instrument with glasses on. The rotary disc on the head has numbers in red on the left side and in black on the right side of the "0" mark. Some instruments may have a different color scheme. The red numbers indicate minus lenses in the viewing aperture, and black numbers indicate plus lenses. Myopia in the patient's lenses is neutralized by the minus lenses and *hyperopia* by the plus lenses in the ophthalmoscope. One can get 15 to 20 diopters of power through these discs. In addition, lenses with plus 8 to plus 10 power can be used to focus on the anterior chamber, margin of the iris, and the lens.

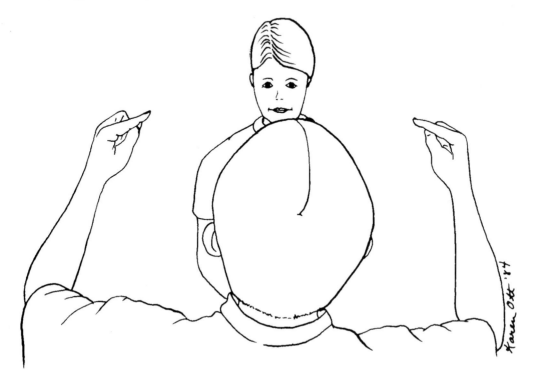

**Figure 11-2.** Confrontation perimetry.

Ophthalmoscopes have devices to give different kinds of beams of light. The control is usually on top or behind the instrument head. Two round apertures (one large, one small), a slit, a grid, and a red-free filter are commonly available. The large round is for large pupils and the small round is for small pupils. The slit is used to recognize the convexity and concavity of retinal lesions. In the presence of a raised or depressed retinal lesion, if the light from the vertical slit is focused on the lesion and the adjoining normal retina, there will be a step-like distortion of the beam at the junction of the normal retina and the lesion. If the distortion is convex pointing towards the observer, the lesion is an elevation. If it bends away from you, it is a defect in the surface of the retina. The grid is used to measure the size of the vessels and other lesions. The green filter (red-free light) makes the blood vessels stand out as dark stripes and allows recognition of small aneurysms and hemorrhages. With fresh batteries, this filter also may help differentiate between melanin (not very black) and old hemorrhage (intense black).

*Techniques for using the ophthalmoscope.* Certain practical points to remember are 1) many children and infants are curious and eventually will look directly into the light if left alone for a time, but if you touch the lid to open the eye, the fight will get tougher. 2) Younger children are best examined when they are lying down. Some older children cooperate better if they are sitting up. 3) Some children may require anesthesia. If the problem is significant enough to warrant such a risk, an ophthalmologist should be looking at the eye. 4) Dilation of the pupil is necessary for a thorough examination of the eye, though a satisfactory examination of the optic nerve head can be accomplished without mydriasis.

For routine office use, one drop of 2.5% phenylephrine in each eye is adequate. For better pupillary dilation, the following procedure is recommended:

**For children less than 9 months of age**: A combination drop of 0.25% cyclopentolate with 2.5% phenylephrine approximately 15 minutes before examination. AVOID atropine drops because of the potential anticholinergic effects.

**For children over 9 months of age**: Tropicamide 1%, phenylephrine 2.5% ophthalmic drops; give one drop of either or both approximately 15 minutes before examination OR a combination drop of 0.25% cyclopentolate with 2.5% phenyephrine approximately 15 minutes before examination.

Although this procedure has been found to be safe when performed in an office setting in infants older than two weeks of age, it is best to explain the need for this examination and potential risks and get an informed consent from a parent.

If the child has seizures, 0.5% Tropicamide applied two or three times over a 10-minute period may work. For children with dark eyes, Tropicamide 1% may work but the waiting period may have to be increased to 20 to 30 minutes.

Start by using a +8 lens, which will show any scars or large deposits in the cornea as black spots in the midst of the red reflex. By changing the lens to +8 or +10, the edge of the iris becomes easily visible. Determine whether the edge is clear and round. In the presence of iridocyclitis, the iris edge will show fine serrations, instead of a smooth round contour.

Examine all infants and young children for "red reflex" using an ophthalmoscope as suggested by Bruckner. Asymmetry in red reflex using the Bruckner method (Bruckner reflex) strongly suggests the presence of risk factors for amblyopia and of intraocular disease. In the original method as described by Bruckner, there were two steps. The first step is to look at the location of the corneal reflex

(Hirschberg test) and the variation in the brightness of the red reflex from the fundi of both eyes viewed simultaneously. The second step is to look at the fixation movement of the eyes on alternate illumination of one eye at a time.

As currently recommended, perform the test before the pupils are dilated. Hold the ophthalmoscope 1 m (approximately one arm length) from the patient and shine the light through the large round aperture of the ophthalmoscope so that both corneas can be illuminated simultaneously. Halogen ophthalmoscope is preferred over battery-operated models. Look through the ophthalmoscope using the lens until both the corneal reflex and the red reflex are in focus. First, assess the position of the corneal reflex in relation to the pupil in each eye. Next, look for asymmetry in the red reflex defined as any noticeable difference in the brightness or color of the red reflex. Asymmetry in brightness is more important than that of color. In the presence of strabismus, the reflex is darker in the fixating eye and lighter, red-yellow or white in the non-fixating eye.

The most recent recommendation by the Red Reflex Subcommittee of the Section of Ophthalmology of the American Academy of Pediatrics is that all infants should have red reflex testing performed within the first two months of life. If it is abnormal (inequality in color or clarity, or if reflection or opacity is present), follow with either a red reflex examination after dilation (see page 126 for details) or examination by an ophthalmologist trained in diagnosing and managing eye problems in young infants.

Occasionally, the normal red reflex is replaced by a "white" or "yellow" reflex, also called the "cat's eye" reflex. A white reflex indicates serious eye disease and requires immediate consultation with an ophthalmologist. Retinoblastoma, toxocara canis, and retrolental fibroplasia can cause a white reflex. Congenital cataract also will give a white reflex instead of the red reflex, but the point of origin of the reflex can be judged by changing the power of the lens. A +10 or +12 lens will be needed to locate the white reflex of a cataract. Dark spots in the red reflex, absent or blunting of the reflex, or white reflex should be followed by quick referral to an ophthalmologist. If the red reflex is crescentic, suspect dislocated lens (as in trauma or Marfan syndrome).

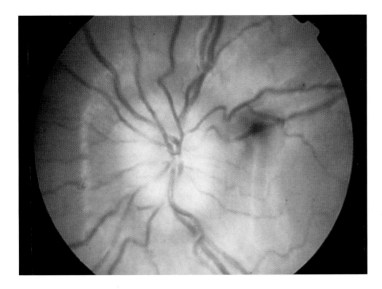

**Figure 11-3.** Papilledema (optic disc swelling) with retinal hemorrhage in a patient with Bechet's disease. (Courtesy of Sharon S. Lehman, MD, Chief Ophthalmology, Nemours Children's Clinic/Al duPont Hospital, Wilmington, DE and Robison D. Harley MD Endowed Chair in Pediatric Ophthalmology, Thomas Jefferson University-Jefferson medical Colege, Philadelphia, PA)

Now look at the *characteristics of the fundus*. Look at the periphery and move slowly toward the optic disc by following the vessels. Take note of the characteristics of the arteries and veins. Finally, look at the macula. The fovea is the center of the macula and is located approximately two disc diameters temporal to the disc. The major points to look for in the macula are 1) pigmented deposits with exudates of toxoplasmosis, and 2) the cherry red spot of Tay-Sachs disease.

Important findings to look for in the fundus of children are related to the retinitis of congenital infections, degenerative diseases, phakomatosis, optic atrophy, and papilledema (**Figure 11-3**). Look for the "jet-black" deposits of retinitis pigmentosa that start in the equatorial region, spreading later to the periphery, and for a yellow-white exudate of congenital syphilis that later turns into pigments all over the fundus. Also look for retinal exudates that appear as faint clusters or masses.

Next, look at the *blood vessels*. The central retinal artery divides into superior and inferior segments. Each of these segments divides into a temporal and a nasal branch. There are veins corresponding to these four arterial branches. Normally, veins are larger than arteries (3:2) and darker. The vessels have a central stripe that is more prominent in the arteries. The arteries and veins are graceful in their course without too many curvatures and acute bends. The veins pass underneath the arteries at the point where the two cross each other.

In hypertensive retinopathy one sees an increase in the reflex stripe along the arteriole, loss of reflex stripe of the veins on either side of A-V crossing, and narrowing of arterioles. Increased tortuosity of vessels in African American patients may indicate sickle cell disease. Perivascular sheathing is seen in vasculitis of various kinds. Hemorrhages along blood vessels are seen in severe papilledema, hypertension, and SLE. Hemorrhages will appear dark when seen through a red-free (green) light. Vascular tumors may be recognized during this portion of the examination. Fullness of the veins and loss of venous pulsation of the optic cup are seen in papilledema.

Next, look at the *optic disc* and characterize the following features: shape, size, color, depth, edge, and vessels. Normally, the disc is round. The central portion of the disc is a shallow, paler area called the "physiological cup." The vessels fan out from the center of the cup. The physiological cup is symmetrical and occupies about 30% of the disc. In glaucoma, the cup extends almost to the periphery and is asymmetric. The vessels are pushed nasally. In primary optic atrophy, the entire disc is white in color, the disc margins are clear, and the vessel undisturbed. In secondary optic atrophy, the disc is pale, there is sheathing of the vessels, and the margin is indistinct.

Edema of the disk may be seen in several conditions including optic neuritis and increased intracranial pressure. The term papilledema (**Figure 11-3**) is used when the disk edema is secondary to increased intracranial pressure. It may be difficult to differentiate between optic neuritis and papilledema. In both of these conditions, the margins of the disc are indistinct and the color hyperemic. Fullness of veins, loss of pulsation of veins, and retinal hemorrhages may be seen in both conditions. The physiologic cup is filled out. In addition to history, two other useful points in differentiating these two conditions are 1) decreased visual acuity in neuritis as opposed to normal vision in papilledema, and 2) presence of inflammatory cells in the vitreous seen in optic neuritis (**Table 11-7**).

## Oculomotor, Trochlear, and Abducent Nerves (Third, Fourth, and Sixth Nerves)

These nerves supply the extraocular muscles and the pupil. Consequently, examination of these nerves involves spontaneous movements of the eyeball and movements on demand. Systematically observe the following:

1. Position of the eyes at rest; squint
2. Movements of the eyes independently of each other
3. Movements of the eyes together (conjugate)
4. Movement of the eyes in relation to the head movements and body movement

Also evaluate:

a. Nystagmus (also see page 270)
b. Double vision
c. Pupils

Some of the clinical clues to lesions of the third, fourth, and sixth nerves are 1) ptosis which is drooping of the eyelids, 2) an eye that is deviated down and out, 3) inability to look outwards, and 4) diplopia.

Younger children are best examined when they are sitting on a parent's lap facing you. Your eyes should be at the same level as the child's. Covering the eyes can frighten the child. Therefore, examine the child with both eyes open before covering one eye at a time. Also, use your own hand or some other nonthreatening device to cover the eyes of the child rather than use any occlusive device. Use of a flashlight or a sparkler toy is bound to make the child focus.

## Testing for (Strabismus) Squint

Look for reflection of the light from the surface of the cornea while the child is looking at an object directly in front of the eye. Normally these reflections should be at comparable points. In the presence of squint, the reflections are at nonconjugate locations. This test is useful in infants with large deviations. To detect deviations of less than 15 degrees, the cover-uncover test (see below) will have to be done.

### Table 11-7. Appearance of Optic Fundus in Three Important Clinical Conditions

|  | Papilledema | Papillitis | Optic Atrophy |
|---|---|---|---|
| Depth | Elevated disc<br>Physiological cup obliterated | Elevated disk<br>Physiological cup obliterated | Shallow |
| Edge | Blurred edge | Blurred edge | Very sharp |
| Vessels | Engorged/no venous pulse | Engorged/no venous pulse | Narrow/few |
| Color | Hyperemic<br>Hemorrhages | Hyperemic<br>Hemorrhages | Pale to white |
| Vision | Good; or enlarged blind spot | Poor vision; or loss of central vision | Reduced vision |

Strabismus (squint) is ocular misalignment. The word *tropia* signifies a manifest misalignment, as in heterotropia. (Orthotropia is the term for absence of ocular deviation.) Esotropia is convergent strabismus and is more likely to be evident while looking at near objects. This is due to inward deviation of the non-fixing eye. Exotropia is divergent strabismus and is likely to be present while looking at distant objects. This is outward deviation of the non-fixing eye.

Tendency for deviation is called *phoria*. Esophoria is the tendency to converge and exophoria is the tendency to diverge. The cover-uncover test is used to test for phoria.

*Cover-uncover test*: With the child looking at an object or a source of light, cover one eye, then the other with cardboard or with a thumb held in front of the eye. Do it slowly and rapidly. *Look at the uncovered eye always.* If there is definite movement of the uncovered eye, phoria is present. When one eye is covered, if the uncovered eye moves to fix on the finger, it was not looking at the object originally. Now, if the covered eye is uncovered (and is found to be moving) to fix on the object, it obviously was deviating when the other eye was looking at the object. This indicates the presence of a tendency (phoria) for squint.

## Independent Eyeball Movements

Next, test for movements of the eyeball in all directions by having the child follow a bright light or sparkler, first with both eyes and then one eye at a time (**Table 11-8 A** and **B**). The third nerve

### Table 11-8A. Actions of eye muscles

| Direction of gaze | To the right | To the left |
|---|---|---|
| UP | Rt Superior Rectus | Lt Superior Rectus |
| | Lt Inferior Oblique | Rt Inferior oblique |
| Lateral | Rt Lateral Rectus | Lt lateral Recrus |
| | Lt Medial Rectus | Rt Medial Rectus |
| Down | Rt Inferior Rectus | Lt Inferior Rectus |
| | Lt Superior Oblique | Rt Superior Oblique |

### Table 11-8 B.  Chart of Paralysis of Individual Eye Muscles

| Muscle | Nerve | Normal action to move the eye | Deviation of Eyeball when weak | Diplopia When looking |
|---|---|---|---|---|
| Internal rectus | III | adduction | Out (external squint) | Toward nose |
| Superior rectus | III | Up with eye in abduction | Down and in | Up and out |
| Inferior rectus | III | Down with eye in abduction | Up and in | Down and out |
| Inferior oblique | III | Up with eye in adduction | Down and out | Up and in |
| Superior oblique | IV | Down with eye in adduction | up and out | Down and in |
| External rectus | VI | abduction | Inward (internal squint) | Toward temple |

*From several sources*

innervates the medial rectus, superior and inferior recti, inferior oblique, levator palpebrae superioris, and the pupillary constrictors. Therefore, if the third nerve is paralyzed, ptosis, pupillary dilatation, and loss of all movements except lateral deviations and downward movement with the eyes in abduction will be present. Paralysis of the fourth nerve (superior oblique muscles) is suggested by the presence of slight upward deviation of the eye in abducted position because of the unopposed action of the inferior oblique muscle. Paralysis of abduction (lateral movement) of the eye suggests a sixth cranial nerve lesion.

To test for rectus and oblique muscles, test the eyes in either abduction or adduction. On abduction of the eye, the superior rectus acts as an elevator and the inferior rectus as a depressor. On adduction of the eye, the superior oblique is a depressor and the inferior oblique is an elevator of the eye. In the midline position, all of these muscles have a rotatory component.

## Conjugate Eyeball Movement

Conjugate deviation of the eyes (both eyes moving parallel) at *rest* with the gaze directed to one side indicates either a corticobulbar irritative lesion on the opposite side or a destructive lesion on the same side. After observing for any conjugate deviation at rest, test for conjugate eye movement on *command*. If it is absent, it denotes injury to the fronto-mesencephalic pathway. In children with head injury, conjugate deviation at rest and inability to produce conjugate movement on command may be seen. Inability to get superior conjugate movement is called "Parinaud syndrome" and denotes a lesion in the corpora quadrigemina.

## Eyeball and Head Movements

The next step is to examine the movement of the eye as the position of the head is changed. With the eyelids held open, rotate the head from side to side. (**Do not perform this test if there is suspicion of cervical spine injury**). A positive doll's eye reflex (oculocephalic reflex) is present if there is conjugate deviation of the eyes in a direction opposite to the direction of movement of the head (head rotated toward right, eyes deviating to left). Such a reflex is absent in normal awake persons but may be present in patients with coma.

In a comatose patient, spontaneous conjugate deviation to one side on the horizontal meridian may mean ipsilateral hemispheric lesion or contralateral pontine lesion. If the eyes are deviated to one side but can be brought beyond midline to the opposite side by passive turning of the head (oculocephalic), hemispheric lesion is the likely cause. If the eyes cannot be brought beyond midline during passive turning of the head, pontine lesion is likely. Conjugate deviation downward suggests mesencephalic lesion. Immobile eyes with absent oculocephalic response may indicate a metabolic cause for coma.

## Double Vision (Diplopia)

Older children with double vision will be able to describe what they experience, but younger children and infants may not be able to do so. In the presence of diplopia (particularly of recent onset), the infant may refuse to open the eye and may lay still with eyes closed. Or, he or she may rotate the head to one side (sixth nerve) or tilt the head (third, fourth nerve).

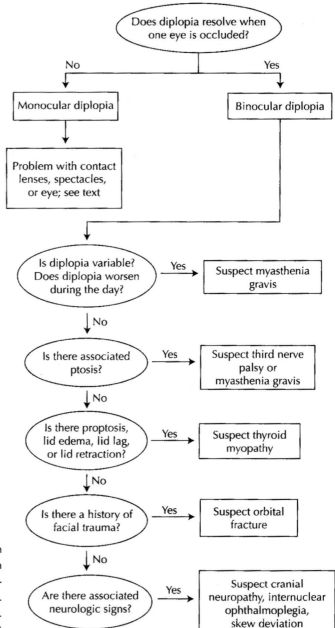

**Figure 11-4.** Clinical algorithm for diplopia. Reproduced with permission from McGee S, Evidence-Based Physical Diagnosis. Philadelphia. 2001. W B Saunders Co. page 684. (Copyright Elsevier 2001)

With both eyes open, ask the child to look at a finger or pencil held around the periphery of the field of vision, first to the patient's right. Find out whether two images are seen. (**Table 11-8B**) A false image appears in the direction toward which the paralyzed muscle usually pulls. Repeat the test with the object to the left of the patient, up and down. A simpler method is to do the cover-uncover test (as in testing for squint) in right, left, up, down, and oblique positions. Any deviation of the uncovered eye in any of these positions suggests diplopia. This test does not require the child's response.

In older children who can cooperate, it is best to ask them to track an object towards each of the six cardinal directions. Ask and find out the direction at which the diplopia is most prominent. Now, inspection of the eye may show which muscle is weak (e.g., lateral rectus on one side). If this is not clear, place a yellow or red filter in front of one eye and ask the patient to identify the more peripheral image in the direction of maximal diplopia. This image will belong to the weak eye. **Figure 11-4** is an algorithm to identify the cause of diplopia.

## *Pupils*

When evaluating the pupils look at 1) shape, 2) size, 3) equality in size between the sides, 4) response to light on the same side, 5) response to light on the opposite side, 6) response to pain, and 7) response to accommodation.

Afferent fibers for the light reflex leave the optic tract and travel via the lateral geniculate body to the pretectal region (**Figure 11-5**). The afferent fibers involved in accommodation reflex course

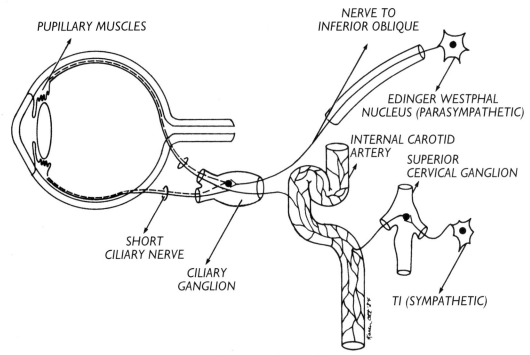

**Figure 11-5.** Nerve supply to the pupil and to the extra ocular muscles.

toward the superior colliculi. The efferent fibers for pupillary control are through parasympathetic and sympathetic fibers. Pupillary constrictors arise in the Edinger-Westphal nucleus and medial nucleus of the third cranial nerve and course along the third nerve to the ciliary muscles. Pupillary dilators originate from the cervical sympathetic ganglion and course along the internal carotid artery. Both parasympathetic and sympathetic fibers course through the ciliary ganglion and short ciliary nerves (**Figure 11-5**).

Small pupils are common in children with pigmented skin and iris. It is often difficult to see the small dark pupil in the center of a dark iris. Using the small aperture of the ophthalmoscope or covering the bulb of the flashlight with yellow cellophane paper and shining the yellow light at an angle may make the pupil more visible.

Very small pupils may be normal but also may indicate head injury, deep coma, pontine lesions, or drug toxicity (e.g., opiates). In Horner syndrome, a small pupil is seen on one side together with ptosis, enophthalmos, and lack of sweating on the ipsilateral side of the face.

Large pupils are seen in third nerve paralysis, fear, anxiety (sympathetic overactivity), drug toxicity (e.g., atropine), and in certain stages of coma. A fixed dilated pupil without reaction to light in a comatose child may be a sign of ipsilateral hippocampal herniation.

Unequal pupil size may be normal. It may be due to a small pupil on one side (local use of drugs, Horner syndrome, or irritative lesion of the third nerve), a large pupil on one side (drugs applied locally, Byrne response to pain stimulus applied to one extremity, complete paralysis of the third nerve on one side), or aniridia on one side.

Pupils fixed in mid-position without response to light but with spontaneous fluctuations in size may be seen in midbrain lesions.

Reaction to light is tested by having the child look away from the major source of light in the room and shining a flashlight on the pupil. Normally, the pupil reacts quickly. At the same time, the opposite pupil also contracts (consensual light response).

To test the accommodation reflex, the child is asked to look at a distant object. Then a finger is held close to his or her nose and the child asked to focus on the finger. Normally, the eyes should converge and the pupils constrict in attempting to look at a close object.

For the ciliospinal reflex, the skin of the neck is pinched. This should cause dilation of the pupils. In Byrne reflex, pinching one lower extremity causes dilation of the pupil on the opposite side.

The interpretation of the reflexes described above is as follows: 1) Loss of direct pupillary response on one side with loss of consensual response on the other side and retention of accommodation reflex is seen in lesions of the optic nerve close to the eyeball. 2) Homonymous hemianopsia without loss of pupillary responses indicates lesions past the point where pupillary fibers leave the optic tract. 3) Loss of direct and consensual responses to light on the same side with retention of accommodation reflex suggests lesions close to the Edinger-Westphal nucleus or ciliary ganglion (Argyll-Robertson pupils). 4) Absolute paralysis of the pupil on one side suggests lesions of the oculomotor nerve. 5) Bilateral absence of pupillary response to light suggests pretectal lesion. 6) Intact ciliospinal reflex suggests intact brainstem. 7) Patients with signs of severe lesions in the mid-brain regions but with intact light reflex probably have a metabolic problem.

The presence of ptosis on one side may mean third nerve palsy, in which case the pupil will be dilated, or Horner syndrome, in which case the pupil will be small. The appearance of ptosis may be spurious because of widening of the palpebral fissure on the opposite side (seventh nerve palsy). Bilateral ptosis is seen in myasthenia.

## Trigeminal Nerve (Fifth Nerve)

The fifth cranial nerve has a motor and a sensory component. There are three divisions of the fifth nerve: ophthalmic, maxillary, and mandibular. The first two are sensory; the third has a sensory and a motor component (**Table 11-9**).

To test for the **motor component**, ask the patient to clench the teeth. Palpate the masseters and the temporalis muscles. Ask the patient to open and close the mouth. If one side is paralyzed, the jaw will deviate to the non-paralyzed side when the mouth is opened.

*Somatic Sensory.* Sensory innervation of the face is given in **Figure 11-6**. Touch and temperature are tested in the usual manner (described on page 282). A child with toothache may pull at the ear because of transmission along the mandibular portion of the trigeminal nerve.

*Corneal Reflex.* In young children, test for corneal reflex by gently blowing air into his or her eye, which causes the eye to blink. The more acceptable method is to twist a small thread out of a cotton ball and touch the cornea with it. Ask the child to look in one direction and approach the cornea from the opposite direction (to avoid a visual blink reflex rather than a corneal blink). Test on both sides.

*Jaw Reflex.* Ask the patient to open the mouth slightly. Place a finger at the tip of the mandible and tap it with a percussion hammer. Normally, there will be a mild contraction of the masseter muscle. An exaggerated reflex indicates upper motor lesion above the fifth nucleus. This reflex may be absent, even in normal individuals.

## Table 11-9. Major Branches of the Trigeminal Nerve and Their Functional Significance

| Branch | Sensory Supply | Motor Supply | Disability if Cut |
|---|---|---|---|
| Ophthalmic | Conjunctiva (except lower lid) | None | Loss of corneal reflex |
| | Lacrimal gland | | Trophic changes in eye |
| | Medial part of skin of nose up to its tip | | Loss of sensation in areas |
| | Upper eyelids | | described under sensory supply |
| | Forehead and scalp, to the vertex | | |
| Maxillary | Cheek, front of temple, lower lids and | None | Loss of sensation in areas |
| | conjunctiva, side of the nose, upper lip, upper | | described under sensory supply |
| | teeth, mucous membrane of nose, upper | | Loss of palatal reflex |
| | pharynx, roof of mouth, soft palate | | |
| Mandibular | Lower part of face | Muscles of | Paralysis of masticators |
| | Lower lip | mastication | Loss of sensation in areas |
| | Tongue, lower teeth and part of ear | | described under sensory supply |
| | Salivary glands | | |

## Facial Nerve (Seventh Nerve)

The anatomy of the seventh nerve is shown in **Figure 11-7**. The seventh nerve is almost entirely a motor nerve. It supplies all the muscles of the face and scalp (except the levator palpebrae superioris) and also the platysma and the stapedius. The chorda tympani, whose course runs partly with the facial nerve, carries taste sensation from the anterior two thirds of the tongue. Parasympathetic presynaptic fibers to the lacrimal, the submaxillary, and submandibular glands also run with the facial nerve.

## Motor Function

While talking to the parents, casually observe the patient's face and the facial expression. In the case of unilateral facial paralysis, the facial furrows are flattened and saliva may accumulate on the affected side. The palpebral fissure may be wider on the affected side, and the eyeball may roll up under the upper eyelid when the child blinks (rather than the upper lid moving down on the eyeball). Blinking may be less forceful on the affected side.

Unilateral facial weakness has to be differentiated from weakness of the depressor anguli oris, which may be congenitally absent (Hufnagel palsy). If the latter is the case, only the lower part of one half of the face below the angle of the mouth is involved.

Look for bilateral facial weakness, which may be part of Guillain-Barre syndrome, various myopathies, and Moebius syndrome.

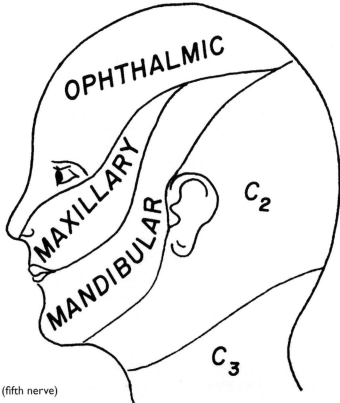

**Figure 11-6.** Sensory supply to the face. (fifth nerve)

If voluntary movements are lost but emotionally induced movements, such as smiling, are intact, suspect supranuclear lesions. In nuclear or peripheral lesions, both voluntary and emotionally-induced movements are lost.

Determine whether only the movements of the lower part of the face are lost (supranuclear lesion) or movements of both upper and lower halves are lost (lower motor). Peripheral lesions affect all facial movements on the affected side. Bell's palsy is one subset of peripheral facial palsy, which is due to lesions distal to the geniculate ganglion.

Some simple tests to evaluate the motor function of the nerve are:

1. Ask the child to close his or her eyes as tightly as possible. Normally, the upper lid will descend with some movement of the eyeball upward. There will be closure of the lids, with lashes buried inward, and lifting of the corners of the mouth upward. In cases of facial paralysis, the upper lid does not close down, even though the eyeball moves upwards (Bell's phenomenon). The eyelashes are not buried in the closure. The angle of the mouth either does not move at all or moves much less than on the unaffected side.

2. Ask the child to whistle—if he or she can understand and try.

3. Ask the child to blow up the cheeks and try to push the air out against closed lips. It is much easier to push air out of the paralyzed side.

4. Ask the child to show the teeth or smile. The face is flat on one side and the pull is toward the unaffected side.

5. Ask the patient to raise the eyebrows and look for asymmetry in wrinkling of the forehead.

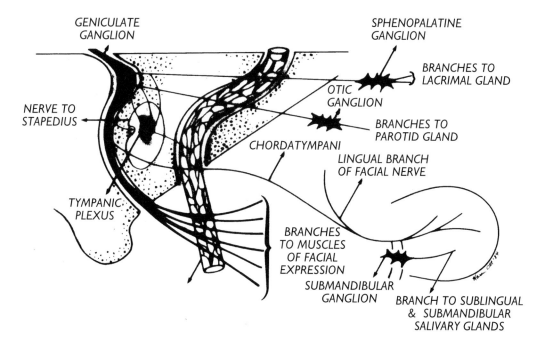

**Figure 11-7.** The anatomy of the seventh nerve.

## Sensory Function

Testing for loss of taste requires patient cooperation. It is rarely needed in children and is also difficult to perform and interpret. Test the sensation of taste over the anterior two thirds of the tongue as follows. Have the child put his or her tongue out as far as possible. Hold the tip with a moist filter paper. Dry half of the tongue with filter paper. With an applicator or a small dropper, carefully place a drop of the following substances over the anterior two thirds of the tongue, one at a time: 5% glucose solution (sweet), 3% sodium chloride (salt), 1% citric acid (sour), and 0.1% quinine hydrochloride (bitter). The child should not draw the tongue in but should indicate the taste with finger clues or by pointing to a set of cards with the names of the tastes written on them. After each drop, the tongue is thoroughly washed, and the next taste is tested. Test the bitter taste last, for obvious reasons.

The taste is lost in lesions along the course of the seventh nerve from the internal auditory meatus to the place where the chorda tympani joins the facial nerve, about 6 mm above stylomastoid foramen.

## Autonomic Functions

In recent lesions of the facial nerve, increased lacrimation and salivation are common.

## Reflexes

Certain motor reflexes of the face are affected in the presence of facial nerve lesions, though most of these reflexes indicate a premature nervous system, regression to an infantile status, or frontal lobe lesions. These are the glabellar reflex and snout reflex. Glabellar reflex is elicited by repeated tapping of the glabellar region. Normally, there will be a blinking response of the lids five to six times and then the response extinguishes. An abnormal response is a persistent blinking response as long as tapping over the glabella is continued. Snout reflex is characterized by pouting of the lips when the area of the philtrum of the upper lip is tapped. This reflex should be absent in normal children after the first two months of life.

Chvostek's sign is elicited by tapping the facial nerve in front of the ears. Marked contractions and spasm in response to tapping suggests hypocalcemia. (This response is not a reflex. This is a response caused by an increased irritability of nerve fibers to mechanical stimulation.)

## Auditory Nerve (Eighth Nerve)

The auditory nerve has two components: one supplying the cochlea and serving auditory functions, and the other supplying the semicircular canals and serving functions of equilibrium of the body. The auditory fibers reach the cochlear nuclei in the pons and the vestibular fibers reach the nuclei in the pons and medulla. From these locations, the secondary tracts decussate partially and terminate in the inferior colliculi and medial geniculate bodies and at the cortical center for hearing, which lies in the temporal lobe.

## *Evaluation of the Auditory Component (Hearing)*

Current practice demands hearing evaluation of all newborns using one of the two available techniques. Infants who do not pass this screening test, or any subsequent tests, should be referred for full medical and hearing evaluation.

Hearing tests are difficult to administer in young infants, in children up to three to four years of age, and in retarded children.

History may give several clues to the nature of the problem. For example, failure to respond to normal sounds (except very loud sounds), excessive response to visual stimuli, delayed speech, and a monotonous voice with normal motor development make one suspicious of nerve deafness. *Inconsistent* response to sounds, delayed speech, avoiding eye contact, ignoring visual clues, and unusual body movements suggests neurodevelopmental problems. Finally, normal but *delayed* response to sounds, with normal reaction to visual stimuli and delayed development in all areas of development, suggests retardation. Family history of early hearing loss is also an important trigger for careful testing.

Let the child sit on a parent's lap facing you. Use the rustling of a piece of paper, the flicking of your nails, a rattle, a small bell, or a tuning fork (256-512 cps) to make noise. Observe the child's face as the noise is made. Hold the object used to make the noise slightly behind the child's ear, first on one side and then on the other. Evidence of intact hearing is a change in the expression of the face, reaction of the pupil, and the child turning to the source of sound.

In older children, use a tuning fork, a watch, or whisper (with the mouth hidden) to make sounds. Ask them whether they hear and, if they do hear, whether there is any difference between one ear and the other.

If there are any abnormalities and suspicion about hearing, obtain both a tympanometry and audiogram or, in the younger infant, an evoked response audiometry. The old tests with a tuning fork, such as Rinne test and Weber test, are of historical interest only. These two tests are based on the comparison of air conduction to bone conduction. If the middle ear is affected, bone conduction is better than air conduction. If the nerve is affected, both air and bone conduction are decreased, but air conduction remains better than bone conduction.

*Rinne test:* Tap a tuning fork (256-512 cps) and hold it next to the ear. If it can be heard, place it on the mastoid. If it can be felt, ask the child to compare. Normally, air conduction is louder and is heard longer. In middle ear disease, bone conduction is louder and is heard for longer periods.

In the *Weber* test, a tuning fork is tapped and held over the forehead in midline. In middle ear disease on one side, the sound is heard louder on the affected side. If there is loss of nerve conduction on one side, the sound is louder on the unaffected side.

## *Abnormal Sounds*

Ringing in the ears (tinnitus) may be due to salicylate toxicity. Hyperacusis is common in facial nerve paralysis. Auditory hallucination may be seen in SLE and in psychosis.

## Vestibular Functions

Children cannot explain the sensation of vertigo. The only clues, therefore, may be unexplained crying, the child trying to bury his or her face, and not wanting to open the eyes. Other clinical clues for vestibular dysfunction are vomiting and/or dizziness with a change of posture, unsteadiness of gait, and nystagmus.

Because children with vertigo may present as dizziness, it is important to rule out other causes such as syncope, orthostatic hypotension, and sensory deficits. Make sure to take a detailed history of ingestion of drugs, ear problems, and other neurological symptoms.

## Nystagmus

Nystagmus is involuntary, conjugate movement of the eyes which may be rhythmic or nonrhythmic, with a fast and a slow component. Nystagmus is defined by the direction of the quick phase. Less frequently it is symmetrical, with rhythmic to-and-fro oscillations called "pendular nystagmus."

To test for nystagmus, ask the child to look at a flashlight or a toy held in front of the eye. Move the object quickly, first to one side and then to the other, also up and down, and ask the child to follow. Keep the flashlight or toy in extreme positions for a few seconds to see if the nystagmus disappears after five or six beats. This is the characteristic of end-point nystagmus, which is physiological. Fatigue nystagmus occurs when the child looks to one side for >30 seconds. This is also transient. Spontaneous nystagmus is seen in children with vestibular and central nervous system diseases.

Nystagmus may be physiologic or pathologic. It may occur at rest or only on movement of the eyes. Nystagmus may be horizontal or vertical, rotary, or mixed. Nystagmus may be fine (less than 1 mm movement), or coarse (over 3 mm movement). When the quick phase is to the direction of the gaze, nystagmus is graded as mild (first degree). If nystagmus is present when the child is looking straight, it is second degree nystagmus. When the quick phase is opposite of the direction of the gaze, it is severe nystagmus (third degree).

The slow component of nystagmus to the affected side is seen in vestibular lesions; whereas, the quick component to the affected side is seen in cerebellar lesions. When the direction of fast component reverses from right gaze to left gaze, it is a cerebellar lesion.

Coarse, slow, searching movements and pendular movements are seen in blind children.

A *caloric stimulation test* to elicit nystagmus helps identify eighth nerve function and is *best performed by specialists who are experienced with interpreting the response in children.* However, the test is described here for the sake of completion. Before the test is done, exclude perforation of the eardrum, tubes placed in the ear surgically, and blocking of the external meatus with wax. Clean the canal if needed. Place the child in a semi-reclining position (30 degrees) with pillows. Hold the child with assistance, since proper positioning of the semicircular canals is essential. Cold water is drawn into a 10-ml syringe with polyethylene tubing. The tubing is placed into the external meatus so that the water, when injected, will be directed at the tympanic membrane. Inject the water very slowly over a period of 30 seconds and observe the eyes carefully. Normally, this should produce slow deviation of the eyes toward the side of injection with the rapid phase of nystagmus away from the side of injection. In other words, if the right vestibular tract is intact and if the right ear is being stimulated, the eyes will deviate slowly to the right with a sudden jump toward the left to bring the eye back to neutral. This response is repetitive, with the eyes again deviating to the right and jumping back to the left. This response is lost if the vestibular nerve is damaged, and may be difficult to elicit if there is brain stem damage.

## Glossopharyngeal, Vagus, and Accessory Nerves (Ninth, Tenth, and Eleventh Nerves)

The glossopharyngeal nerve carries sensory fibers for the posterior third of the tongue, and motor fibers for the stylopharyngeus and middle constrictors of the pharynx. The only clue to unilateral paralysis of the ninth nerve may be a slight flattening of the arch of the palate on the affected side at rest.

The vagus nerve is the motor for the soft palate, pharynx, and larynx. Its parasympathetic portion supplies the respiratory, cardiovascular, and gastrointestinal systems.

The accessory nerve is a purely motor nerve supplying the sternocleoidomastoid and the trapezius muscles.

The following findings suggest lesions of the ninth and tenth nerves:

1. Presence of stridor in the absence of mechanical obstruction suggests denervation of the larynx and vocal cords (recurrent laryngeal nerve paralysis).
2. Hoarse voice suggests recurrent laryngeal nerve paralysis.
3. Aphonia.
4. Loss of swallowing reflex with drooling and choking.
5. Nasal regurgitation when swallowing liquids suggests palatal weakness.
6. Ineffective cough reflex.
7. Inability to pronounce words such as egg (which sounds as "eng") and words ending with a k sound.
8. Palatal reflex--in unilateral paralysis, the palate may droop on the affected side and not move on phonation. Palatal reflex is tested by touching the soft palate with a tongue blade. This produces elevation of the soft palate and retraction of the uvula (the sensory nerve is the ninth and the motor nerve is the tenth for this reflex).
9. Gag reflex (afferent nerve is the ninth nerve and motor is the tenth nerve for this reflex). The stimulus is touching the base of the tongue or the pharyngeal wall with a tongue blade. The normal response is elevation of the pharynx and tongue retraction.
10. Loss of sensation of taste in the posterior one third of the tongue.

The eleventh nerve supplies the sternocleidomastoid and the trapezius muscles. Ask the patient to shrug the shoulder against resistance (elevate shoulder). This tests the upper part of trapezius. To test the lower fibers of the trapezius, ask the patient to lie prone with the arms abducted 90 degrees and rotated laterally. Ask the patient to adduct the scapula against resistance. The movement should take place between the scapula and the thorax. The sternomastoid is tested by asking the patient to rotate the head to one side when resistance is applied against this movement at the chin.

If torticollis is present, which implies rotation of the chin to a direction opposite that of the direction of rotation of the occiput, make sure that there is no head tilting or spasmodic involuntary movement of the head. Torticollis and head tilting are seen in athetoid cerebral palsy, hiatus hernia, rheumatoid arthritis with cervical spine involvement, enlarged cervical lymph nodes, retropharyngeal abscess, mastoid disease, vocal cord tumors, paralytic torticollis, and as compensation for visual field defects and diplopia.

### Hypoglossal Nerve (Twelfth Nerve)

The twelfth nerve is a purely motor nerve supplying muscles of the tongue and depressor muscles attached to the hyoid bone. Look at the normal position of the tongue at rest when the mouth is slightly open. If the tongue is in midline, ask the patient to put the tongue out. In the presence of unilateral paralysis, the tongue deviates toward the unaffected side. This may be difficult to interpret if there is facial weakness. Hold a pencil vertically from the midline of the nose and compare the position of the tongue in relation to this midline. Also ask the child to push against a tongue blade, first on one side and then on the other, to look for inequality in power. Finally, look for fasciculations (seen best on the under surface of the tongue), and for wasting.

Examination of the rest of the central nervous system including motor system, sensory system, reflexes, and neurodevelopmental reflexes follows.

# MOTOR SYSTEM

The five areas to be examined in evaluating the motor portion of the nervous system include:
- Strength
- Tone
- Coordination
- Involuntary movements
- Bulk (muscle mass)

### Strength

There are two kinds of strength: *kinetic*, in which the muscle is used to move a joint through a range against resistance, and *static*, in which the muscle is used to keep a joint in one position against the force used by the examiner to move the joint in the opposite direction. The strengths are almost equal, although in extrapyramidal conditions, a loss of kinetic strength but retention of static strength may be seen.

Muscle testing can be performed for quick screening, or as a detailed examination as would be performed by neurologists and physical therapists. In the case of young children, one may have to rely on the parents' history and observations such as unequal Moro reflex, poor swinging of one arm while walking, excess wear of the front of the shoe, and resistance to examination.

Some of the simple methods to test important large muscles are as follows:*

1. Anterior neck flexors: Ask the patient to lift the neck off the pillow from a lying down position.
2. Deltoid: Ask the patient to abduct the shoulders to 90 degrees.
3. Elbow flexors (biceps and brachialis): Have the patient flex the elbow against resistance.
4. Hip flexors: Have the child lie supine with the knee flexed. The child is asked to flex the thigh against resistance.
5. Hip extensors: Ask the child to climb stairs; ask the child to stand up from a sitting position in a chair.
6. Quadriceps: Test the child's ability to extend the knee with the patient sitting at the edge of a table.
7. Hamstring: With the patient lying prone, test the ability to flex the knee.
8. Gastrocnemius: Ask the child to walk on tiptoes.

If possible, it is important to grade strength of each individual muscle. This is particularly important to assess progress. Grading is from 0 to 5 as shown in **Table 10-2**.

It is also important to differentiate between weaknesses produced by upper motor neuron (UMN) lesion, lower motor neuron (LMN) lesions, and diseases of muscle (**Table 11-10**). Spasticity, exaggerated stretch reflexes, and a positive Babinski sign suggest UMN lesions. Upper motor neuron lesions are associated with other neurological signs depending on the level of the lesion as well. For example, crossed motor findings suggest lesions at the brain stem. Seizures, speech problems, and hemianopia suggest cortical lesions.

*For detailed descriptions of testing of muscles, refer to Daniels L and Worthingham C. Muscle Testing Techniques of Manual Examination. 3rd ed. Philadelphia: Saunders; 1972.*

## Table 11-10. Differential Diagnosis of Weakness*

| Location of Lesion | Motor Examination | | | | |
| | Muscle Tone | Atrophy or Fasciculations? | Sensory Changes | Muscle Stretch Reflexes | Other Findings |
|---|---|---|---|---|---|
| Upper motor neuron | Spasticity | No | Sometimes | Increased | Babinski sign |
| Lower motor neuron | Hypotonia | Yes | Usually† | Decreased/absent | |
| Neuromuscular junction | Normal or hypotonia | No | No | Normal/decreased | Ptosis, diplopia |
| Muscle | Normal | No‡ | No | Normal/decreased | Myotonia |

**These characteristics are specific but not sensitive, and thus are helpful when present, not when absent.*

*†Sensory findings are in distribution of spinal segment, plexus, or peripheral nerve.*

*‡Atrophy may be a late finding.*

*Reprinted with permission from: McGee S. Evidence-based Physical Diagnosis. Philadelphia: WB Saunders Co; 2001. p. 734. (Copyright Elsevier 2001)*

Hypotonia and absent stretch reflexes suggest peripheral nerve lesions. Fasciculations and atrophy also may indicate LMN lesions.

In UMN lesions, the distribution of weakness gives a clue to the side of the lesion and associated findings give a clue to the location of the lesion.

In LMN type of weakness (**Table 11-11** and **Figures 11-8** and **11-9**), the physician has to determine whether the lesion is at the peripheral nerve (neuropathy), at the plexus (plexopathy), or at the spinal segment (radiculopathy). Peripheral neuropathy is common in children. The other two locations are less common. In lumbosacral radiculopathy due to disc herniation, which is rare in children, straight leg raising (the physician lifts the extended leg of the patient slowly and gently as far as possible thus flexing the hip) elicits pain radiating down the back of the ipsilateral leg. Pain at the hip or buttocks it NOT a positive response. In plexopathy, distribution of weakness corresponding to both a peripheral nerve and adjacent segments will be seen.

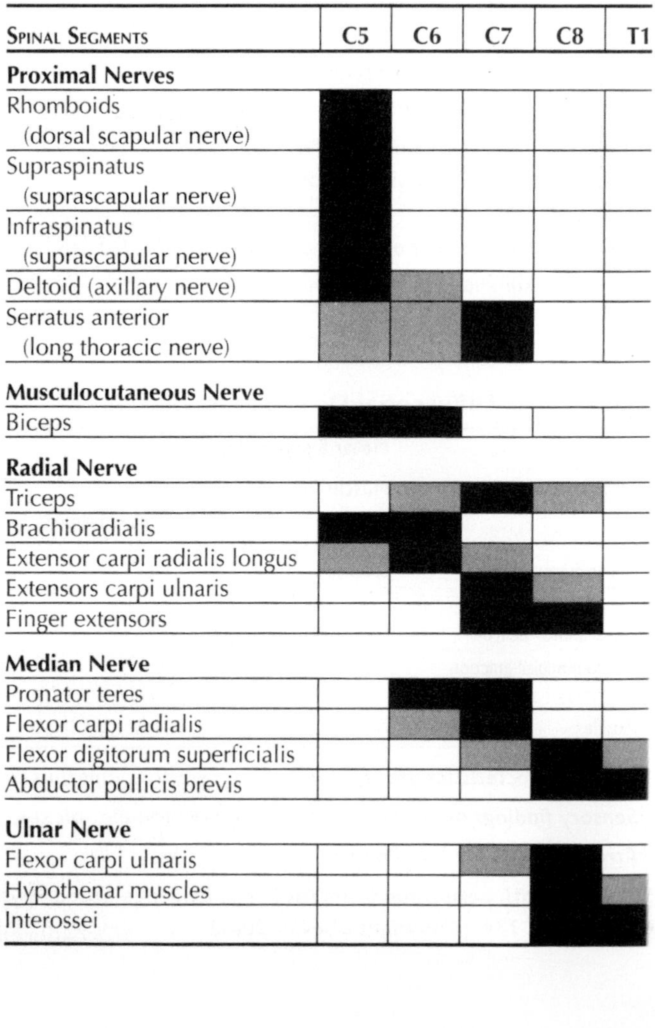

**Figure 11-8.** Innervation of muscles of the arm. Black shade indicates spinal levels that usually contribute nerve fibers to the muscle; grey shade indicated spinal levels that sometimes contributes innervation. Reproduced with permission from McGee S, Evidence-Based Physical Diagnosis. Philadelphia. 2001. W B Saunders Co. page 796. (Copyright Elsevier 2001)

| SPINAL SEGMENTS | C5 | C6 | C7 | C8 | T1 |
|---|---|---|---|---|---|
| **Proximal Nerves** | | | | | |
| Rhomboids (dorsal scapular nerve) | ■ | | | | |
| Supraspinatus (suprascapular nerve) | ■ | | | | |
| Infraspinatus (suprascapular nerve) | ■ | | | | |
| Deltoid (axillary nerve) | ■ | ▦ | | | |
| Serratus anterior (long thoracic nerve) | ▦ | ▦ | ■ | | |
| **Musculocutaneous Nerve** | | | | | |
| Biceps | ■ | ■ | | | |
| **Radial Nerve** | | | | | |
| Triceps | | ▦ | ■ | ▦ | |
| Brachioradialis | ■ | ■ | | | |
| Extensor carpi radialis longus | ▦ | ■ | | | |
| Extensors carpi ulnaris | | | ■ | ▦ | |
| Finger extensors | | | ■ | ▦ | |
| **Median Nerve** | | | | | |
| Pronator teres | | ▦ | ■ | | |
| Flexor carpi radialis | | ▦ | ■ | | |
| Flexor digitorum superficialis | | | ■ | ■ | ▦ |
| Abductor pollicis brevis | | | | ■ | ■ |
| **Ulnar Nerve** | | | | | |
| Flexor carpi ulnaris | | | ▦ | ■ | |
| Hypothenar muscles | | | | ■ | ▦ |
| Interossei | | | | ■ | ■ |

In certain situations, it may be difficult to decide whether muscle weakness is real or is due to malingering. The presence of spontaneous reflex movements, such as contractions of the latissimus muscle during cough, offer a simple way for ruling out malingering. A test specifically applicable to differentiation between hemiplegia and hysterical paralysis is performed as follows. With the patient lying on his or her back, place the palms of your hands under the heels of the patient. Now, ask the patient to lift one leg off the table and then the other. In the presence of true hemiplegia, when the patient lifts the paralyzed leg off the table, you can feel the counter pressure of the nonparalyzed side on your palm kept under the heel. If a patient with hysterical paralysis is asked to lift the so-called paralyzed side, you will not feel any counter pressure of the normal leg because the patient is making no effort to lift the leg. This is called "Hoover sign."

Another clue is obtained when you ask the patient to contract a muscle and then apply resistance to this movement. If the muscle is not truly paralyzed (malingering), when the resistance is withdrawn, there will be no movement. In true paralysis there will be follow-through movement.

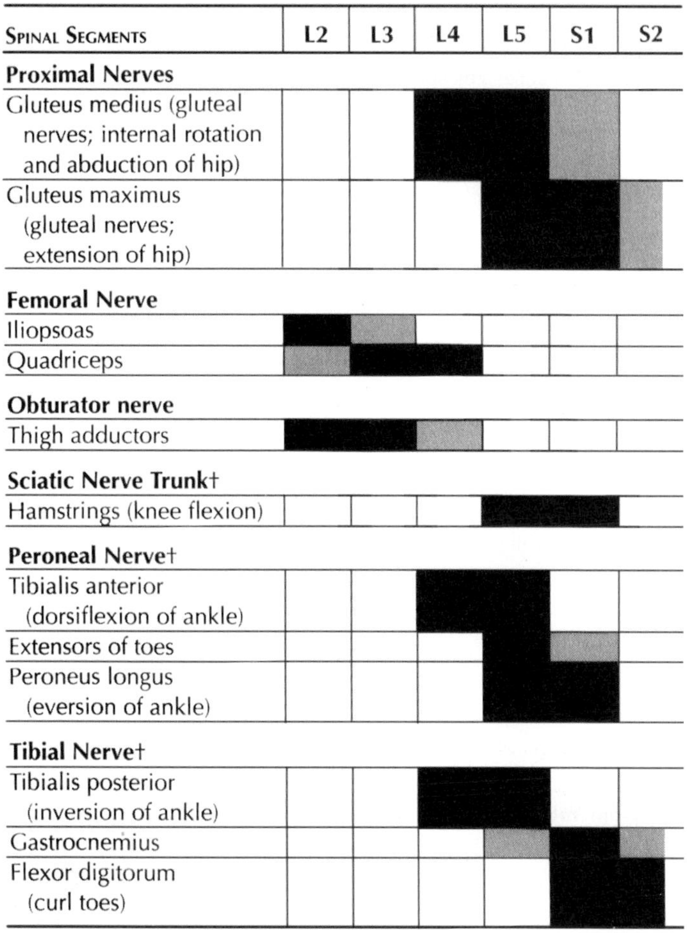

| SPINAL SEGMENTS | L2 | L3 | L4 | L5 | S1 | S2 |
|---|---|---|---|---|---|---|
| **Proximal Nerves** | | | | | | |
| Gluteus medius (gluteal nerves; internal rotation and abduction of hip) | | | ■ | ■ | ▨ | |
| Gluteus maximus (gluteal nerves; extension of hip) | | | | ■ | ■ | ▨ |
| **Femoral Nerve** | | | | | | |
| Iliopsoas | ■ | ▨ | | | | |
| Quadriceps | ▨ | ■ | ■ | | | |
| **Obturator nerve** | | | | | | |
| Thigh adductors | ■ | ■ | ▨ | | | |
| **Sciatic Nerve Trunk†** | | | | | | |
| Hamstrings (knee flexion) | | | | ■ | ■ | |
| **Peroneal Nerve†** | | | | | | |
| Tibialis anterior (dorsiflexion of ankle) | | | ■ | ■ | | |
| Extensors of toes | | | | ■ | ▨ | |
| Peroneus longus (eversion of ankle) | | | | ■ | ■ | |
| **Tibial Nerve†** | | | | | | |
| Tibialis posterior (inversion of ankle) | | | ■ | ■ | | |
| Gastrocnemius | | | | ▨ | ■ | ▨ |
| Flexor digitorum (curl toes) | | | | | ■ | |

**Figure 11-9.** Innervation of muscles of the leg. Black shade indicates spinal levels that usually contribute nerve fibers to the muscle; grey shade indicated spinal levels that sometimes contributes innervation. Reproduced with permission from McGee S, Evidence-Based Physical Diagnosis. Philadelphia. 2001. W B Saunders Co. page 805. (Copyright Elsevier 2001)

## Tone

Tone of a muscle is indicated by its resistance to passive movement. The tone is either normal, reduced (hypotonia), or increased (hypertonia, spasticity, rigidity). Exclude bone deformity or tendon contracture as the cause of the resistance, if resistance is present.

In severe hypotonia, resistance to passive movement may be very little or none, allowing the limbs to be placed in various grotesque positions, as in myopathies or myelomeningocele. Exclude hyperextensible joints as the cause of excessive movements of the joints. Hypotonia may be found in a primary muscle disorder, in peripheral nerve lesions, in disease of anterior horn cells (polio), and in cerebellar lesions. Sudden and episodic hypotonia may signify akinetic seizure or syncope due to various causes.

## Spasticity

Spasticity is characterized by increased tone of the muscles with exaggerated tendon reflexes. The increased tone depends on the velocity of movement (resistance is more with faster movement) and is different between flexors and extensors. In spasticity, limitation of range of movement is only mild to moderate, and contracture is possible. Resistance occurring as soon as the passive movement is started and changing with speed of movement characterizes spasticity. Also, when the joint is passively extended and close to full extension, the tone of the muscle increases dramatically. This results in the joint snapping into full extension just like a pocket knife (clasp-knife). Typically this is seen with the knee joint.

**Table 11-11. Segmental Innervation of Muscles***

| Spinal Level | Muscles |
| --- | --- |
| **Arm** | |
| C5 | Elbow flexors (biceps, brachialis) |
| C6 | Wrist extensors (extensor carpi radialis longus and brevis) |
| C7 | Elbow extensors (triceps) |
| C8 | Finger flexors (flexor digitorum profundus of middle finger) |
| T1 | Small finger abductors (abductor digiti minimi) |
| **Leg** | |
| L2 | Hip flexors (iliopsoas) |
| L3 | Knee extensors (quadriceps) |
| L4 | Ankle dorsiflexors (tibialis anterior) |
| L5 | Long toe extensors (extensor hallucis longus) |
| S1 | Ankle plantar flexors (gastrocnemius, soleus) |

*Most muscles are innervated by nerves from more than one spinal root. This table simplifies this innervation to standardize the description of spinal cord injury.*

*Reprinted with permission from: McGee S, editor. Evidence-based Physical Diagnosis. Philadelphia: WB Saunders Co; 2001. p. 742. (Copyright Elsevier 2001)*

*Rigidity* also is characterized by resistance to passive stretching. However, the resistance is uniform throughout the range, irrespective of the speed of movement, and allows a full or nearly full range (similar to the experience of bending a metallic flexible pipe and aptly called "lead-pipe" type). There is no difference between the flexors and extensors. There is no persistent contracture. The tendon reflexes are normal.

In addition, look for any unusual patterns when the child tries to move any part of the body. In cerebral palsy and following brain injury, the child may have some coarse voluntary movements, but these follow a set pattern. For example, when the child is asked to extend the great toe against resistance, the lower limb may adduct at the hip and extend at the knee and at the ankle--this is an "extensor synergy" pattern. Similarly, when the child is asked to open the fingers, the shoulder adducts, the elbow flexes, and the wrist flexes and pronates. This is the "flexor synergy" pattern.

In cerebral palsy, one has to differentiate between the spastic type and the athetotic-extrapyramidal type (dyskinetic). **Table 11-12** summarizes Dr. Gillette's suggestions for differentiating between these two types of cerebral palsy.

Increased muscle tone (hypertonicity) also may be due to reflex spasm of muscles secondary to pain (for example, spasms of hip flexors in synovitis of the hip and in iliopsoas abscess, and spasm of cervical muscles in meningeal irritation). Increased tone due to disease of the muscle itself has to be ruled out as well.

## Coordination

A child steadying the upper arm against the chest while trying to carry out hand activity probably has unsteadiness of hands and lack of coordination. Other clues for poor coordination in children are frequent falls, dropping objects, bumping into furniture, poor penmanship, and clumsiness. For proper coordination of muscle movement, the muscle must be strong, agonists and antagonists should act together, proprioceptive impulses from the muscles and joints should be received by the cerebellum and cortex, and body orientation should be intact. Lesions disrupting any of these areas will affect coordination.

### Table 11-12. Differences Between Spastic and Dyskinetic Types of Cerebral Palsy

| Spasticity | Athetoid-Extrapyramidal (Dyskinetic) |
| --- | --- |
| Exaggerated stretch reflex; clonus | No clonus; more of continuous resistance to passive stretch |
| Tone greatest in arm flexors and leg extensors | Tone greatest in extensors throughout |
| Contractures common and appear early | Contractures occur later |

*Reprinted with permission from: Gillette H. Systems of Therapy in Cerebral Palsy. Springfield (IL): Chas. C. Thomas; 1974.*

## Tests for Coordination

1. *Finger-nose test:* In this test, the patient touches his or her nose with a finger, then touches the tip of your finger held in space, and then touches the nose again. *Intention tremor (kinetic tremor)* appears when the patient is attempting the finger-nose test but subsides at rest. Presence of intention tremor may signify a cerebellar lesion. In addition, one may see *dysmetria* (inability to coordinate for distance) and past pointing (consistently missing your finger on the same side), both indications of cerebellar lesion. In chorea, the coordination is normal, but is periodically *interrupted* by the involuntary movements.

2. *Rapid alternating movement:* The patient is asked to repeatedly pronate and supinate the forearm by slapping the thigh with the palm and back of the hand alternately. The other method is to ask the child to repeatedly touch the tip of the index finger with the tip of the thumb as fast as possible. The same test is done on the foot by asking the child to repeatedly do tapping movements with his or her forefoot against your palm held close to the foot. Inability to perform rapid alternate movement is called "dysdiadochokinesis" and is present in cerebellar lesions and spasticity. Normally, children above five years of age should be able to perform rapid alternate movements.

3. *Rebound test of Holmes:* The patient flexes the elbow against resistance by the examiner. Now the examiner suddenly withdraws the resistance. In the presence of problems in controlling and checking muscle contraction, the arm flexes uncontrollably and even may hit the face. Positive rebound test implies a cerebellar lesion.

4. *Ability to maintain posture: For the upper extremities,* this is tested by asking the patient to extend the arms in front, with the fingers slightly separated. Tremor, chorea, and athetosis are recognized during this maneuver. In hemichorea, the affected limb will tend to drift and the patient will bring it back up. Romberg's test is used to evaluate the *lower extremities.* This test may help distinguish between cerebellar lesions and posterior column lesions as the cause of problems in maintaining posture. The test consists of the patient standing with the feet together and the eyes closed. If he or she cannot maintain this posture without swaying for at least 60 seconds, the test is considered positive. Some swaying may be seen even in normal children. Increased swaying may be seen in cerebellar disease and vestibular disease. The main difference is that in sensory ataxia, the patient will sway and fall within 10 to 15 seconds. There are differences of interpretations of this sign. Some would consider any swaying as abnormal. Others consider extreme swaying with danger of the patient falling down as positive.

5. Other methods of testing for coordination include asking the child to run, to climb stairs fast, to ride a bicycle, to tie the shoes, to write, and to draw a person.

## Involuntary Movements

Some examples of abnormal involuntary movements are:

1. *Tic:* Tics are *purposeless* but *repetitive* movements. They do not interfere with normal activities of a child and disappear during sleep. They get worse when others are watching. The areas usually affected are the eye muscles, facial muscles, and upper limb muscles.

2. *Fasciculation*: Rapid twitching movements of bundles of fibers that leave a furrow on the skin over the muscle are called "fasciculations." Some mistakenly call it "fibrillation." True fibrillation is an event occurring in the individual muscle fiber and cannot be seen clinically by the naked eye. Fasciculation occurs in conditions associated with dysfunction of anterior horn cells, for example, poliomyelitis and Werdnig-Hoffmann disease. In the latter disease, the tongue is a good place to look for fasciculation.

3. *Chorea*: Chorea is *purposeless* but *nonrepetitive* movements. These are aggravated by activity and emotional stress. There is usually hypotonia and poor coordination in various activities such as eating and writing. Children with chorea may run into objects and hurt themselves. Coordination is intact, but interrupted by sudden involuntary movement. Some of the classic signs of chorea include inability to keep tongue protruded (the tongue goes in and out of the mouth and hence is called the "trombone" tongue), and inability to maintain grasp with fingers (hence called milkmaid's hands).

4. *Myoclonus*: Myoclonus is intermittent contractions of a single muscle or groups of muscles resulting in quick jerky motion of a limb. It is made worse by voluntary activity and emotional stress. This usually occurs in association with lesions of the brain stem nuclei and reticular formation.

5. *Athetosis*: Slow, rhythmic, writhing movements of the extremities and the face are brought on by voluntary activity and emotional stimuli. The limbs take characteristic postures. The movements involve the distal muscles more than the proximal muscles (as seen in tetany).

6. *Dystonia*: This is characterized by fluctuations in tone and involves the proximal muscles of the extremities resulting in strange postures and torsion spasms. If resistance is applied to a movement, the spasm gets even worse. It disappears in sleep (e.g., cerebral palsy and reaction to drugs such as phenothiazines).

7. *Tremor*: These are rapid rhythmic oscillations of a part of the body (usually the hands) with movements of the agonists and antagonists of equal amplitude. Tremors may be present at rest or elicited by asking the child to extend his or her arms in front (see pages 54 & 231).

## Bulk (Muscle Mass)

Wasting and atrophy of muscles are seen in severe malnutrition, lower motor-neuron disease, or disuse of a limb. Regional wasting is obvious in certain diseases, such as poliomyelitis, but it may be difficult to assess if it is only minimal.

Observe for symmetry or asymmetry of wasting. Also note whether it is proximal wasting (myopathies) or wasting of distal muscles (peripheral neuritis). In conditions associated with wasting of muscles from early childhood, the affected limb may be smaller or shorter. Hypertrophy may occur with excess use (such as in the upper arms of paraplegics who walk with crutches or adolescent boys and girls who perform weight lifting) or in diseases, such as myotonia congenita or congenital hemihypertrophy. Pseudohypertrophy is seen in Duchenne muscular dystrophy and usually is localized to the gastrocnemius. Loss of fat as in lipodystrophy may make muscles look hypertrophic.

# SENSORY SYSTEM

It is often difficult to examine the sensory system (**Figures 11-10** and **11-11**) in children. Infants get frightened, distracted, and fatigued easily and cannot cooperate. Therefore, patience and ingenuity are needed. Besides, even if the child cooperates, he or she may be correct 50% of the time by chance. If time permits, it may be necessary to examine the child on more than one occasion to get reasonable cooperation and obtain essential findings. On each occasion one may have to confine oneself to testing a single sensory modality.

The modalities to be tested may be classified under four headings:

- Superficial Sensory:
  - Touch
  - Pain
  - Temperature:
  - Cold, hot
- Deep Sensory:
  - Pressure
  - Joint position sense
  - Vibration sense
- Cortical Sensory:
  - Stereognosis
  - Discrimination
  - Extinction
- Special Sensory:
  - Smell
  - Taste
  - Hearing
  - Vision

Some definitions: Complete loss of sensation is *anesthesia*. Diminished ability to appreciate a sensation is *hypesthesia*. *Hypalgesia* is decreased sensitivity to painful stimuli. *Allodynia* indicates increased sensitivity to tactile stimuli, whereas *hyperpathia* is increased sensitivity to painful stimuli.

## Superficial Sensory

Equipment needed for testing include a cotton ball or soft tissue paper, broken wooden applicator stick, and a metal tube for hot and cold water. *Sharp pins, which come included with reflex hammers, should not be used to test painful stimuli.*

Method: Ideally, the child's eyes should be closed (another frightening experience for small children) as you touch the skin gently, moving from one area of the body to another in an organized fashion. For example, start with the neck and move to the shoulder, outer aspect of the upper arm, outer aspect of the forearm, outer aspect of the palm, inner aspect of the palm, and inner aspect of the forearm. Complete this on one side and then go to the opposite side. Such an organized approach will ensure

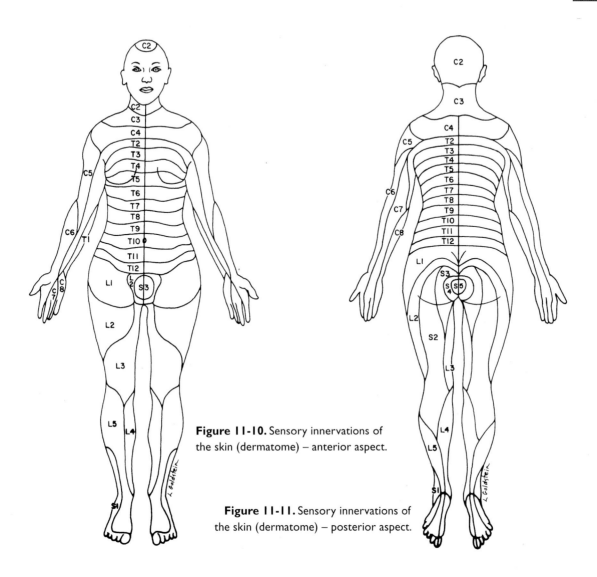

**Figure 11-10.** Sensory innervations of the skin (dermatome) – anterior aspect.

**Figure 11-11.** Sensory innervations of the skin (dermatome) – posterior aspect.

covering all the areas (don't forget the perianal area supplied by S2-S4). This is time consuming and may have to be completed at more than one examination. The child has to indicate whether he or she felt the touch by saying "now." During this procedure, you should not give any clues as to whether you are touching. In other words, do not ask, "Do you feel?" with every touch.

To test for pain, a similar approach is used with the stimulus being the tip of a broken wooden applicator stick. Both the dull end and the sharp end should be used. The child should be instructed to respond by saying "sharp" or "dull," every time he or she feels the sensation. This is done to avoid having the child respond to the pressure aspect of the sensation. If the child cannot respond verbally, facial expression and withdrawal of the limb is used as an indication of intact pain sensation.

To test for temperature sensation, use two tubes, one filled with cold water and the other with hot water. The water should not be excessively hot or cold. The test should be done as described above. The skin is touched first with one tube, then the other, randomly alternating the sequence, and asking the child to respond by saying "hot" or "cold." Again, the response should be spontaneous each time the child feels something touch the skin, not on questioning by the examiner.

*Interpretation*: Loss of sensation on one side of the body (hemianesthesia) is rare and may be seen following a head injury. The cut-off point exactly at the midline suggests psychogenic causes, because in hemianesthesia due to neurological damage, the cut-off point is just lateral to the midline. In spinal cord injury, the level of anesthesia has to be remembered in relation to the injured vertebra since the number of the vertebra does not correspond to the spinal cord segment. The levels to be remembered are:

| Vertebra | Spinal Segment |
|----------|----------------|
| CI | CI |
| C7 | C8 |
| T10 | T11 |
| T12 | L3 |
| LI | End of cord |

To test for anesthesia in spinal cord injury, first examine from above downward, then from below upward. If the point at which sensations are not felt is higher when tested from below upward than when examined from above downward, incomplete cord lesion is indicated. In myelomeningocele, the level is never strictly defined. It is patchy and uneven between the halves of the body. Loss of sensation for pain and temperature with retention of sensation of touch, position, and vibration sense in the upper limb is seen in syringomyelia. Hyperesthesia is seen in transverse myelitis, peripheral neuritis, reflex sympathetic (neurovascular) dystrophy, herpes zoster, and in children with hemiplegia and hemianesthesia, during the recovery phase of head injury.

## Deep Sensory

Deep sensations originate from muscle spindle and other nerve endings in muscles, tendons, and joints. Vibration sense usually is included with these proprioceptive sensations. The nerve impulses travel along the spinocerebellar tracts to the cerebellum. Others constitute the afferent arc of the stretch reflex and still others travel through posterior columns and the medial lemniscus to the thalamus, and thence to the parietal lobe. Parts of these nerve fibers and connections thus are involved in other functions, such as tendon reflexes and sense of position. Tendon reflex tests the peripheral arc of this system. Sense of position tests the spinocerebellar tract; whereas, special tests of proprioception test the entire system (to be described in the following paragraphs).

Deep sensory tests have to be explained adequately to children. Before the test is done, the child should have a good explanation and then be tested with the eyes open. The child should be old enough to understand and follow directions (usually older than three years of age).

To test for proprioception, the child should sit with eyes closed. Move the toes up and down passively and suddenly stop in an up or down position. The child should be able to say whether the toe is up or down. Also, during this procedure, the toes should be held on the lateral aspects, not held by the nail and the pulp, since the sense of touch may give clues. Finally remember children can say "up" and "down" and be correct 50% of the time purely by statistical chance.

Other tests for proprioception are 1) ask the child to touch the tips of corresponding fingers of both hands in space with eyes closed, and 2) arrange the finger of one hand in space in varying positions (eyes closed) and ask the child to put the finger of the opposite hand in the same position.

Test for vibration sense by using a tuning fork of 128 vibrations per second. The fork is placed over various bony prominences, sometimes with vibrations and sometimes without, and the child is asked to say whether or not he or she feels the vibrations.

*Interpretation*: Loss of proprioception and of vibration sense indicates posterior column lesions, such as in spinocerebellar ataxia. Loss of proprioception also is seen in parietal lobe lesions. If the loss of sensation affects only a portion of a limb, the lesion is most likely at the peripheral nerve, or its root. If it involves an entire limb and/or the trunk, find out whether the sensory loss involves both halves of the body (polyneuropathy and spinal cord lesion). Is there dissociation (syringomyelia and Brown-Sequard syndrome)? Is there a definite cut-off level for the sensory loss (spinal cord injury)? Is the face affected (brain stem and thalamic lesions)?

## *Cortical Sensory*

- Stereognosis
- Two-point discrimination
- Texture
- Tactile extinction

*Stereognosis* is tested at the bedside by asking the child to close his or her eyes and placing common objects in his or her hands, such as a coin, a key, or blocks (from the Denver kit), and asking the child to name the object. For more precise testing, one has to use standard geometric shapes, such as cubes and spheres, and these methods are well described in texts listed in the references.

*Discrimination of two points* is tested using a paper clip or hairpin. The child must first understand with the eyes open what "one" and "two" mean. Now the test is done with the eyes closed. Touching the child with one or two points should be done at random. Both points should touch simultaneously when testing is done for two points. The distance between the two points should be narrow in certain areas, such as fingertips (2 mm), and wider (20 mm) in areas such as the forehead.

*Textures* can be tested using silk, wool, and plastic.

*Extinction* is tested as follows: the child is asked to close the eyes and you touch two parts of his or her body--both cheeks, both hands, one hand and one cheek, or one hand and one foot--simultaneously and with equal pressure. The child is asked to name or point to the areas that were touched. When the cheek and the hand are touched, if the child recognizes that the cheek was touched but not the hand was touched, suspect extinction of distal stimulus.

*Interpretation*: Loss of stereognosis and of two-point discrimination suggests parietal lobe syndromes. Extinction of distal stimulus (when the face and the hand are touched) also is seen in parietal lobe deficits.

# REFLEXES

Reflexes can be grouped under four headings:
- Superficial
- Deep
- Developmental (infantile automatisms)
- Autonomic

## Superficial (Cutaneous) Reflexes

These are involuntary contraction of muscles following stimulation of the skin.
- Plantar
- Cremasteric
- Abdominal
- Anocutaneous
- Palmar

### Plantar Reflex (Babinski)

The reflex arc runs through the tibial nerve to the spinal cord (L4-S1).

*How to elicit*: Stimulate the sole of the foot by pressing along the plantar surface using a blunt instrument, such as the handle of the reflex hammer or a key, or the end of a ball-point pen. Start near the heel along the lateral border of the foot and carry the stimulus over to the base of the metatarsals, ending near the ball of the great toe.

*Normal response*: Plantar flexion of the great toe is the normal response. Other toes also may flex and adduct. In children, particularly ticklish ones, the entire leg may be withdrawn.

*Abnormal response*: Dorsiflexion of the great toe with fanning of other toes is an indication of a pyramidal lesion. *Babinski test is considered positive if the great toe dorsiflexes with or without fanning of the other toes.* In some cases, there may be dorsiflexion of the ankle and withdrawal of the entire extremity. This suggests that the afferent area for eliciting this reflex has enlarged. Therefore it may be possible to elicit the Babinski response by using one of the following methods:

1. Method of Oppenheim: pressing firmly with thumb and stroking along the anterior border of the tibia.
2. Method of Gordon: Squeezing the calf.
3. Method of Gonda: Flexing and twisting any toe.
4. Method of Bing: Stroking the big toe along the lateral side. (This test may be useful when examining patients in a leg cast, such as after an automobile accident.)

### Cremasteric Reflex

This reflex is tested in males by scratching the upper medial aspect of the thigh with a blunt instrument.

*Normal response*: Contraction of the cremasteric muscle with elevation of the scrotum on the same side.

*Abnormal response*: This reflex is lost in lesions above L-2.

## Bulbocavernosus Reflex

This reflex is elicited by gentle squeezing of the tip of the glans penis or clitoris.

Normal response: Contraction of the bulbocavernosus muscle as palpated by touching the skin behind the scrotum or the anal sphincter by placing the index finger in the anal canal.

Abnormal response: Absence of this reflex suggests spinal cord lesions above the S2 level or diseases of the pelvic nerves.

## Abdominal Reflex

This is elicited by stroking the four quadrants of the abdominal wall with a blunt instrument, such as a key or ball-point pen.

Normal response: Contraction of the abdominal wall at the stimulated quadrant, as shown by the movement of the umbilicus toward the quadrant stimulated.

Abnormal response: Loss of abdominal reflex, which indicates pyramidal lesion above T-8.

## Anocutaneous Reflex

This is stimulation of the perianal skin by a sterile sharp object.

*Normal response*: Contraction of the external anal sphincter, with resultant in-drawing of the anal opening (called the anal wink response).

*Abnormal response*: Loss of this reflex is seen in lesions involving S-2, S-3, and S-4.

## Palmomental Reflex

This is elicited by scratching or tapping the thenar eminence of the hand.

*Normal response*: No movements in the face.

*Abnormal response*: Contraction of the mentalis and orbicularis oris muscles on the ipsilateral side. Abnormal response indicates bilateral frontal lobe lesion.

## Hoffman's Sign

The child's hand is held at the wrist, palm facing down, and hanging loosely. Grasp the tip of the middle finger with your thumb and index finger. Give the nail of the middle finger a snap with your thumb.

*Normal response*: No movement of the child's thumb.

*Abnormal response*: If the reflex is present, the thumb on the same side flexes and adducts into the palm. All of the other fingers also flex. Presence of abnormal response indicates a pyramidal lesion above C-7.

# Deep Reflexes

Ideally these are called "muscle stretch reflexes," not tendon reflexes. These are involuntary contractions of muscles caused by a brisk stretch of the muscles. The reflex is elicited only in response to fast stretch. Therefore, the tap should be with maximum speed, and at the same time, not painful.

### Biceps Reflex (C5-C6)

Hold the child's arm with the elbow in flexion and supported by one of your hands. The thumb of the supporting hand is held over the insertion of the biceps tendon, and the thumb is tapped with a reflex hammer. A normal response is flexion of the biceps, with or without flexion at the elbow.

### Triceps (C6-C8)

With the arm flexed 90 degrees at the elbow, support the forearm. A sharp tap over the triceps tendon causes contraction of the triceps, with or without elbow extension.

### Brachioradialis (C5-C6)

While supporting the child's forearm, with his or her arm between pronation and supination, tap the tendons over the lateral aspect of the radius approximately one to two inches from the radial styloid. Normal response is flexion of forearm and supination.

### Knee Reflex (L2-L4)

The various positions in which to test knee reflex are 1) patient sitting at the edge of the table with the knees hanging free and loose; 2) patient lying supine, with knees supported by your hand, relaxed, and flexed to 30 or 40 degrees; and 3) in newborns, flexing the knee and placing the foot flat over your abdomen.

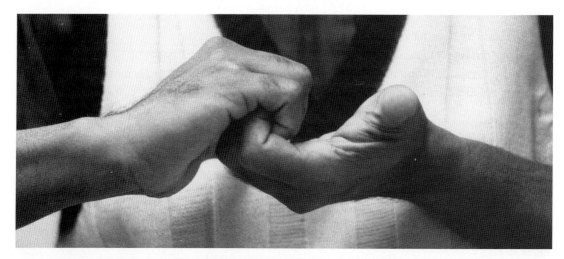

**Figure 11-12.** Jendrassik's maneuver to augment knee reflex.

Tapping the patellar tendon with a reflex hammer produces visible contractions of the quadriceps. Response is extension at the knee. This reflex is sometimes difficult to elicit. Divert the child's attention by talking about a subject of interest to the child. This reflex can be augmented by asking the child to close his or her eyes tightly, or to hook the fingers and then to pull them apart when asked (**Figure 11-12**) (Jendrassik's maneuver). To get the best response from this maneuver, tap the tendon within the first few milliseconds of the child's effort.

## Ankle Reflex (S1, S2)

The best position is for the child to be prone with the knee flexed 90 degrees. Now, hold the toes down so as to produce slight tension in the calf muscles (**Figure 11-13**). Another position is with the child lying supine, hip flexed and externally rotated, and the knee flexed with the foot lying over

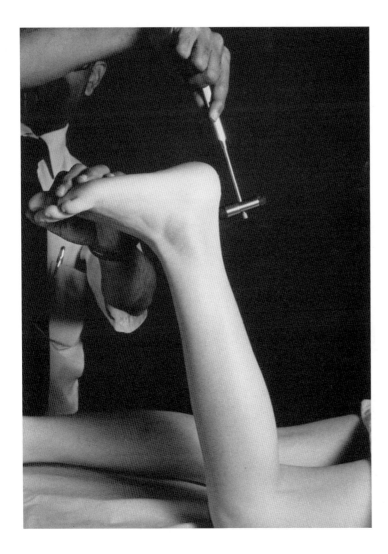

**Figure 11-13.** Testing ankle reflex with the patient in prone position.

the anterior aspect of the other leg (**Figure 11-14**). Now press firmly against the sole of the foot to dorsiflex the ankle and tap the tendoachilles. A third method is to tap at the ball of the foot. The normal response is plantar flexion.

## Interpretation of All Tendon Reflexes

Exaggerated responses are seen with spasticity (pyramidal lesions). Decreased deep tendon reflexes are seen in myopathies. Absent reflexes are more characteristic of peripheral nerve lesions.

### Clonus

Clonus is characterized by rapid movements of a particular joint due to alternating contractions of agonists and antagonists. This is brought about, if present, by sudden stretching of a tendon (such as tendoachilles) and maintaining the stretch.

Ankle clonus is elicited as follows: With the child in the supine position, flex his or her knee. Hold the forefoot with your other hand and dorsiflex with a quick movement and maintain in that position. If clonus is present, the foot will go through plantar flexion-dorsiflexion movements repeatedly.

In children with cerebral palsy, such a clonus may be elicited just by the ball of the foot touching the floor, making it impossible for these children to walk.

Patellar clonus is elicited using the following method: The child is in the supine position with the knee in extension. Hold the superior border of the patella and quickly push toward the foot (caudal), and hold. If clonus is present, the patella will move up and down repeatedly (caudal-cephalic movement).

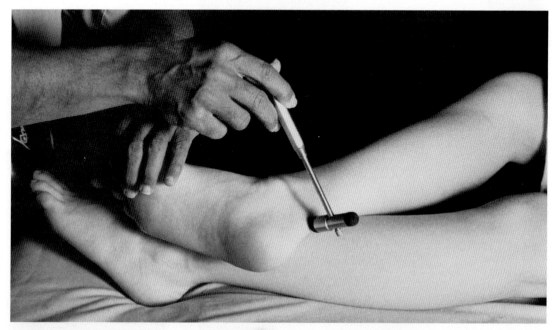

**Figure 11-14.** Testing ankle reflex with the patient supine and the knee in partial flexion.

The significance of clonus is the same as marked hyperreflexia, and is seen in pyramidal lesions. Also, fewer than three or four beats of the ankle and knee may be elicited in any normal child, particularly if the child is tense and holds his or her muscles tight.

## Signs of Meningeal Irritation

With the child supine and flat, passive flexing of the neck causes the knees and hips to flex, drawing the legs towards the chest (*Brudzinski sign*).

*Kernig sign* is tested with the child supine. The hips and knees are first flexed and the knee is extended. If the patient resists extension of the knee beyond 135 degrees, the Kernig sign is present.

*Neck stiffness* is caused by muscle spasm secondary to irritation of the inflamed meninges and nerve roots in the cervical region. Stretching of irritated *distal* spinal cord and nerve roots causes Kernig's sign, and stretching of the *proximal* nerve roots causes Brudzinski's sign.

Stretching of the neural elements of the *entire spinal cord* is a more sensitive test. This is achieved by flexing the neck passively (by the examiner), with the child sitting and the knees in full extension (**Figure 11-15**). In addition to the classic tripod sign, one can see clearly that the child cannot flex the neck, and the angle between the plane of the nape of the neck and the vertical is less than 45 degrees.

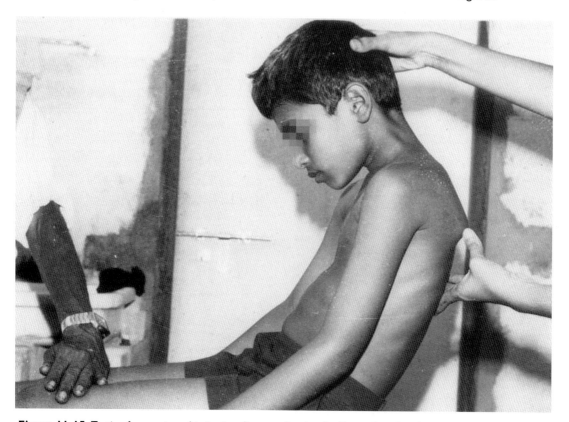

**Figure 11-15.** Testing for meningeal irritation. See text for details. (Reproduced with permission from Archives of Diseases in Childhood. 1993; 68: 215-18)

## Some Primitive Reflexes

These are present in children with congenital or acquired cortical diseases such as head trauma and encephalitis. They indicate frontal lobe lesions. These are the *palmomental reflex* and the *glabellar reflex* described on pages 268 & 285.

Grasp reflex is elicited by the clinician placing his or her index and middle fingers on the thenar eminence of the child's hand and gently taking it between the thumb and index finger. A positive response is when the child's fingers involuntarily grasp your fingers and the grip tightens as you try to withdraw (frontal lobe release).

# NEURODEVELOPMENTAL REFLEXES

All infants go through stages of neurodevelopmental integration before assuming a standing posture and beginning to walk. These include various body righting and balancing (automatic) reflexes that help to keep the balance while walking. Some of these reflexes are mediated at the spinal cord level, some at the brain stem level, some at the midbrain level, and some at the cortical level (**Table 11-13**). They evolve from the caudal toward the cephalic level of control. (For a more detailed description, see Fiorentino's "Testing Methods for Evaluating CNS Development" published in 1979.)

## Table 11-13. Developmental Reflexes

|         | Reflex | Mediated at |
|---------|--------|-------------|
| Group A | Flexor withdrawal | Spinal cord level |
|         | Extensor thrust | |
|         | Crossed extensor | |
| Group B | Asymmetric tonic neck | Brain stem level |
|         | Symmetric tonic neck | |
|         | Positive supporting | |
|         | Tonic labyrinthine | |
| Group C | Neck correcting body | Midbrain |
|         | Labyrinthine right reflex | |
|         | Optical righting reflex | |
| Group D | Various balancing reflexes | Cortical/cerebellar |
| Group E | Automatic movement reactions | Stretch receptors of the neck |
|         | Moro reflex | |
| Group F | Parachute reflex | Semicircular canals |
|         | Landau reflex | |

# Timing of Developmental Reflexes

In the natural course of development, *spinal cord reflexes* are present immediately after birth and disappear within one to two months. *Brain stem* reflexes are primitive reflexes that start appearing at about the second week of life and should disappear by the sixth month. As long as spinal cord reflexes and brain stem reflexes are dominant, children cannot walk and cannot even crawl. (In essence, they will be lying supine in various positions.) Persistence of these reflexes after this time indicates brain damage *in utero* or in early life. These reflexes reappear in children who, after normal progression, regressed to a more primitive level after a cerebral insult, such as a head injury, meningitis, or anoxia (drowning).

Most *midbrain reflexes* start appearing at about the fourth month of age but become suppressed by cortical influences after two years. Persistence of midbrain reflexes after two and a half years of age is abnormal. These abnormalities are seen in children with cerebral palsy and after cerebral insult. Children with dominant midbrain reflexes after two and a half years of age can crawl easily, but walking may be difficult without protective devices. Children who do not develop the midbrain reflexes may not be able to walk at all, except on all fours.

Absence of *cortical reflexes* beyond two and a half years is abnormal, though this is not incompatible with walking. These are balancing reflexes, and they contribute to safety in walking.

# Spinal Cord Reflexes

## Flexor Withdrawal

*How to elicit?* Pinch the sole of the foot (without tickling) with the child supine, the head in neutral position, and legs in extension.

*What is the anticipated response?* Dorsiflexion of the foot with uncontrolled flexion at the knee is a positive response. The avoidance response of older normal children is considered a negative reaction.

*What is normal?* Flexion response described above until two months of age and avoidance response in older children is normal.

*What is abnormal?* Persistence or reappearance of slow uncontrolled flexion response after two months of age is abnormal.

## Extensor Thrust

*How to elicit?* With the child supine, stimulate the sole of the foot *of the flexed leg* by pinching the sole.

What is the anticipated response? A nondeliberate extension with adduction is considered a positive reaction.

*What is normal?* The above response is normal up to two months of age.

*What is abnormal?* The above response persisting or recurring after two months of age is abnormal.

## Crossed Extensor

*How to elicit?* With the child supine and both lower limbs in extension, stroke the plantar aspect of the foot.

*What is the anticipated response?* Flexion followed by extension and adduction of the opposite lower limb is a positive response.

*What is normal?* The response described above is normal until two months of age.

*What is abnormal?* Persistence of the response described above after two months of age is abnormal.

## Brain Stem Reflexes

### Asymmetric Tonic Neck Reflex

*How to elicit?* With the child in the supine position and the arms and legs extended, turn the head to one side.

*What is the anticipated response?* Extension and stiffening of arms and legs on the side toward which the face is turned, together with flexion of the arms and legs of the opposite side (occiput side), is considered a positive response (**Figure 11-16**).

*What is normal?* This reflex is seen normally up to four to six months of age.

*What is abnormal?* Persistence of this reflex after six months of age is abnormal.

### Symmetric Tonic Neck Reflex

*How to elicit?* Sit in a chair and support the child prone on your thighs. Passively flex the neck. After observing the response of the arms and legs to passive flexion, extend the neck.

*What is the anticipated response?* When the neck is flexed, the arms flex and legs extend. When the neck is extended, the arms extend and legs flex. These are considered a positive response.

*What is normal?* A positive response as described above is normal until four to six months of age.

*What is abnormal?* Response as described above after six months of age is abnormal.

### Positive Supporting Reaction

*How to elicit?* Pick up the child by the axilla and bounce several times so that the feet touch the floor.

*What is the anticipated response?* When the feet are in contact with the floor, hold the child in a vertical position. Look for increase of adductor and extensor tone in the legs and ability of the child to bear weight. Look for sustained position in plantar flexion with adduction. This is a positive response.

*What is normal?* Positive supporting reaction to bear weight normally is present at birth and disappears by two or three months.

*What is abnormal?* Sustained plantar flexion with increased tone of adductors after four months of age is abnormal. Positive supportive reaction reappears at six months of age in preparation for walking, but not with significant adduction or plantar flexion.

### Tonic Labyrinthine Reflex

*How to elicit?* Examine the tone of the flexors and extensors of the arms and legs with the child in a prone and supine position and the head in midline.

*What is the anticipated response?* A positive response occurs when flexor tone dominates when the child is prone and extensor tone dominates when the child is supine.

*What is normal?* Response as described above until four months of age is normal.

*What is abnormal?* Response as described above after four months of age is abnormal.

## Midbrain Reflexes

### *Neck on Body Correcting Reflex*

*How to elicit?* With the child lying supine, turn the head toward one side.

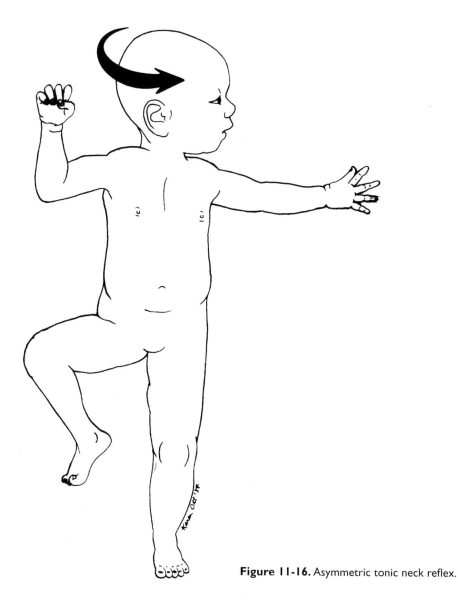

**Figure 11-16.** Asymmetric tonic neck reflex.

*What is the anticipated response?* Positive neck righting reaction is rotation of the body nonsegmentally in the same direction.

*What is normal?* This nonsegmental reflex is present at birth and disappears by two months of age. The mature segmental rotation of the thorax followed by the pelvis appears after two months.

*What is abnormal?* Presence of nonsegmental response after six months, or the absence of segmental response after six months of age is abnormal.

## *Labyrinthine Righting Reflexes*

*How to elicit?* With the child blindfolded, support him or her in space in a prone position. Repeat the same test by suspending the child in space in a supine position. Next, hold the child by the pelvis in the vertical position and tilt the body to one side and then the other.

*What is the anticipated response?* Positive responses for the four positions are as follows: With the child prone or supine, the head rises to a normal position with the face vertical and the mouth horizontal. With the child in a vertical position, the head tilts back to the neutral position with the face vertical and the mouth horizontal.

*What is normal?* Positive response to prone position is normal after two months of age throughout life. Positive responses to other positions come on normally at about six to nine months of age. They are suppressed by cortical influences after two and a half years of age.

*What is abnormal?* Absence of the positive response after two months of age in the prone position, and absence of the response to other positions between six months and two and a half years of age are abnormal.

## *Optical Righting Reflex*

The test is performed the same way as described for the labyrinthine righting reflex and is interpreted the same way, but the labyrinthine righting reflex is tested with the eyes closed and the optical righting reflex with the eyes open.

## Cerebral Cortical and Cerebellar Reflexes

These reflexes test the balancing ability of the child and are influenced by the cerebral cortex and cerebellum.

*How to elicit?* With the child sitting or standing, first push him or her to one side (taking care that the child does not fall to the opposite side in the event these reflexes are not developed); then repeat on the other side.

*What is the anticipated response?* If the child is sitting, the arm on the side toward which he or she is falling extends, the fingers open, and the neck corrects so that the head is brought to neutral position. If the child is standing, the same response is seen. In addition, the knee on the side toward which the child is falling flexes, the opposite knee extends and tries to cross over toward the direction of the momentum.

Now, with the child standing and held by the axilla, gently push him or her forward and then backward. If the child is pushed forward, the neck extends to bring the head to neutral and the child takes forward steps to catch up with gravity; if the child is pushed back, the neck flexes and the child takes backward steps.

*What is normal?* Positive responses as described above for balance in the sitting position should appear by six to eight months of age. Reflexes for balance in the standing position should appear by 12 to 15 months of age.

*What is abnormal?* Absence of balancing reflexes for sitting after eight months of age, and absence of balancing reflexes for standing after 15 months of age are abnormal; asymmetric responses are also abnormal.

## Automatic Movement Reactions

### Moro Reflex

How to elicit? Produce a sudden noise away from the visual field of the infant. Another method is to support the child in a semi-sitting position. Suddenly drop the upper part of the body and catch it at once so that the infant's body is not dropped all the way to the table.

*What is the anticipated response?* Sudden extension and abduction at the shoulder is quickly followed by flexion at the shoulder and the elbow in a movement like an embrace. The fingers open during this reflex.

*What is normal?* Presence of this response is normal in newborns and infants up to four months of age.

*What is abnormal?* Persistence of this response after four months of age is abnormal.

### Parachute Response

How to elicit? Hold the child by the waist and tilt him or her forward as dropping on the face.

*What is the anticipated response?* Extension and abduction of the upper limbs with extension of the fingers as if to break a fall occurs.

*What is normal?* This response should be present in most normal infants after six to eight months of age.

*What is abnormal?* The absence of this response after eight months is abnormal; unilateral response is abnormal.

### Landau Reflex

How to elicit? Suspend the child in space (carefully) in a prone position by supporting the thorax.

*What is the anticipated response?* The neck spontaneously extends with some stiffening of the back and lower extremities.

*What is normal?* Presence of this reflex between the ages of six months and two and a half years is normal.

*What is abnormal?* Failure of this reflex to develop by 10 to 12 months is abnormal.

## Significance and Uses of Neurodevelopmental Reflexes in Pediatric Practice

1. Abnormal responses in these categories suggest brain damage (e.g., cerebral palsy, post-head injury, and post-meningitis).

2. Persistence of reflexes mediated by the brain stem and spinal cord after four to six months of age signifies brain damage.

3. Delay in the appearance of reflexes mediated at the midbrain and cortical level after the appropriate age signifies brain damage.

4. Asymmetric responses (such as lack of parachute response on one side and unilateral Moro) signify hemiplegia.

5. These reflexes may mature at a slower pace in children with cerebral palsy (e.g., Landau reflex may not appear until age two years).

6. Older children with head injury and infectious or anoxic brain insult may lose their advanced reflexes and regress to reflexes at a primitive level. They then go through the various stages during the recovery period.

These reflexes also are useful as indicators of prognosis for walking in children with cerebral palsy. For example, strong asymmetric tonic reflex, crossed-extensor reflex, and Moro together with absence of parachute response, indicate poor prognosis for walking.

These reflexes can be used in physical therapy for the treatment of cerebral palsy and acquired brain damage. For example, rolling an infant over a large beach ball will elicit a parachute response, if present. This will help open a spastic adducted thumb, since opening of the palm and extension of fingers is part of this response. The child with severe persistent tonic labyrinthine reflex may get equinus deformity if he or she is allowed to remain in the supine position most of the day. This deformity occurs because extensor tone is increased in a supine position in the presence of active tonic labyrinthine reflex. If this child is treated in a prone position most of the day, flexor tone is accentuated as part of the same reflex.

# ASSOCIATED MOVEMENTS

*(Also see page 241 for newer definitions of reduced selective motor control.)*

A normal child freely swings his or her arms during walking. In the presence of pyramidal or extrapyramidal disease, this movement is lost. A paralyzed upper arm hangs loosely by the side of the body and does not move during walking.

When a child attempts rapid, repetitive activity with one hand or foot, there may be spontaneous movement of the corresponding part of the opposite limb until five to six years of age. This associated movement is called the "mirror movement." After the age of five years, mirror movements indicate cerebral disease, such as cerebral palsy.

## Autonomic Nervous System and Reflexes

Symptoms associated with disorders of the autonomic nervous system include the following: dizziness and syncope (due to hypotension or arrythmia), postural hypotension, cold extremities due to vasomotor instability, recurrent vomiting, bloating and constipation due to dysmotility of the gastrointestinal tract, hypo- or hyperhydrosis (sudomotor), and loss of bladder control (after five years of age).

To assess the autonomic nervous system, examine the heart rate, heart rhythm, blood pressure, and orthostasis. Also, examine the skin and sphincters. The two most important points to observe in the *skin* are 1) vasomotor instability, color changes, and allodynia, as in reflex sympathetic (neurovascular) dystrophy and 2) lack of sweating, as in Horner syndrome.

The *anal sphincter* is examined to see if the opening is normal and contracted or patulous. A rectal examination will tell about sphincter tone. Anocutaneous reflex is tested by pricking the perianal skin with a sterile sharp object. A normal response is a brisk contraction of the external sphincter.

Since the *bladder* cannot be adequately examined clinically, obtain a good history. History of dribbling, lack of awareness of full bladder, lack of desire to void, and inability to hold urine suggests neurogenic bladder.

In the presence of bowel and bladder sphincter problems, examine the motor and sensory systems carefully to rule out lesions of the spinal cord (such as myelomeningocele or lipomeningocele).

## Minimal Neuromotor Dysfunctions

In the follow-up examination of premature babies, subtle neurological abnormalities may be found even though routine neurological examination is normal. Touwen's system of examination groups these abnormalities under four headings: posture and muscle tone, reflexes, balance and coordination, and facial and eye movements. If abnormalities are detected in one or two of these areas, the child is said to have mild minimal neuromotor dysfunction (MND-1), and if there are abnormalities in two or more systems, the child is said to have moderate minimal neuromotor dysfunction (MND-2) (k value of > 0.7). The details of this examination are as follows:

1. Posture is assessed during lying, sitting, standing, and walking. The tone of the muscle is assessed at the ankle. Consistent mild deviation in muscle tone and/or consistent mild deviation in posture are considered positive.
2. Abnormal intensity or asymmetry of response in the knee AND ankle reflexes.
3. Presence of age-inadequate performance of one of the following tests for coordination and balance: finger-nose test, diadochokinesis, Romberg test, standing on one leg, and walking along a straight line.
4. Presence of associated movements of the face and eye muscles during performance of diadochokinesis or finger apposition test.

# BIBLIOGRAPHY

American Academy of Pediatrics, Section on Ophthalmology. Red reflex examination in neonates, infants and children. Pediatrics. 2008;122(6):1401-4.

Axelrod FB, Chelimsky GG, Weese-Mayer DE. Pediatric autonomic disorders. Pediatrics. 2006;118(1):309-21.

Baird HW, Gordon EC, Oppe TE. Neurological Evaluation of Infants and Children. In: Clinics in Developmental Medicine, nos. 84/85. London: William Heinemann Medical Books; 1983.

Chusid JG. Correlative Neuroanatomy and Functional Neurology. 17th ed. Los Altos: Lange Medical Publications; 1979.

Fily A, Truffert P, Ego A, Depoortere MH, Haquin C, Pierrat V. Neurological assessment at five years of age in infants born preterm. Acta Paediatr. 2003;92(12):1433-7.

Fiorentino MR. Reflex Testing Methods for Evaluating CNS Development. 2nd ed. Springfield (Il): Charles C. Thomas; 1979.

Plum F, Posner JB. The Diagnosis of Stupor and Coma. 3rd ed. Philadelphia: FA Davis Co; 1980.

Sanger TD, Chen D, Delgado MR, Gaebler-Spira D, Hallett M, Mink JW, Taskforce on Childhood Motor Disorders. Definition and classification of negative motor signs in childhood. Pediatrics. 2006;118(5):2159-67.

Teasdale G, Jennett B. Assessment of coma and impaired consciousness. A practical scale. Lancet. 1974;2(7872):81-4.

Tongue AC, Cibis GW. Bruckner test. Ophthalmology. 1981;88:1041-4.

Vincent J, Thomas K, Matthew O. An improved clinical method for detecting meningeal irritation. Arch Dis Child. 1993;68(2):215-18.

# APPENDIX 11-1. EYE EXAMINATION GUIDELINES*

Eye Examination Guidelines*

## Ages 3-5 Years

| Function | Recommended Tests | Referral Criteria | Comments |
|---|---|---|---|
| Distance visual acuity | Snellen letters<br>Snellen numbers<br>Tumbling E<br>HOTV<br>Picture tests -Allen figures<br>-LEA symbols | 1. 20-ft line with either eye tested at 10 ft monocularly (ie, less than 10/20 or 20/40)<br>or<br>2. eyes, even within the passing range (ie, 10/12.5 and 10/20 or 20/25 and 20/40) | 1. Tests are listed in decreasing order of cognitive difficulty; the highest test that the child is capable of performing should be used; in general, the tumbling E or the HOTV test should be used for children 3-5 years of age and Snellen letters or numbers for children 6 years and older.<br>2. Testing distance of 10 ft is recommended for all visual acuity tests.<br>3. A line of figures is preferred over single figures.<br>4. The nontested eye should be covered by an occluder held by the examiner or by an adhesive ocduder patch applied to eye; the examiner must ensure that it is not possible to peek with the nontested eye. |
| Ocular alignment | Cross cover test at 10 ft (3 m)<br>Random dot E stereo test at 40cm | Any eye movement<br>Fewer than 4 of 6 correct | Child must be fixing on a target while cross cover test is performed. |
|  | Simultaneous red reflex test (Bruckner test) | Any asymmetry of pupil color, size, brightness | Direct ophthalmoscope used to view both red reflexes simultaneously in a darkened room from 2 to 3 feet away; detects asymmetric refractive errors as well. |
| Ocular media clarity (cateracts. tumors. etc) | Red reflex | White pupil, dark spots, absent reflex | Direct ophthalmoscope, darkened room. View eyes separately at 12 to 18 inches; white reflex indicates possible retinoblastoma. |

## 6 years and older

| Function | Recommended Tests | Referral Criteria | Comments |
|---|---|---|---|
| Distance visual acuity | Snellen letters<br>Snellen numbers<br>Tumbling E<br>HOTV<br>Picture tests -Allen figures -LEA symbols | 1. 15-ft line with either eye tested at 10 ft monocularly (ie, less than 10/15 or 20/30)<br>or<br>2. eyes, even within the passing range (ie, 10/10 and 10/15 or 20/20 and 20/30) | 1. Tests are listed in decreasing order of cognitive difficulty; the highest test that the child is capable of performing should be used; in general, the tumbling E or the HOTV test should be used for children 3-5 years of age and Snellen letters or numbers for children 6 years and older.<br>2. Testing distance of 10 ft is recommended for all visual acuity tests.<br>3. A line of figures is preferred over single figures.<br>4. The nontested eye should be covered by an occluder held by the examiner or by an adhesive occluder patch applied to eye; the examiner must ensure that it is not possible to peek with the nontested eye. |
| Ocular alignment | Cross cover test at 10 ft (3 m)<br>Random dot E stereo test at 40 cm | Any eye movement<br>Fewer than 4 of 6 correct | Child must be fixing on a target while cross cover test is performed. |
|  | Simultaneous red reflex test (Bruckner test) | Any asymmetry of pupil color, size, brightness | Direct ophthalmoscope used to view both red reflexes simultaneously in a darkened room from 2-3 feet away; detects asymmetric refractive errors as well. |
| Ocular media clarity (cateracts. tumors. etc) | Red reflex | White pupil, dark spots, absent reflex | Direct ophthalmoscope, darkened room. View eyes separately at 12 to 18 inches; white reflex indicates possible retinoblastoma. |

* Assessing visual acuity (vision screening) represents one of the most sensitive techniques for the detection of eye abnormalities in children. The American Academy of Pediatrics Section on Ophthalmology, in cooperation with the American Association for Pediatric Ophthalmology and Strabismus and the American Academy of Ophthalmology, has developed these guidelines to be used by physicians, nurses, educational institutions, public health departments, and other professionals who perform vision evaluation services.

Source: American Academy of Pediatrics, Section on Ophthalmology. Red reflex Examination in Neonates, Infants and Children. Pediatrics. 2008;122(6):1401-4. And **Committee on Practice and Ambulatory Medicine, Section on Ophthalmology, American Association of Certified Orthoptists, American Association for Pediatric Ophthalmology and Strabismus and American Academy of Ophthalmology.** Eye examination in Infants, Children, and Young Adults by Pediatricians. Pediatrics. 2003;111(4) 902-7.

# SECTION IV

# SPECIAL EXAMINATIONS

Chapter 12

# SPECIAL EXAMINATIONS

# A. PHYSICAL DIAGNOSIS OF THE NEWBORN

*By Stephen Pearlman, M.D.*

## INTRODUCTION

The newborn physical examination presents some unique challenges and differs in several aspects from the examination of the older child. It is extremely important to be thorough and methodical to ensure that nothing important is missed on your examination. Therefore, completely undress the infant and use a standard routine of examination. For the sake of simplicity, this chapter is written as if the examination of a newborn proceeds from head to toe, but in reality, the examination should proceed from the least to the most invasive parts.

It is helpful to keep the infant calm during the critical part of the examination. A proper environment is conducive to a good physical examination. The room temperature should be comfortable, the light should be adequate, and the external noises should be minimal. Prioritize and perform those aspects of the examination that require the infant to remain quiet, such as the cardiac evaluation, before you carry out the components that may disturb the infant, such as examination of the hip.

The initial assessment should be done within 24 hours of birth. The baby should have follow-up examinations on subsequent days in the hospital, including the day of discharge.

## HISTORY

Paying careful attention to the maternal history will enable you to perform a better physical examination. Questioning the mother about chronic illness is important. If there is a history of maternal diabetes there may be short-term complications, such as hypoglycemia causing jitteriness, but there also is an increased risk of congenital anomalies of the nervous, renal, cardiac, and skeletal systems. Another chronic condition, maternal SLE, may cause heart block.

Taking a good history for infections, particularly sexually transmitted diseases, is useful because some are associated with congenital infections and associated typical physical findings. Herpes infection during pregnancy may cause microcephaly and skin blisters.

Assessment of drugs and medications taken during pregnancy is essential. Some drugs, if taken early in pregnancy, have teratogenic effects leading to birth defects in the fetus. Maternal drug abuse may lead to neurological abnormalities such as irritability, seizures, and altered sensorium due to withdrawal.

Knowledge of the complete history of the pregnancy, labor, and delivery also provides useful clues for the physical examination. For example, advanced maternal age should make one more alert for signs of Trisomy 21. A history of shoulder dystocia makes one check carefully for signs of clavicular fracture and brachial plexus injury. Duration of pregnancy helps the examiner ascertain whether he or she is dealing with a preterm, term, or post-term infant.

# PRENATAL DIAGNOSIS

Evaluations done by high-risk obstetricians provide helpful information that can be used to improve our physical examination. Most pregnant women undergo a diagnostic ultrasound during gestation. Prenatal ultrasound provides information regarding the growth of the fetus and the presence of congenital anomalies. Some particularly complex anomalies may require a higher level of scrutiny by performing magnetic resonance imaging on the fetus.

It is important to ask if the mother has had genetic studies done during pregnancy. These are done based on advanced maternal age or when the findings on prenatal ultrasound suggest a genetic disorder. Results of prenatal evaluation provide useful data to guide your physical examination.

# GESTATIONAL AGE ASSESSMENT

One of the first assessments that should be done on any newborn is gestational age, which is arrived at by a combination of physical attributes and neurologic signs such as the Ballard test (**Figure 12A-1**). Become familiar with one of the methodologies used to evaluate the gestational maturity and perform it on each newborn until you are able to do so in a consistent and reliable way. This is important because better anticipatory care can be provided when the gestational age is known. For example, if a newborn has respiratory distress, it would be useful to know if the infant was born preterm (<37 weeks gestational age). Furthermore, it is valuable to plot the growth measurements of weight, length, and head circumference against the gestational age on standard growth curves (**Figure 12A-2**). This is helpful because it permits the caregiver to classify the newborn as either small (<10th percentile), appropriate (10th-90th percentile), or large (>90th percentile) for gestational age.

There are many factors that determine fetal growth. Poor growth can result from maternal conditions such as hypertension or smoking, uteroplacental insufficiency caused by factors such as chronic abruptio placenta, and fetal conditions such as chromosomal disorders or congenital infections. The determinants of fetal growth are quite complex and one also must consider maternal factors such as pre-gravid weight, weight gain during pregnancy, and if the mother has a job that requires a great deal of standing causing reduced uterine blood flow. Macrosomia or excessive growth is common in infants born to diabetic mothers. An infant who is small for gestational age without any obvious explanation for poor growth requires an evaluation for the presence of congenital infection and chromosomal defects.

**Neuromuscular Maturity**

| | -1 | 0 | 1 | 2 | 3 | 4 | 5 |
|---|---|---|---|---|---|---|---|
| Posture | | | | | | | |
| Square Window (wrist) | >90° | 90° | 60° | 45° | 30° | 0° | |
| Arm Recoil | | 180° | 140°-180° | 110°-140° | 90°-110° | <90° | |
| Popliteal Angle | 180° | 160° | 140° | 120° | 100° | 90° | <90° |
| Scarf Sign | | | | | | | |
| Heel to Ear | | | | | | | |

**Physical Maturity**

| | -1 | 0 | 1 | 2 | 3 | 4 | 5 |
|---|---|---|---|---|---|---|---|
| Skin | sticky friable transparent | gelatinous red, translucent | smooth pink, visible veins | superficial peeling &/or rash. few veins | cracking pale areas rare veins | parchment deep cracking no vessels | leathery cracked wrinkled |
| Lanugo | none | sparse | abundant | thinning | bald areas | mostly bald | |
| Plantar Surface | heel-toe 40-50mm: -1 <40 mm: -2 | >50mm no crease | faint red marks | anterior transverse crease only | creases ant. 2/3 | creases over entire sole | |
| Breast | imperceptible | barely perceptible | flat areola no bud | stippled areola 1-2mm bud | raised areola 3-4mm bud | full areola 5-10mm bud | |
| Eye/Ear | lids fused loosely:-1 tightly:-2 | lids open pinna flat stays folded | sl. curved pinna; soft; slow recoil | well-curved pinna; soft but ready recoil | formed &firm instant recoil | thick cartilage ear stiff | |
| Genitals male | scrotum flat, smooth | scrotum empty faint rugae | testes in upper canal rare rugae | testes descending few rugae | testes down good rugae | testes pendulous deep rugae | |
| Genitals female | clitoris prominent labia flat | prominent clitoris small labia minora | prominent clitoris enlarging minora | majora & minora equally prominent | majora large minora small | majora cover clitoris & minora | |

**Maturity Rating**

| score | weeks |
|---|---|
| -10 | 20 |
| -5 | 22 |
| 0 | 24 |
| 5 | 26 |
| 10 | 28 |
| 15 | 30 |
| 20 | 32 |
| 25 | 34 |
| 30 | 36 |
| 35 | 38 |
| 40 | 40 |
| 45 | 42 |
| 50 | 44 |

**Figure 12A-1**. Maturational assessment of gestational age.
Reprinted from: Ballard JL, Khowy JC, Wedig K, Wang L, Eilers-Walsman BL, Lipp R. New Ballard Score, expanded to include extremely premature infants. J Pediatr. 1991;119(3):417-23. With permission from Elsevier.

# PHYSICAL EXAMINATION

## Newborn

Before examining any newborn baby, make certain that you have cleaned your hands thoroughly. Many hospitals also require the use of gloves when handling babies.

### General Appearance

Using your observations to obtain an initial impression of the well being of the neonate will be your guide as you examine specific body parts and systems. Look for details of the overall appearance of the infant.

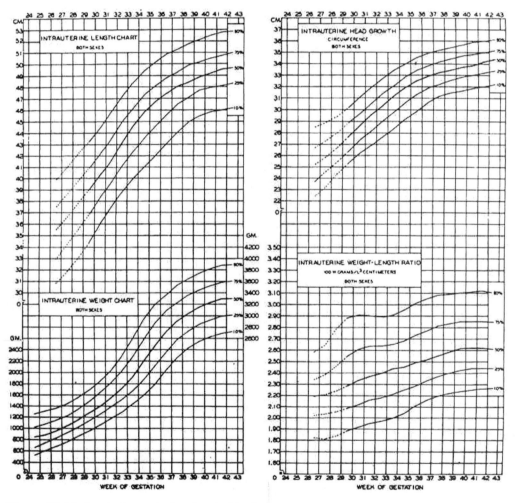

**Figure 12-A2.** Standard growth chart for the Newborn.
Reprinted from Battaglia FC, Lubchenco LO. A practical classification of newborn infants by weight and gestational age. J Pediatr. 1967; 71(2):159-63. With permission from Elsevier.

Are there any signs of distress such as grunting (forced expiration against a partially closed glottis), flaring of the alae nasi, or use of the accessory muscles of respiration causing retractions? Is the baby pink? Answering these questions will give one a sense of wellness of the baby's cardiorespiratory system.

Is the baby asleep, alert, or hyperalert? What kind of posture does the infant have lying quietly in the bed and what is the quality of the cry? These observations give an overview of the functionality of the newborn's nervous system.

If your assessment begins in the delivery room, the Apgar score should be performed. This simple system quantifies the well being of the newborn at birth. **Table 12A-1** illustrates the five components of the score, each being assigned a value of 0 or 2. The Apgar score should be assigned at one and five minutes. In cases where it remains <7 at five minutes, it should be assigned every five minutes until it is >7. In cases where the newborn requires resuscitation, the Neonatal Resuscitation Program emphasizes that only color, heart rate, and breathing should be assessed until the infant has been stabilized.

## Head

The normal shape of the head is oval. Moulding of the head due to intrauterine positioning or vaginal delivery results in a misshapen head which should resolve in a few days. If the head is permanently misshapen, consider the possibility of craniosynostosis. This diagnosis is made by obtaining skull radiographs.

Bleeding into various compartments under the scalp leads to swelling that is or will be both visible and easily palpable. **Figure 12A-3** demonstrates the potential spaces of the scalp where bleeding may occur. Caput succedaneum (edema of the scalp skin) is very common after vaginal birth. Its location corresponds to the presenting part, most often the occiput, and crosses the suture lines. Cephalohematoma most often is seen in one parietal region and does not cross the suture line because the blood is subperiosteal. As opposed to caput which resolves in a day or two, a cephalohematoma may calcify along the periphery, giving you the impression of a depressed skull fracture. These resolve over days to weeks but the calcifications may persist for months. Subgaleal hemorrhage, which is bleeding under the aponeurosis, is far less common. This hemorrhage crosses suture lines but is much more firm than the caput. The subgaleal space is large and hemorrhage may be associated with other signs of blood loss (pallor, tachycardia, etc.).

## Table 12A-1. Apgar Score

| Sign | 0 | 1 | 2 |
| --- | --- | --- | --- |
| Color | Blue or pale | Acrocyanotic | Completely pink |
| Heart Rate | Absent | Less than 100/min | Greater than 100/min |
| Reflex irritability | No response | Grimace | Cry or active withdrawal |
| Muscle Tone | Limp | Some flexion | Active motion |
| Respiratory | Absent | Weak cry; hypoventilation | Good strong cry |

*Source: Apgar V. A proposal for a new method of evaluation of the newborn infant. Curr Res Anesth Analg 1953; 32 (4): 260-267.*

Measure the head circumference and plot on a standard graph of newborn measurements (normal range is 30.5 cm to 35.5 cm in term infants). A small head (microcephaly) suggests an early neonatal insult such as congenital infection. A large head (megacephaly, macrocephaly) may be associated with congenital hydrocephalus. Transillumination may be helpful in diagnosing hydrocephalus in babies with an increased head size before obtaining a neuroimaging study.

Begin to gently palpate the cranium, feeling the fontanels and suture lines (see **Figure 6-1**, page 109). If the baby is resting quietly, the fontanels should be open and flat. When a baby is crying, the fontanels may be tense and slightly bulging. The anterior fontanel is diamond shaped and measures 4 to 6 cm at its largest diameter. The posterior fontanel is triangular and is the size of a fingertip. Large fontanels may be a normal variant but could suggest a skeletal dysplasia, chromosomal anomaly, hypothyroidism, or hydrocephalus. Small fontanels may be normal or a feature of hyperthyroidism, craniosynostosis, or microcephaly. A small anterior third fontanel is found in babies with Down syndrome or congenital hypothyroidism.

Defects of the skin overlying the skull called "cutis aplasia" may be an isolated finding or may be associated with syndromes such as Trisomy 13.

Palpation of the head also may reveal craniotabes or softening of the skull. These soft depressible areas give you the impression of a "ping pong ball" when pushing gently on the skull. This may be a normal variant or may be seen in osteogenesis imperfecta and congenital syphilis.

It is rarely necessary to auscultate the anterior fontanel unless an arteriovenous malformation, which may be associated with a bruit, is suspected.

Newborns have a variable amount of hair at birth. The color should be fairly uniform and concordant with the baby's race. Blonde hair in a dark skinned baby may represent albinism. A white forelock may be associated with deafness and mental retardation (Waardenburg's syndrome).

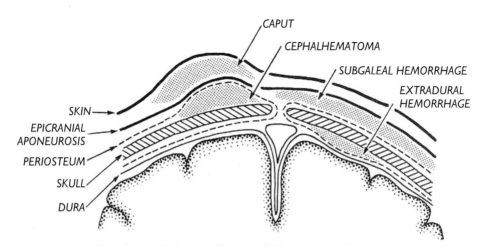

**Figure 12A-3.** Sites of extracranial and extradural hemorrhages in the newborn.
From Volpe JJ. In: Neurology of the Newborn. 4th ed. Philadelphia: WB Saunders; 2001, p. 814. Copyright Elsevier.

## Eyes

Inspect the eyes for their position, size, and shape. Lateral upward slanting eyes with epicanthic folds are seen in Down syndrome. Downward slanting eyes are seen in Treacher-Collins syndrome. Absence of the eyes (anophthalmia) and cyclops are rare but devastating conditions. Decreased intercanthal distance may be seen in fetal alcohol syndrome and other disorders of midbrain development, such as holoprosencephaly.

Occasionally, the baby will have his or her eyes open. If not, rocking the baby gently from side to side or holding the baby in a vertical upright position may cause him or her to open the eyes. If not, you may need to employ an aide to retract the lids. This is more easily done when the baby is relaxed, which may be accomplished by having the baby suck on a pacifier or your gloved finger. Inspect the eyes for subconjunctival hemorrhage which may have resulted during the delivery process. These hemorrhages resolve spontaneously but may alarm parents. Injection of the conjunctiva associated with a discharge is seen in conjunctivitis; this is rare in the immediate newborn period. The sclerae are generally white. A blue sclera is indicative of osteogenesis imperfecta.

Also inspect the iris for color, continuity, and papillary margins. Parents frequently will ask about the baby's eye color which may change as the baby matures. Small white spots in the periphery of the iris called "Brushfield spots" are seen in Down syndrome, although these may be a normal variant. Coloboma (black hole or a defect in the continuity) of the iris may be seen in cat eye syndrome or CHARGE association.

Examination of the newborn's eyes with an ophthalmoscope can be challenging. Look for the red reflex (see pages 126, 256 & 299). Holding the ophthalmoscope six to 12 inches from the baby, look for the orange-red reflection of the light. Its absence suggests clouding of the cornea as seen in congenital cataracts and glaucoma. Retinoblastoma, a rare tumor of the eye, causes the red reflex to be absent (leukocoria). Whenever the normal red reflex is absent, consult a pediatric ophthalmologist who will examine the baby using an indirect ophthalmoscope following pupillary dilation (also see page 256 in Chapter 11 for vision screening).

Many babies will have some retinal hemorrhages after vaginal delivery. These may be seen more readily by an ophthalmologist after dilation of the pupils. Babies born after traumatic delivery will have numerous flare hemorrhages throughout the retina. Babies with symmetrical intrauterine growth restriction defined as having a birthweight, length, and head circumference of less than the 10th percentile, require examination of the eye following pupillary dilation by a qualified ophthalmologist to look for evidence of chorioretinitis due to congenital infection with cytomegalovirus or toxoplasmosis.

## Ears

Inspect the ears for their presence, size, shape, and orientation. Anotia or absence of the ear can be seen in Treacher-Collins syndrome. Preauricular skin tags or pits may be isolated findings but are common in Goldenhar syndrome. Normal ear position is defined by an imaginary line joining the medial canthi and perpendicular to the vertical axis of the head. If the helix lies below this line, the ears are considered low set as seen in Rubinstein-Taybi or Smith-Lemli-Opitz syndromes. Malformed auricles are seen in Down syndrome and CHARGE association.

Hearing can be grossly assessed by observing if the baby startles in response to a loud noise. Current recommendations from the American Academy of Pediatrics state the need for a universal hearing screen on all newborns prior to discharge from the hospital by employing either the evoked otoacoustic emissions or the auditory brainstem response (see page 269).

Otoscopic evaluation is difficult to perform in the newborn because the external canal is frequently occluded by vernix. It is rarely necessary to perform this procedure.

## Mouth

It is important to visually inspect the mouth and palpate for evidence of a cleft palate. After palpation, it is helpful to leave your finger in the baby's mouth to assess the quality of the suck. A newborn should be able to generate suction between the tongue and palate causing your finger to feel stuck to the palate. This also may help calm the baby, facilitating the rest of the examination.

Cleft palate and lip may be isolated or part of a syndrome. Pierre Robin is a common syndrome which includes a cleft palate, micrognathia, and glossoptosis.

Inspection of the mouth may show a large tongue. Macroglossia, an enlarged tongue, can be seen in Beckwith-Weidemann syndrome, hypothyroidism, and the mucopolysaccharidoses. Ankyloglossia or "tongue tie" occurs when the frenulum under the tongue is short, preventing protrusion of the tongue. Inspection of the mouth also may reveal retention cysts on the alveolar ridge or on the palate, which are called "Epstein's pearls."

Natal teeth (rare presence of teeth at birth) should be removed by a dentist with pediatric experience to prevent the risk of aspiration.

If palpation of the palate is difficult or if there is concern about structures that are more posterior such as the uvula, it may be necessary to examine the throat utilizing a light source and a tongue depressor. This requires a second individual to help keep the baby from moving. A bifid uvula is associated with a submucous cleft palate.

## Nose

Newborns are obligate nose breathers. Any baby who becomes cyanotic or distressed when the mouth is closed should be evaluated for patency of the nares. Choanal atresia is diagnosed by the inability to pass a feeding tube through the nares. Positional deformities of the nose are the result of the birth process. Dislocation of the triangular cartilage can occur, producing a septal deviation.

Nasal flaring is a sign of respiratory distress in the newborn period. Swelling in the medial canthus due to nonfunctional nasolacrimal ducts is common during the first few days of life.

## Neck

Webbed skin in the back of the neck may suggest Turner syndrome. Redundant nuchal skin can be found in syndromes such as Trisomy 21.

Masses can be found in the neck. Thyroglossal duct cysts are found on the midline and branchial cleft cysts are lateral and anterior to the sternocleidomastoid muscle. Goiter may be seen in the newborn and often can be diagnosed by the prenatal ultrasound. Extension of the neck makes these lesions easier to palpate. Cystic hygroma are spongy masses found in the posterior triangle of the neck but they may invade the airway causing respiratory distress.

Palpation over the clavicles for evidence of a mass, crepitus, or tenderness provides evidence of fractures that may occur during delivery.

Prominence of the xiphoid process of the sternum or pectus carinatum is considered a normal variant. Pectus excavatum (depression of the sternum) may be seen in newborns, particularly those with respiratory distress, or may be associated with several syndromes. A tension pneumothorax or paralysis of the hemidiaphragm may lead to chest asymmetry. Retractions caused by the use of accessory muscles of respiration are prevalent in babies with respiratory difficulties. Suprasternal retractions suggest upper airway obstruction. Retractions that are intercostal, subcostal, or substernal likely indicate lower airway disease.

Note the nipples for their location and size. Supernumerary nipples may be associated with syndromes. At birth, the breast bud may be enlarged (up to 3-4 mm) and the nipple may produce a watery white fluid referred to as witch's milk. This is physiologic and is due to the effects of maternal hormones. The nipples become reddened and engorged in neonatal mastitis.

The chest circumference is about 1 to 2 cm smaller than the head circumference and normally measures 28.5 to 33.5cm. The anterior-to-posterior diameter of the chest is increased in the presence of significant air trapping.

Percussion of the newborn chest is not easy to interpret. Dullness may be noted when consolidation or fluid exists. However, a chest radiograph usually helps make the diagnosis of pneumonia, pleural effusion, or congenital malformations. Hence, chest films are an integral part of the physical examination of the newborn chest in any infant with suspected lung pathology.

Auscultate the chest while the infant is calm. Often this can be accomplished by allowing the baby to suck on your finger or a pacifier. Place a warmed stethoscope over both axillae first where the breath sounds are best heard. The normal respiratory rate is 30 to 60 breaths per minute. Many newborns demonstrate periodic breathing with pauses of up to 10 seconds. Tachypnea with rates over 70 are usually an indication of respiratory distress, especially if associated with retractions, nasal flaring, grunting, and cyanosis. Isolated tachypnea suggests cardiac pathology.

Breath sounds should be equal on both sides of the chest. Diminished sounds on one side suggest a pneumothorax, pneumonia, or a space-occupying lesion such as a congenital diaphragmatic hernia. Stridor, most commonly heard during inspiration, suggests upper airway obstruction as in tracheomalacia. In the newborn, it is common to hear sounds transmitted from the upper airway. The best way to distinguish between upper airway and lung sounds is to listen with the stethoscope near the baby's mouth and nares. Rales are discontinuous crackling sounds often heard immediately after delivery. Rarely, bowel sounds may be heard when auscultating the chest (more commonly on the left), which suggests the diagnosis of diaphragmatic hernia. In intubated infants, asymmetry of the breath sounds denotes either a malpositioning of the endotracheal tube in the right mainstem bronchus or a pneumothorax. Transillumination of the chest may help differentiate between the two. When a light source is placed in each axilla, the side with the pneumothorax will light up.

## Cardiovascular System

Inspection should start with noting the baby's color. Central cyanosis is seen when the mucus membranes of the mouth demonstrate a blue or purple coloration together with the rest of the body. Thoroughly evaluate central cyanosis since it indicates either pulmonary or cardiovascular pathology. In the absence of signs of respiratory distress, a cardiac problem is more likely. Polycythemia is another cause of central cyanosis. Peripheral cyanosis (acrocyanosis) is very common in the newborn period and rarely indicates a cardiorespiratory pathology.

A hyperdynamic precordium often is seen shortly after birth; however, if it is persistent, it suggests cardiac pathology.

Palpation of the precordium is important. The normal heart rate is between 100 and 180 beats per minute. The point of maximal impulse (PMI) normally is found in the fourth left interspace just medial to the midclavicular line. A significant change in the location of the PMI suggests situs inversus, dextrocardia, pneumothorax, or masses such as a diaphragmatic hernia. Thrills also may be palpated and often are associated with heart murmurs.

Palpate the peripheral pulses. All the pulses will be diminished in left-sided obstructive lesions, such as aortic stenosis or hypoplastic left heart syndrome. These infants demonstrate shock and their color is more ashen than cyanotic. Stronger pulses in the upper rather than the lower extremities suggest a coarctation of the aorta. Pulses with a bounding quality due to a widened pulse pressure are associated with a patent ductus arteriosus. Follow palpation of the pulses with blood pressure measurements. Newborn blood pressure varies with birth weight and gestational age. Mean systolic values on day 1 range between 40 and 70 mm of mercury and diastolic range between 25 and 40 mm of mercury. These values increase rapidly during the first 5 days of life to 60 to 80 mm systolic and 35 to 50 mm diastolic.(For details on values for the 95th percentile and correlations with birth weight and gestational age, please refer to Determinants of Blood Pressure in infants admitted to Neonatal Intensive care Units: A prospective multicenter study. Zubrow AB, Hulman S, Kushner H, Falkner B. J.Perinatol 1995: 15: 470-479 or one of the Neonatology Handbooks)

The skin also should be palpated to determine the capillary filling time, see page 74, which is normally one to two seconds. This is accomplished by lightly pressing on the skin over the pulp of the fingers to produce blanching and measuring the time needed for the capillary bed to refill. Filling times of more than three seconds indicate hypoperfusion (also see pages 39 & 74).

To perform cardiac auscultation, the neonate should be calm and quiet. Therefore, this part of the examination along with auscultation of the lungs is best done early in the course of evaluation. The cardiac rhythm should be regular with fluctuations that occur with respiration. Premature beats, both atrial and ventricular, are fairly common in the immediate newborn period. These extra beats are generally benign and disappear over the first few days after birth. When it is difficult to distinguish the normal sinus arrhythmia from a truly abnormal rhythm due to premature beats, an electrocardiogram is helpful.

Evaluating the components of heart sounds in the newborn is difficult because of the fast rate. The first heart sound is best heard at the apex, whereas the second heart sound is heard at the left second intercostal space. Using an appropriate size stethoscope, begin auscultation at the apex and then inch along the left and right sternal borders. Splitting of the second heart sound is difficult to appreciate immediately after birth. By 24 to 48 hours, as the pulmonary vascular resistance drops, splitting should be apparent.

Heart murmurs due to turbulent blood flow commonly are heard during the initial examination of the newborn because of the thin chest wall and transitional circulatory physiology. So called "innocent murmurs" are soft, vibratory, and are sometimes intermittent. Pathologic murmurs associated with a thrill are louder, and are heard over a wider area of the chest and beyond the first few days of life. The finding of a murmur should be evaluated in the context of the rest of the examination. In the absence of cyanosis, respiratory distress, blood pressure abnormalities, or rhythm disturbances, it is probably best to observe the baby and perform sequential examinations, avoiding unnecessary testing.

## Abdomen

The abdomen of the newborn is slightly protuberant. Babies are abdominal breathers and hence one should look for synchrony between the movement of the abdominal wall and the respiratory movements of the chest. Excessive distension of the abdomen occurs in intestinal obstruction, ileus, or from enlargement of the abdominal viscera. It is of particular concern if the bowel loops are visible, suggesting obstruction. Conversely, a scaphoid abdomen suggests a decrease in abdominal contents as seen in patients with congenital diaphragmatic hernia. Dilated veins over the abdomen are an indication of venous distension.

Inspect the umbilical cord, which is made of Wharton's jelly, for the presence of one umbilical vein and two umbilical arteries. Infants with a single umbilical artery have an increased risk of renal malformations and vesicoureteral reflux. The umbilical cord stump falls off by approximately two weeks of life. Delayed separation of the umbilical cord may suggest an immunologic defect. Redness, edema, a foul odor, or a discharge from the umbilicus suggests infection (omphalitis).

Bulging of the abdominal wall in the midline may be due to diastasis of the rectus abdominis muscle. External masses such as omphalocele, gastroschisis, or umbilical hernia should be readily apparent to the examiner.

It may be beneficial to auscultate the abdomen before palpation so that the infant remains calm. Bowel sounds should be heard over the abdomen shortly after delivery unless the mother has received medication that affects intestinal motility (e.g., magnesium sulfate).

Palpate using gentle counter pressure between the examining hand and the other hand, which is placed posteriorly. Using this bimanual technique, the liver edge is generally felt 1 to 3.5 cm below the right costal margin; the spleen tip, if palpable, is found no more than 1 cm below the left costal margin and the lower pole of each kidney in the pelvic gutter. When palpating for the liver and spleen, it is helpful to start in the right lower quadrant and gradually ascend until the liver edge, which is sharp and soft, is noted or the rounded edge of the spleen is palpated. The most common intraabdominal masses, such as hydronephrosis from urinary tract obstruction and cystic lesions of the kidney, are usually renal in origin.

It is challenging to assess abdominal tenderness in the newborn. If an inflammatory process such as necrotizing enterocolitis is suspected, it is useful to have the baby suck a pacifier and flex his or her legs to promote relaxation of the abdominal musculature. Note for any resistance to palpation, facial grimacing, and crying.

### Genitourinary System

Examination of the female external genitalia begins with the inspection of the labia. The labia majora are pigmented and reddish in color at the initial examination. In darker skinned babies, the labia are more pigmented than the rest of the skin. They should completely cover the labia minora in the term infant. Gently separate the labia majora to assess patency. There may be clear white mucus in the vagina during the first few days after birth. There may be some blood-tinged discharge starting on the second or third day of life and lasting for several days due to withdrawal from maternal estrogen.

The vagina and urethral orifice also should be inspected. An abnormal membrane covering the vaginal opening may lead to hydrometrocolpos, which may present as a mass in the lower abdomen requiring surgical intervention. Ovarian enlargement due to a cyst or torsion may be detected by prenatal ultrasound. Postnatally, suspected ovarian masses should be assessed by ultrasound since rectal examination of the newborn may result in trauma.

Palpate the inguinal area and labia for evidence of a hernia, although these are uncommon in females. If present the mass should be reducible by gentle compression.

Examination of male genital area begins with inspection of the phallus, which measures about 2.5 to 3.5 cm in length. The prepuce adheres tightly to the glans penis but should be gently retracted to bring the urethral orifice into view. The urethral opening should be at the tip of the penis. When the urethral orifice is located on the glans, ventral surface of the shaft, or in the perineum, it is called "hypospadias." The more severe forms of hypospadias, where the opening is on the shaft or in the perineum, are associated with renal malformations and therefore require radiographic and ultrasound studies of the urogenital tract. Chordee, resulting from incomplete development of the foreskin, leads to a caudal curvature of the penis and is associated with hypospadias.

The scrotum appears pigmented with rugae and a midline raphe. The scrotum in dark skinned babies often is more pigmented than the rest of the skin. The testes are commonly palpable in the scrotum or may be retracted in the inguinal canal. Retractile testes should be able to be gently advanced into the scrotal sac. If not, suspect undescended testes, which will need appropriate follow-up.

Scrotal enlargement suggests either a hydrocele or a direct inguinal hernia. Although hydroceles transilluminate and hernias should be reducible, this distinction may be difficult to assess and scrotal ultrasound may be helpful. Ninety percent of inguinal hernias occur in males. Rarely, newborns are born with a unilateral cyanotic testis indicative of torsion of the testicle. The testis feels hard and rubbery, and unlike torsion seen in older patients, is painless. This is an intrauterine event and thus the testis is generally nonviable. Scrotal ultrasound with Doppler studies to ascertain blood flow is an important diagnostic tool and a pediatric urologist should be consulted.

Functionally, 95% of newborn infants void during the first 24 hours. Delay beyond 24 hours may suggest obstruction of the urinary tract, but this must be considered in the context of any pertinent physical findings (e.g., enlarged kidney) or significant history (e.g., oligohydramnios).

Ambiguous genitalia or intersex is a condition in which the newborn's gender cannot be determined due to masculinization of the female (e.g., clitoromegaly) or feminization of the male (e.g., undescended testes, severe hypospadias). The causes of intersex are complex and there may be associated life-threatening electrolyte disturbances. These cases require involvement of specialists in genetics, pediatric endocrinology, and pediatric urology. Families of these infants also need a great deal of counselling. This condition is a true medical emergency.

The anus should be inspected for patency. Ninety-nine percent of infants pass meconium within the first 48 hours. Imperforate anus may not be obvious on physical examination and radiologic studies may be necessary. Anal or rectal atresias may have an accompanying fistula through which stool may pass. The opening to the fistula can be found in the normal anal location or may open closer to the external genitalia (anterior displacement), or in a female, into the vagina (rectovaginal fistula). The distance from the anus to the scrotum or posterior fourchette of the vagina is divided by the distance from the coccyx to the scrotum or posterior fourchette. A ratio of <0.34 in females or <0.46 in males indicates anterior displacement of the anus. These cases require the expertise of a pediatric surgeon.

## Extremities

Inspection of the limbs begins with observation of their overall size and shape. They should be symmetric in appearance. Unequal size suggests a congenital malformation or growth, such as hemangioma or lymphangiomas. Also, the limbs should move spontaneously and the joints should have full range of motion. Unusual flail limbs and multiple joint contractures should be recognized. Limb reduction deformities can be seen in amniotic band syndrome or as a result of maternal cocaine use. Oligohydramnios or uterine malformations limit total movements, leading to positional deformities at birth. Some may have multiple joint contractures called "arthrogryposis." This also may be due to an underlying neuromuscular disorder. Inspect the hands and feet to ensure that there is a full complement of fingers and toes. Extra digits (polydactyly), fused digits (syndactyly), or curved digits (clinodactyly) may be isolated findings or be seen with other anomalies or syndromes. Extra digits have a familial tendency and are more common in African Americans.

A single transverse palmar crease (simian crease) often is associated with chromosomal disorders or other congenital malformations. It also may be seen in 5% to 10% of normal newborns.

Palpation of the pulses in the extremities is also important and has been discussed previously in the cardiovascular section.

The nails should be well developed at birth. Ingrown nails embedded in the skin at birth are common, but these grow out with time. Nail hypoplasia is seen in genetic disorders affecting ectodermal development.

Screening for developmental dysplasia of the hip (DDH) is a critical component of the newborn exam.

Some laxity of the joint capsule secondary to maternal hormonal effect is common. A dislocatable hip is found in five of 100 live births, but a fixed dislocation is less common. A fixed dislocation is seen more often after breech delivery and in infants with a family history of DDH. Initial screening is based on two maneuvers–Barlow's and Ortolani's (see page 76 for details). Babies with suspected DDH need a dynamic ultrasound of the hip joint performed by a skilled pediatric radiologist. The American Academy of Pediatrics recommends hip ultrasound in certain high risk groups, such as females born in the breech position.

Hyperextensibility of the joints may occur in a single joint or affect multiple joints. This may be due to severe hypotonia or to connective tissue disorder. Genu recurvatum refers to a knee joint that is hyperextensible. This is seen with increased frequency in females, breech deliveries, connective tissue disorders, or chromosomal anomalies. Classic clubfoot (talipes equinovarus) is seen when there is a tight hyperextension and incurvation of the foot (**Figure 12A-4**). It may be an isolated deformity (unilateral or bilateral), or may be associated with other joint or neurologic abnormalities.

## *The Spine*

The spine can be examined while the infant is lying prone or when being supported by your hand in the ventral suspension. The newborn's spine appears straight when the infant is lying prone. Obvious lesions, such as meningocele, cannot be missed. Pigmentation changes or a tuft of hair associated with a sacral dimple raises suspicion of a spina bifida occulta or a tethered spinal cord. Palpate the spine for any masses in the paraspinal areas where soft tissue tumors, such as lipomas, may occur.

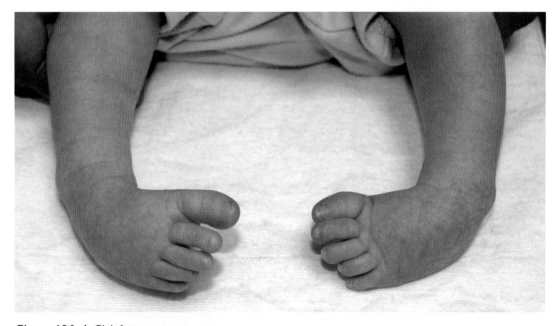

**Figure 12A-4.** Club feet.

Pay particular attention to the sacral area where dimples may occur. Radiographic or ultrasonic studies are warranted when these observations are made.

## The Skin

The newborn's skin should be soft, smooth, and opaque. Post-term infants may have skin that is dry, cracked, and peeling, particularly on the hands and feet. The underlying color should be pink. A dark rosy color suggests polycythemia, whereas pallor is indicative of anemia. Jaundice should not be present on the first examination (<24 hours) unless a pathologic condition exists. Petechiae are common on the presenting part following vaginal delivery. Petechiae that are present elsewhere on the body, or increase on sequential examination, suggest thrombocytopenia or coagulopathy.

Certain rashes are common in the newborn period. Erythema toxicum, with firm yellow-white papules or pustules surrounded by an erythematous flare, is benign and occurs in about half of term newborns (**Figure 12A-5**). Neonatal pustular melanosis with evanescent superficial pustules and hyperpigmented macules is benign as well, and is seen much more frequently in African American infants. Milia, seen as multiple yellow or pearly white 1-mm papules on the nose, chin, cheeks, and forehead, and sucking blisters on the hands and forearm are also common benign findings of newborn skin.

Alteration in pigmentation and a variety of birthmarks are common. Mongolian spots, blue or gray flat lesions over the buttocks and lower back, often are seen in darker skinned neonates. The salmon patches (nevus flammeus) are flat pink lesions commonly seen over the glabella, eyelids, lips, and nuchal area and become more obvious when the baby is cold or crying. They are often symmetric. Port-wine stains, however, are larger, darker, and unilateral. Transient changes in the color of the skin commonly are due to poor autonomic control. Cutis marmorata (marble skin) is a lacy reticulated red or blue pattern over most of the body surface. This is commonly seen in newborns exposed to cold temperatures, but it disappears with advancing age. Cutis marmorata may persist in infants with genetic

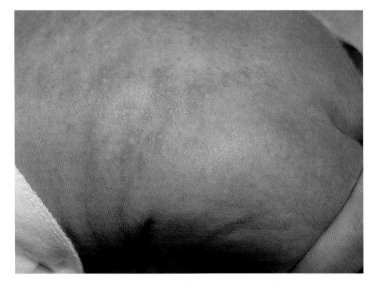

**Figure 12-A5.** Erythema toxicum.

syndromes, such as Down syndrome and Trisomy 18. When an infant is placed on his or her side, if the upper portion becomes pale and the lower half becomes red with a clear demarcation across the body longitudinally, it is called the "harlequin sign." This resolves with a change in the baby's position.

## Neurologic System

Neurologic evaluation is affected easily by the level of alertness. Therefore, it is best to perform this examination prior to feeding time, when the baby is most responsive. Many components of the neurologic examination have been assessed previously as part of the evaluation of other organ systems. General factors such as tone, level of alertness, and vital signs have been noted already, and are a reflection of the baby's neurologic status. Alertness and tone are linked and should be evaluated before too much manipulation has been done. Normal newborns sleep much of the time. It is normal for the baby to arouse easily to environmental stimuli such as light, sound, and touch but fall back to sleep afterwards. Muscle tone is primarily flexor, with the lower extremities being more flexed than the upper extremities. Tone also is assessed with many of the maneuvers done as part of the Ballard assessment of gestational age. Babies should demonstrate symmetric spontaneous movements of all four extremities as well.

Many newborn infants are slightly jittery or demonstrate myoclonic jerks. These may be difficult to distinguish from seizure activity, which can be quite subtle in the newborn period. Evaluate repetitive movements that are not easily stopped by light touch with an electroencephalogram. Associated abnormal eye movement increases the suspicion of seizures.

Assess the cranial nerves as part of the neurologic examination. The olfactory nerve can be assessed by placing a strong smelling substance, such as a peppermint, under the nose and observe for a grimace, startle, or sniffing. The pupillary light reflex should be present in babies born beyond 32 weeks of gestation (also refer to the Bruckner test in Chapter 11, page 256). Extraocular eye movements can be assessed by direct observation. Test for doll's eye reflex by rotating the head from side-to-side and looking for movement of the eyes away from the direction of rotation. Conjugate gaze should be present, but some degree of disconjugate gaze usually is present in the newborn period. The trigeminal nerve is involved in closing the mouth during sucking, and thus evaluating the suck is an essential part of the examination. The facial nerve may be damaged during delivery leading to hemiparesis of the face. This leads to an inability to close the eye on the side of the damage, the mouth being pulled to the contralateral side during crying, and the nasolabial folds being asymmetric. Facial nerve damage must be distinguished from absence of the depressor angularis oris, which manifests as an asymmetric crying facies affecting only the angle of the mouth and not the entire half of the face. The absence of the depressor angular oris has a familial tendency and can be associated with cardiac malformations.

Assessing the quality of the cry is important. A weak cry may indicate neurologic depression or muscular weakness. A high pitched cry suggests neurologic dysfunction or drug withdrawal. The auditory nerve is assessed best by observing if the baby has a startle response to loud noises. The ninth and tenth cranial nerves are involved in swallowing, and the eleventh nerve controls contraction of the sternocleidomastoid muscle. The hypoglossal nerve (twelfth) supplies the tongue and is evaluated by observing the baby's suck-swallow.

The deep tendon reflexes are assessed best when the infant is relaxed. The patellar, Achilles, and brachial reflexes should all be present and symmetrical. The plantar response is not reliable in the newborn since withdrawal to the stimulus may lead to an extended great toe. Checking for ankle clonus is perhaps a better way to check for extrapyramidal signs in the newborn period. However, six or seven beats may be seen even in normal children; therefore, look for sustained clonus.

There are several primitive reflexes that are apparent in the immediate newborn period. These are described in the section on the neurological examination on page 284.

## Preterm Infant

Since the onset of assisted ventilation for preterm infants in the early 1970s, there has been a dramatic improvement in the survival of preterm infants. Therefore, pediatricians should be familiar with the similarities and differences in examination compared with that of term infants.

Infants born before 37 weeks are considered preterm. Gestational age assessment should be part of the initial evaluation (see earlier section on gestational age assessment). Furthermore, infants should be weighed, measured, and have their growth parameters plotted against their estimated gestational age to see if their growth is appropriate. This information assists caregivers in providing better care, and helps focus the physical examination as gestational age and growth status determine to which conditions infants are prone. For example, preterm infants have a high incidence of surfactant deficiency leading to respiratory distress. This section will highlight important differences in the physical findings of the preterm infant compared with the term infant.

## General

Preterm infants have less subcutaneous fat deposition. Their muscle tone and level of activity are diminished compared with that of term infants. Myoclonic jerks are more common. Signs of respiratory distress, such as cyanosis and grunting respirations, often are seen in preterm infants.

## Skin

Very early preterm infants (23-26 weeks of gestation) have skin that is thin and translucent, revealing the blood vessels beneath. The skin also is covered with lanugo on the back, shoulders, scalp, forehead, and extremities. Creases on the plantar surface of the feet are absent. The skin thickens, lanugo decreases, and creases gradually form as gestation progresses. These physical characteristics are part of the gestational age assessment.

## Head

The skull is softer in the preterm newborn. Bruising of the scalp is common but moulding is not because the head is smaller than the birth canal. There is less hair than in the term newborn, making the subcutaneous blood vessels prominent.

## Eyes

The eyelids may be fused in extremely preterm infants (23-24 weeks gestational age). The pupillary light reflex usually is absent before 32 weeks of gestation and red reflex is less prominent due to membranous remnants of the uveal tract.

## Ears

The external auricles of the preterm infant have less cartilage, making them less likely to return to a normal position after being folded. This test is part of the gestational age assessment as well.

## Chest and Lungs

The chest wall of a preterm infant is more compliant than that of a term infant. Use of accessory muscles of respiration (retractions) is common as the infant attempts to compensate for poor diaphragmatic movement. Sternal retractions give the appearance of pectus excavatum. In the presence of surfactant deficiency or other causes of respiratory distress, breath sounds often are diminished. Grunting, or exhaling against a partially closed glottis, is an attempt to maintain the functional residual capacity of the lung.

## Heart

Murmurs are more common in preterm infants because the chest wall is very thin and there are hemodynamic changes that differ from those of the term infant. Preterm infants are at equal risk for having congenital heart disease as term infants. Patent ductus arteriosus in the preterm infant, due to the immaturity of the normal mechanism for ductal closure, often is present in the first week of life. This presents with a systolic heart murmur along the left sternal border, a widened pulse pressure, and bounding peripheral pulses.

## Abdomen

The examination of the preterm abdomen is notable for its decreased musculature, making the underlying organs easily palpable. Necrotizing enterocolitis (NEC) is the most common gastrointestinal abnormality in preterm infants. The physical signs associated with NEC are abdominal distension with or without visible bowel loops, decreased bowel sounds, and abdominal tenderness.

## Genitalia

Preterm males frequently have undescended testes. In preterm females, the labia minora and clitoris are prominent. Physical maturity of the genitalia is part of the gestational age assessment.

## Neuromuscular

Preterm infants have diminished muscle tone and decreased activity. Various aspects of the neuromuscular examination are evaluated as part of the gestational age assessment. Seizure activity may be subtle in preterm infants and difficult to diagnose. Physical findings of seizure include lip smacking, repetitive flexing of extremities or mouth movements, yawning, or autonomic instability. Preterm infants are at increased risk for intraventricular hemorrhage. While often clinically silent, physical findings such as a bulging fontanel, increased head circumference, or alterations of muscle tone or levels of consciousness may be seen.

## Multiple Gestations–Special Considerations

There has been a marked increase in multiple gestations due to advanced maternal age and assisted reproductive technologies. Multiple gestations frequently deliver prematurely and have lower birthweights than their singleton counterparts. Monozygotic twins are at increased risk for twin-to-twin transfusion. If this occurs, one twin is plethoric and the other pallid. Other aspects of the examination are similar to those of singleton infant.

# BIBLIOGRAPHY

Avery ME, Taeusch HW. Avery's Diseases of the Newborn. Philadelphia: WB Saunders; 2005.

Behrman RE, Kliegman RM. Nelson Textbook of Pediatrics. 17th ed. Philadelphia; WB Saunders; 2007.

Fletcher MA. Physical Diagnosis in Neonatology. Philadelphia: Lippincott-Raven Publishers; 1998.

Jones KL. Smith's Recognizable Patterns of Human Malformation. Philadelphia: WB Saunders; 2006.

Spitzer AR. Intensive Care of the Fetus and Neonate. St. Louis: Mosby; 2005.

Thureen PJ, Deacon J, O'Neill P, Hernandez J. Assessment and Care of the Well Newborn. Philadelphia: WB Saunders; 2005.

# B. EXAMINATION OF THE ADOLESCENT

## GENERAL APPROACH

An adolescent may feel ambivalent about being seen in a pediatrician's office for examination, and the parents also may have doubts as to whether their teenager should continue with the pediatrician or move to an internist. The pediatrician has to make sure that the physical set-up of the office and the emotional climate make patients and parents comfortable with their presence in the office.

A "teenage" waiting area that is partially partitioned off from the toys and games in the section used by younger children, and with appropriate reading material, can be helpful. There should be adequate room for privacy. Examining tables of adequate size and availability of stirrups for pelvic examination are important as well.

The patient and parent should determine whether a parent should be present in the examining room. The physician should broach the question of the parent's presence but not resolve it, unless asked to do so. It is important to have a female attendant in the room while examining female adolescents.

The examination is an anxiously anticipated occasion for a teenager. It is essential that the doctor maintain conversation directed to the mechanics and nature of what is being done and explain all the normal and abnormal physical findings using simple language. After the patient has dressed, allot time for discussion, preferably in a relaxed consultation room. Confer with the teenager alone first for review of the examination and an opportunity for a private, confidential exchange. The parent then can be invited to join the discussion.

## HISTORY TAKING

It is best to take the history directly from an adolescent patient. The parent, if present, may feel free to interject or remind. Insight can be gained into the relationship between the two by observing the frequency and appropriateness of the parent's contribution.

Particularly appropriate history to be explored for this age group includes: rate of growth; development of secondary sexual characteristics; onset and regularity of menstruation; weight gain or loss; appetite; sleep patterns; energy levels; peer and family relationships; school and work activities; academic satisfaction; skin blemishes; recurrent sore throat; recurrent chest, abdominal, or head pain; awareness of skipped or rapid heartbeat; extremity pain or swelling; genital discomfort or discharge; and presence of tumors, growths, or "swollen glands."

Much can be learned about the patient's personality, self-image, and relationships during the history taking process. Does he or she seem self-confident? Depressed? Hostile? Articulate? Does he or she look at you or avoid eye contact? Can he or she speak frankly and openly? Does he or she have unexpressed fears regarding his or her own health or of a family member or a friend? If so, why? Careful listening to the patient can provide clues to the possible origin of such symptoms as chest or abdominal pain or headache. Listen to all complaints seriously and evaluate carefully.

A common complaint is that of being "tired," of just not having much energy. Careful history taking may reveal that the patient is in tenth grade, growing rapidly, taking a full academic load, worried about college entrance examinations, playing in the school band, on the basketball team, working at a part-time job some evenings and weekends, trying to do more than the body is capable of doing and not getting adequate duration of sleep.

Provide an opportunity to discuss sexuality, smoking, alcohol, and drug use. This is best done during private, confidential time with the patient. The parent can be included, without breaching confidentiality, if the patient so requests. It is important to establish boundaries of confidentiality and legal issues before taking this part of history.

Specific questionnaires to help with structured interviews are available. One such instrument is called HEADSS. This acronym stands for home, education, activities (employment), drugs/depression, and sexual behavior. The second S is for suicide. This format helps lead gradually from easy issues, such as home and school, to sexuality and suicide. This tool is an excellent screening instrument and touches on major adolescent issues. One other variation of this instrument adds another S to ask the adolescent about his or her strengths (**Table 12B-1**). Yet another variation uses S to remind about safety practices and risk-taking behavior.

Also refer to the screening questionnaire in Chapter 2 (**Table 2-8**).

### Table 12B-1. The HEADSS: Psychosocial Interview for Adolescents

#### Examples of Questions

**Home**: Where do you live? Who else is living at home? Any new people living in the home?

**Education**: What is your favorite subject? What are your grades? Have you changed schools recently? Do you feel safe at school?

**Activities**: What do you do for fun? Are you in any clubs or teams? Do you have a job? If so, what kind? How many hours a week?

**Drugs:** Do you have friends who drink alcohol or take drugs? Have you also tried?

**Sex**: Have you dated anyone? Have you ever had sex? History of pregnancy and abortion? Do you practice protected sex?

**Suicidality**: Have you been so sad that you wanted to hurt yourself? Are you sad now?

**Strength**: What do you think your strengths are? Who are your strong supporters?

*Source: Katzenellenbogen R. HEADSS: The "review of systems" for adolescents. Virtual Mentor. 2005;7(3).*

# PHYSICAL EXAMINATION

Examination of various systems has been described in the previous chapters. In this section, the focus will be on the striking changes of sexual maturation that mark the transition from the prepubertal state to adulthood. The primary characteristics are best described in relation to growth of the breasts in females, the genitals in males, and the development of pubic hair in both. The secondary characteristics relate to growth velocity, body mass and shape, and hair.

## External Sexual Characteristics

The work by Marshall and Tanner in England, first published in the late 1960s, has become the standard to assess sexual maturation of adolescents. They established criteria, which have been modified only slightly over the years, for staging the phases of primary sexual development. **Figure 12B-1** shows the normal stages (so-called Tanner stages) of secondary sexual characteristics for boys and girls. Testicular development in the male and breast enlargement in the female almost always precede the appearance of pubic hair.

Data based on the Third National Health and Nutrition Examination Survey (NHANES III) show that in the USA, the mean age at onset of pubic hair was 9.5 years for African American girls, 10.3 years for Mexican American girls, and 10.5 years for Caucasian American girls. Ages for breast development were 9.5 years, 9.8 years, and 10.3 years for African American, Mexican American, and Caucasian American girls, respectively. Ages for menarche were 12.1 years, 12.2 years, and 12.7 years for African American, Mexican American, and Caucasian American girls, respectively (**Table 12B-2**).

**Table 12B-2. Mean Ages (in Years) at Onset of Pubic Hair, Breast Development, and Menarche for 3 Racial/Ethnic Groups of US Girls: NHANES III, 1988-1994**

| Puberty Milestone | Non-Hispanic White | | Black | | Mexican American | |
|---|---|---|---|---|---|---|
| | Mean Age (95% CI) | Mean Age* | Mean Age* (95% CI) | Mean Age* | Mean Age (95% CI) | Mean Age* |
| Pubic hair† | 10.6 (10.4, 10.9) | 10.5 | 9.5 (9.2, 9.8) | 9.5 | 10.3 (10.1, 10.6) | 10.3 |
| Breast development† | 10.3 (10.0, 10.5) | 10.3 | 9.5 (9.3, 9.8) | 9.5 | 9.7 (9.4, 9.9) | 9.8 |
| Menarche† | 12.6 (12.4, 12.8) | 12.7 | 12.2 (12.0, 12.4) | 12.1 | 12.2 (12.0, 12.5) | 12.2 |
| Menarche‡ | 12.7 (12.5, 12.8) | 12.7 | 12.4 (12.2, 12.5) | 12.3 | 12.5, 12.6) | 12.5 |

CI indicates confidence interval.

*Estimated with application of weights for the examination sample of NHANES III.

†Estimated using probit model for the status quo data of the puberty measurements.

‡Estimated using failure time model for the recalled age at menarche.

*Reprinted from: Wu T, Mendola P, Buck GM. Ethnic differences in the presence of secondary sex characteristics and menarche among US girls: the third national health and nutrition examination survey, 1988-1994. Pediatrics. 2002;110(4):752-7. (With permission from the American Academy of Pediatrics)*

Almost 50% of African American girls aged nine years had breast development compared with 24.5% of Mexican American girls, and 15.8% of Caucasian American girls. Also, the appearance of pubic hair was noted early in African American girls compared with non-Hispanic white and Mexican American girls. The lower end of the normal range for onset of puberty is between seven and eight years for girls and nine years six months for boys.

By 13 years of age, 100% of girls from all ethnic groups had pubic hair and breast development and by age 15 years, 100% of girls from all ethnic groups had attained menarche (**Table 12B-2**).

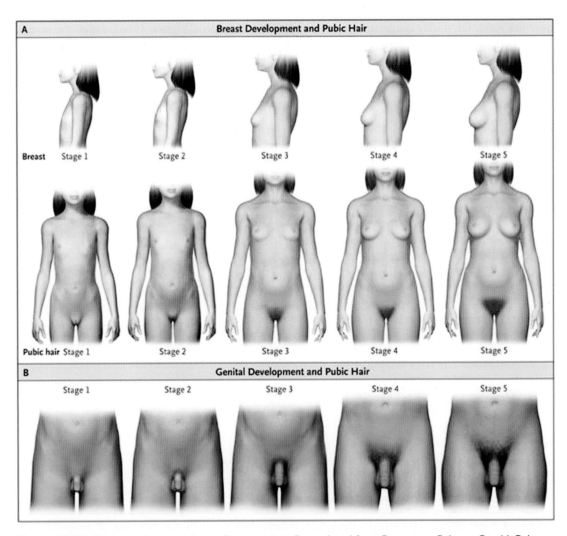

**Figure 12B-1.** Puberty rating according to Tanner stages. Reproduced from Precocious Puberty Carel J-C, Leger J. N Eng J Med 2008; 358 (22): 2366-77.(Copyright 2008.Massachusetts Medical Society. All rights reserved)

Menarche usually occurs at Tanner Stage III or later. Rarely, however, it can occur before the appearance of any significant development of primary characteristics. Primary amenorrhea may be defined as failure of menarche by the 16th birthday. There are regional and geographic variations, and local norms should be used where available and applicable.

Normal development usually proceeds in an orderly fashion, following the approximate sequences suggested in the tables. Marked disparities in the sequences of staging, particularly if accompanied by disturbances in stature or weight, should raise suspicion of endocrinologic abnormalities. As examples, the presence of significant amounts of pubic hair for a length of time in the male, without the expected changes in the genitalia, may be associated with Klinefelter syndrome or with an excessive degree of adrenal androgen secretion. Although breast development usually begins before the appearance of pubic hair in females, patients with stage V breasts and no pubic hair should be evaluated for the possibility of testicular feminization syndrome. On the other hand, a female who has had pubic hair for a considerable length of time and no breast development may have a failure of gonadal hormone secretion.

## Breasts

The areola of the male breast develops in a manner similar to the female up to Tanner Stage II. Small (1 to 3 cm), round, cyst-like breast-buds may be palpable, directly underlying the nipple. They may even be tender. But they are physiologic and disappear later in puberty. An excess of tissue (gynecomastia) is usually physiologic and can be a source of embarrassment.

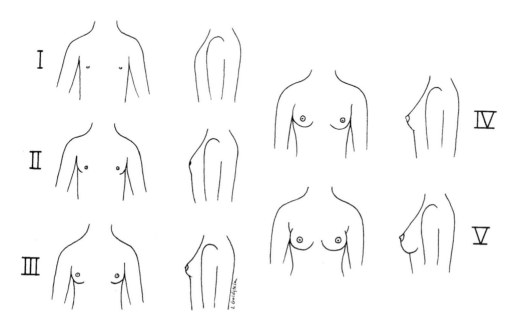

**Figure 12B-2.** Stages of breast development (after Marshall and Tanner)

have completed their growth by the time they have been menstruating for two years and grow only an additional 2 to 5 cm after menarche. For the male, markers for the end point of growth are not as well-defined, though the transition from Tanner Stage IV to Stage V is a good physical diagnostic end point. Physiologically, growth ends with the closure of the skeletal epiphyses.

Girls begin and end their growth spurt at an earlier chronologic age than boys. As a result, at about eighth grade (or about age 13), the average female is taller than the average male, a predicament that may be embarrassing to the tall girl or the short boy. By tenth grade (age 15), most females have just about achieved their final height, while most males are heavily into their growth spurt and often outgrow their female counterparts.

A normal child may shoot up to a higher percentile or lag back at a lower one during the growth spurt. The patient who achieves sexual maturation early may seem quite tall as a 14-year-old-boy or as an 11-year-girl. They may stop growing, however, at these early ages and be passed in physical stature by most of their peers. Any attempt at making a prediction of ultimate height during adolescence must take into consideration the stage of sexual maturation and the skeletal epiphyseal development.

## Body Mass and Shape

The composition of body mass (lean [muscle] versus fat) undergoes change in adolescence. Traditionally, "baby fat" is known to lessen early in puberty in both boys and girls. In girls, it does so until menarche, after which fat, as a percentage of body mass, again increases. In boys, fat mass continues to decrease and lean mass increases so that, at maturation, fat is a far greater percentage of body composition in girls than in boys.

Upper/lower body-span ratio is determined with the patient standing. The distance from the top of the head to the symphysis pubis is the upper (U), and the distance from the symphysis to the floor is the lower (L). U/L is about 1.0 immediately prepubertal, diminishes to 0.9 in early puberty as the extremities grow more rapidly, and returns to 1.0 in later puberty. Arm span is measured as the distance between the fingertips of outstretched arms and is usually equal to or only minimally greater than total height. Marked variations in the U/L or arm-span ratio may suggest endocrine-mediated growth disturbance.

## Hair (also see Chapter 9)

Body hair becomes widely distributed during adolescence. Facial, extremity, chest, axillary, and perianal hair appear under androgenic stimulation, and therefore appear more profusely in the male. Excessive growth of body hair in females is hirsutism and may be physiologic or suggestive of abnormalities related to excessive androgen or insufficient estrogen production (Cushing, polycystic ovary syndrome). Children who have blond-colored hair in early childhood tend to darken somewhat. Look for premature graying or whitening of the hair, particularly of the scalp (early sign of thyroid disease; associated with pernicious anemia, vitiligo, neurofibromatosis, Waardenburg syndrome). Early hair loss may be physiologic as in premature balding, or associated with fungal skin infection or alopecia areata.

# BIBLIOGRAPHY

Grumbach MM, Styne DM. Puberty: ontogeny, neuroendocrinology, physiology, and disorders. In: William's Textbook of Endocrinology. 10th ed. Philadelphia: WB Saunders; 2003.

Hoffmann A, Editor. Adolescent Medicine. Menlo Park (CA): Addison-Wesley; 1983.

Katzenellenbogen R. HEADSS: The "review of systems" for adolescents. Virtual Mentor. 2005;7(3).

Marshall WA, Tanner JM. Variations in the patterns of pubertal changes in boys. Arch Dis Child. 1970;45(239):13-23.

Marshall WA, Tanner JM. Variations in patterns of pubertal changes in girls. Arch Dis Child. 1969;44(235):291-303.

Sanfilippo JS, Muram D, Dewhurst J, Lee PA, Editors. Pediatric and Adolescent Gynecology. 2nd ed. Philadelphia: WB Saunders; 2001.

Wu T, Mendola P, Buck GM. Ethnic differences in the presence of secondary sex characteristics and menarche among US girls: the Third National Health and Nutrition Examination Survey, 1988-1994. Pediatrics. 2002;110(4):752-7.

# C. DEVELOPMENTAL AND BEHAVIORAL ASSESSMENT

Pediatricians play a central role in early identification of developmental and behavioral/emotional problems in children. This is part of routine well-child care. In addition, this is an important area of concern during the follow-up of children with chronic illness and physical disabilities, and high-risk newborns. The burgeoning field of developmental and behavioral assessment is not strictly within the scope of this book. Therefore, we will give an overview of the role of pediatricians in developmental assessment. The reader is referred to standard texts and monographs for details.

Developmental examinations differ in two major respects from examination of other systems. These differences are 1) assessment of functions rather than of a disease process, and 2) the need for input from other professionals to complete the assessment.

There are differences of opinion on the use of the words "assessment" and "evaluation." The Council on Children with Disabilities, in the Section on Developmental Behavioral Pediatrics of the American Academy of Pediatrics, avoids the use of the term "assessment" and recommends three stages in the process of developmental evaluation. The first is surveillance to recognize children at risk using simple interviewing and observation techniques. The second is screening in which standardized tools are used to identify and refine the recognized risks. The third stage is a detailed evaluation to identify and manage the specific developmental disorder.

Developmental surveillance is a continuous process that has to be practiced at every visit to the pediatrician's office, particularly at the well-child visits. This includes eliciting parental concerns, documenting developmental history at every visit, observing the child carefully for any clues, identifying risk factors, and maintaining an accurate record. If there is any concern on the part of the parent or the physician, a developmental screening should be performed to address the specific concern using appropriate instruments (to be described later). When the above two steps identify a child as being at risk for a developmental disorder, a full diagnostic developmental assessment must be planned. Trained professionals in several related fields will be needed to complete this process. Referral to a pediatrician trained in this field or to a center specializing in the management of children with developmental disabilities is appropriate at this stage.

Child development denotes the orderly emergence of "interdependent skills of sensory-motor, cognitive-language, and socio-emotional" functioning. Developmental assessment, therefore, should include screening for early identification of problems, definitive assessment using standardized tools, as indicated, and integration of this information with data obtained through medical history, family and social history, and physical examination. Finally, as the child is growing and developing, *sequential observation (multiple points over time) is more important than assessment at a single point in time.*

The brain grows in its size and complexity from early intrauterine life. Its structure and functions are influenced by several factors including genetic, environmental, socioeconomic, and nutritional, before and after birth. Disruptions can occur at any time at any one of the anatomic structures and at any one of the neurodevelopmental functions (motor, cognitive, emotional) with long-term consequences. Neurodevelopmental dysfunctions may manifest themselves as delays or deviations from normal development. These may in turn present themselves to the clinician as physical limitations, behavioral or emotional problems, or academic underachievement.

Every mother has some concern or other about her child's development, behavior or emotions, social skills, or academic performance. However, only a small proportion of mothers bring their psychosocial concerns to the attention of their physicians. In addition to the developmental problems, pediatricians are seeing more and more children with psychiatric problems, such as anxiety disorders, depression, substance abuse, and conduct disorders. It is, therefore, essential that pediatricians are knowledgeable in screening children in their practice for developmental and behavioral/emotional problems.

Reliable, validated screening tests are available to evaluate the various components of the neurodevelopmental functions. They may be broadly divided into Screening Tests (**Table 12C-1**) and Standardized Measurement tests (**Table 12C-2**). Many of these tools require special training in administering and scoring. Management of these children also requires special knowledge, and specialized resources. Therefore, once a problem is recognized, it is best to refer the child to a pediatrician with specialized training, knowledge, and resources to manage these children. This may be one with specialized training and certification either in behavioral and developmental pediatrics or neurodevelopmental disabilities.

Even if a general pediatrician is interested in the field, pressures of office practice do not allow sufficient time for developmental assessment. The pressure to schedule patients into time slots and

### Table 12C-1. Developmental Screening Tools

**General Screening Tools**

Battelle Developmental Inventory Screening Tool, 2nd Edition—Birth to 95 Months

Bayley Infant Neurodevelopmental Screen—3-24 Months

Child Development Inventory—18 Months to 6 Years

Denver II-Developmental Screening Test—0-6 Years

**Language and Cognitive Screening Tools**

Capute Scales—3-36 Months

Early Language Milestone Scale—0-36 Months

**Motor Screening Tools**

Early Motor Pattern Profile—6-12 Months

**Autism Screening Tools**

Checklist for Autism in Toddlers—18-24 Months

the poor reimbursement for these visits are major roadblocks even to an interested physician. Finally, some pediatricians may not feel comfortable managing these patients. Therefore, one approach is to refer all children with suspected developmental or behavioral problems to a specialist in this field.

However, parents bring their concerns to the pediatrician first. Paying attention to these concerns and identifying developmental problems will have an enormous impact on the future development of these children. This leads to better physician-parent/patient relationships, which is rewarding. It is indeed expected that every pediatrician screen every child in his or her practice for developmental and behavioral problems. Fortunately, several simple screening tools are available. They are in the form of pre-visit questionnaires the parent or the patient can complete. Trained office personnel can administer some of the tools. These have to be supplemented with a diagnostic interview and a physical assessment.

The focus of the chapter will be on taking a good developmental history and performing basic assessment using a few sample screening tests. The reader is referred to more detailed texts to learn about standardized measurement tools.

# TAKING HISTORY

Allow adequate time to complete a thorough history and perform a physical examination. There should be adequate privacy and lack of interruptions. It is best to read the answers to the pre-visit questionnaire and use them to start a discussion.

The questions should be open-ended. Allow adequate time for the parent or child to reflect and answer, even if it seems like an eternity. Listen deeply. Be attentive to verbal and nonverbal clues.

## Table 12C-2. Some Examples of Specific Tests

**Tests of General Intelligence:**
> Stanford-Binet Intelligence Scale
> Wechsler Intelligence Tests (for different age groups)

**Tests of Academic Achievement/Education:**
> Wide Range Achievement Tests
> Peabody Individual Achievement Test

**Tests of Specific Sensor, Motor, and Cognitive Function:**
> Boston Naming Test for Language
> California Verbal Learning Test for Verbal Memory
> Rey's Complex Figure Test for Nonverbal Memory
> Purdue Pegboard Test for Motor Proficiency

**Tests of Behavior/Personality**
> Achenbach Child Behavior Checklist
> Conners Parent/Teacher Ratings

Demonstrate that you are listening by your words and posture and encourage them with statements of approval.

The initial interview most often will be with one or both parents and the child. Obtain history from both parents and from the child, as a group, and separately. When appropriate, particularly with an adolescent, it is important to talk to the child without the parent. Parents are more likely to give better information on externalized behavior, whereas children are more likely to be able to explain their feelings and internal states. Generally, parents are more reliable on the sequence of events until the child is 10 years old. After that age, there is very little difference in the details of current problems. It is also important to get history from as many sources as possible. For example, history obtained

## Table 12C-3. Pre-visit Questionnaire

Child's name: _____ Date of birth:_____

Today's date:_____

Child currently lives with: _____Mother            _____Father

_____Another person (who?)_____

Do parents have any disagreements about the raising of this child?_____Yes          _____No

Does anyone else care for the child on a regular basis?          _____Relative          _____Babysitter

_____Child Care Center

Do you have concerns about this child care arrangement?          _____Yes          _____No

Are you concerned about your child with regard to any of the following issues?

| | | | |
|---|---|---|---|
| _____sleeping | _____problems at meals | _____temper tantrums | _____disobedience |
| _____vision | _____speech | _____thumb sucking | _____appetite |
| _____general development | _____shy, clinging | _____toilet trainin | _____hearing |
| _____activity level | _____gets upset too easily | _____soiling | _____wants too much attention |
| _____sad or unhappy | _____wetting the bed | _____relationship with brothers and sisters | |
| _____feelings hurt easily | _____relationships with other children | _____discipline methods | |

Have there been any important changes in your family recently?

_____child care arrangements _____new baby _____death or illness of a family member

_____marital problems, divorce or separation _____moving _____financial stresses

_____other_____

| | | |
|---|---|---|
| Do you have any other concerns about this child you wish to discuss? | _____Yes | _____No |
| Are there any problems in the family related to alcohol or other drugs? | _____Yes | _____No |
| Do you have any concerns about your child's behavior or progress at school or preschool? | _____Yes | _____No |
| Are you ever afraid you might lose control and hurt your child? | _____Yes | _____No |
| In the past week how many days have you felt depressed? | _____ | |
| In the past year have you had 2 weeks or more during which you felt sad, blue, or depressed or lost pleasure in things that you usually care about or enjoyed? | _____Yes | _____No |

*From: Perrin EC. Behavioral screening. In: Parker S and Zuckerman B, editors. Behavioral and Developmental Pediatrics. Boston: Little, Brown Co; 1995. p. 23. (Reprinted with permission from Wolters Kluwer)*

from the babysitter, school teacher, or a grandparent may be very helpful. Such outside sources may be contacted only with the permission of the family and also from the child, if he or she is over the age of 16 years.

Start the interview with proper introductions, a statement about source of referral, reasons for the consult, and about confidentiality issues. It is best to clarify everyone's expectations at this time. The interview may be structured, semi-structured, or based on a specialized questionnaire. At the end of the visit, summarize the main findings in a way the family and the child can understand and suggest a plan of action. This is a good time to emphasize the strengths and the positives and also allow time for questions by the parents and the child.

In addition to a detailed history of the present concerns, obtain a thorough medical history, past medical history, family history, socioeconomic history, prenatal history (illness, medications, trauma, alcohol, exposure to radiation and chemicals), and perinatal history (nature of delivery, gestational age, birth weight, Apgar score, and neonatal illness). More detailed history includes information about the family unit and how it functions, family stability and domestic violence, if any, mental health of household members, school performance, and friends. There are two samples of questions in **Tables 12C-3** and **12C-4**. The first can be used as a pre-visit questionnaire and the second as a guide for a semi-structured interview.

Questions such as "Please tell me your concerns about your daughter's sleep habits" or "tell me what you heard about your son's behavior in school, which worried you" or "about his school work that is of concern you" or "what are the new things your child can do since the last visit?" are open ended and should help start the conversation. Another way to start is to read the answers to the pre-visit questionnaire and ask questions about the concerns raised by the parent or the child. An example of this questionnaire is the Pediatric Symptoms Checklist (**Table 12C-5**). This is a 35-item list that the parent can complete while waiting or before the visit. Each item is scored with a 2 for "often," 1 for "sometimes," and a 0 for "never." A score of 28 or more suggests a possible dysfunction and the need for an indepth assessment and a referral.

Doctor Henry Cecil suggests the following outline for organization of an emotional and behavioral history:

1. Child's assets and liabilities based on:
   a. Primary reaction pattern (see the next paragraph)
   b. Secondary (adaptive) reaction pattern (in older children)
   c. Level of sensory motor integration
   d. Physical status, physiologic function, and health condition
   e. Social responsiveness--in older children, history of relationship with siblings, peers, and adults; progress toward self-care and reaction to discipline
   f. Nature and degree of disordered functioning or developmental deviations
2. Family assets and liabilities based on:
   a. Past history of rearing this child. Start with history of pregnancy including details such as whether this was a wanted child, whether there was stress during pregnancy, etc.
   b. Current state of child-rearing behavior with this child (continued on page 340)

### Table 12C-4. Psychological Questions for Use in Clinical Pediatric Office Practice*

**FAMILY**

1. Who is in your family and who lives with you in your home?

**Household Stability**

2. How many times has your family moved?

3. Have there been any changes in your family lifestyle since the last time we met?

4. How are you and your child coping with this change?

**Marital Conflict and Divorce**

5. Are you and your spouse able to work together with your child?

6. How do you handle disagreements in raising your children between yourselves?

7. When things get out of hand, how far do they go?

**Crisis**

8. Has your family ever been through a major crisis?

9. How did you deal with that crisis?

**Parental Mental Health**

10. Have you or any of the members of your family ever suffered from a mental illness or substance abuse problem?

11. Are you aware of any effects that this problem may have had on your child or his or her care?

**SCHOOL**

12. How does your child like school and his or her teachers?

    *How do you like school and your teachers?*

13. How did your child do in first grade?

**Academic Achievement**

14. What grades does your child get on his or her report card?

    *What grades did you get on your report card?*

15. Has your child ever stayed back a grade?

16. Has your child ever been in special education classes?

**School Attendance**

17. Have you ever had difficulty getting your child to go to preschool or school?

18. Has your child ever missed more than 10 days of school in 1 year? What was the reason?

19. Has your child ever cut school? How often?

    *Have you ever cut school? How often?*

**PEER RELATIONSHIPS**

20. How does your child get along with peers?

**Friends**

21. Does your child have a best friend? (In adolescence, a group of good friends?)

    *Do you have a best friend?*

**Bullies and Victims**

22. Does your child seem to enjoy picking on, bothering, or bullying weaker children?

    *Did you ever like to pick on or bother another kid?*

23. Does your child always seem to get picked on?

*Are you a kid who always gets picked on?*

## ACTIVITY

24. What does your child like to do?

*What do you like to do?*

25. Is there something your child is really good at doing?

*Is there something you are really good at doing?*

## EMOTIONAL HEALTH

26. What emotions do you see in your child these days?

*Everyone feels sad or angry at times. How about you?*

27. Has your child suffered the loss of someone important to him or her?

28. Has your child ever been treated for an emotional problem?

## MISCELLANEOUS TOPICS

### Poverty

29. Have you ever been on welfare or been unable to financially support your family?

### Injury

30. Has your child ever had to go to the emergency room for treatment of an injury? How many times?

### Substance Abuse

31. Do you ever drink alcohol? If yes, then:

   C  Have you ever felt the need to cut down on your drinking?

   A  Have people ever annoyed you by criticism of your drinking?

   G  Have you ever felt guilty about your drinking?

   E  Have you ever taken a morning eye opener to steady your nerves or get rid of a hangover?

32. Do you think your child is drinking alcohol or using drugs?

*Have you ever tasted beer, wine, or alcohol?*

*How old were you when you began to drink alcohol?*

### Risk-taking Behavior

33. Is there anything that your adolescent is doing or has done to him- or herself that has you really concerned?

### Suicide

34. Has your teenager ever tried to intentionally hurt him- or herself?

*Did you ever feel so upset that you wished you were not alive or that you wanted to die?*

*Did you ever do something that you knew was so dangerous that you could have gotten hurt or killed?*

*Did you ever intentionally try to kill yourself?*

---

*Questions in regular type are questions for parents. Questions in italics are questions for children. **Reprinted with permission from: Hack S and Jellinek MS. Historical clues to the diagnosis of the dysfunctional child and other psychiatric disorders in children. Pediatr Clin North Am. 1998;45(1):25-48. (Copyright: Elsevier 1998)***

    c. Mother's (father's) sources of support

    d. Mother's life situation apart from child rearing

    e. Mother's and father's experience in being reared

Many of these items are self-explanatory. Understanding of the primary reaction pattern (item la) of a child and his or her adaptive response (secondary pattern) is an important subject that all pediatricians should master and deserves further explanation. This will be of great use in counseling mothers during routine office visits.

Most mothers know instinctively that babies differ in their style and quality of response to environmental stimuli. There are intrinsic patterns of behavior for each child, and it is the interaction of these with the characteristics and behavior of the caretaker that determines child-rearing practices and outcome. Dr. Stella Chess (1959) organized these predictable patterns of behavior of children in nine categories. These patterns are: 1) Activity/Passivity: Some children are by nature very active; others are quiet and do not move around that much. One can ask the mother how active the baby is when she tries to bathe the baby or change a diaper and get an idea of behavior in this area. 2) Regular/Irregular: Some babies wake regularly every morning and ask for their food at about the same time. Others are very irregular. Questions to elicit information on sleep-wake cycles, hunger frequency, regularity in urination and bowel movement will give answers to understand this aspect of a child's behavior. 3) Approach/Withdrawal is shown by the initial reaction to a new stimulus. Does a child approach new people, new toys, and new food quickly or is it usually a negative or cautious approach the first time? 4) Adaptive/Nonadaptive: The ability of the child to relate to a new situation after the initial contact may be adaptive or not. Some children may be nervous the first time they see a new person or taste a new food. But they quickly relate to the situation on repeated contacts. Others take a few days or weeks to adjust to a new stimulus even if it is presented many times in a predictable fashion. 5) Low threshold/High threshold: The threshold describes the intensity level of stimulation necessary to evoke a discernable response (auditory, visual, cutaneous sensory stimuli). One of the simplest ways of learning the threshold level of the baby is to find out how soon after wetting the diaper does he or she cry to be changed. Some babies will scream as soon as they wet the diaper. Others will stay in wet diapers for a long time without a whimper and get diaper rash if the mother is not sensitive to the subtle clues given by the child. This is a good example for how parental behavior can be affected by the child's threshold for stimuli. 6) Intense/Mild: The energy content of the response may vary in degree. Some babies are mild in their response to various stimuli. Some are intense and let you know without doubt. Questions on how intensely a baby responded to a new food, a wet diaper, or a new face will give clues to this aspect of behavior. 7) Positive/Negative: Some babies are smiling all the time and friendly. Others cry more often and are unfriendly. Everybody wants to carry a smiling baby, and therefore a happy infant gets many opportunities for socialization. The crying, unfriendly baby is often left alone and lacks socialization. A quiet, high-threshold, unfriendly baby is likely to be a neglected child, particularly if the mother is not a sensitive person. An active, low-threshold, intense baby is likely to be abused. The importance of taking a history of these aspects of behavior is obvious when evaluating children with emotional problems who fail to thrive, who have poor maternal-child bonding, and who are subject to child abuse. 8) Attention Span/Persistence: The attention span measures the difficulty with which an

## Table 12C-5. The Pediatric Symptom Checklist

|  | Never | Sometimes | Often |
|---|---|---|---|
| 1. Complains of aches or pains | | | |
| 2. Spends more time alone | | | |
| 3. Tires easily, little energy | | | |
| 4. Fidgety, unable to sit still | | | |
| 5. Has trouble with a teacher | | | |
| 6. Less interested in school | | | |
| 7. Acts as if driven by a motor | | | |
| 8. Daydreams too much | | | |
| 9. Distracted easily | | | |
| 10. Is afraid of new situations | | | |
| 11. Feels sad, unhappy | | | |
| 12. Is irritable, angry | | | |
| 13. Feels hopeless | | | |
| 14. Has trouble concentrating | | | |
| 15. Less interest in friends | | | |
| 16. Fights with other children | | | |
| 17. Absent from school | | | |
| 18. School grades dropping | | | |
| 19. Is down on him- or herself | | | |
| 20. Visits doctor with doctor finding nothing wrong | | | |
| 21. Has trouble sleeping | | | |
| 22. Worries a lot | | | |
| 23. Wants to be with you more than before | | | |
| 24. Feels he or she is bad | | | |
| 25. Takes unnecessary risks | | | |
| 26. Gets hurt frequently | | | |
| 27. Seems to be having less fun | | | |
| 28. Acts younger than children his or her age | | | |
| 29. Does not listen to rules | | | |
| 30. Does not show feelings | | | |
| 31. Does not understand other people's feelings | | | |
| 32. Teases others | | | |
| 33. Blames others for his or her troubles | | | |
| 34. Takes things that do not belong to him or her | | | |
| 35. Refuses to share | | | |

*Reprinted with permission from: Hack S and Jellinek MS. Historical clues to the diagnosis of the dysfunctional child and other psychiatric disorders in children. Pediatr Clin North Am. 1998; 45(1):25-48. (Copyright Elsevier 1998)*

*Denver II is not a diagnostic test.* It is not an intelligence test either. Doctor Frankenburg who developed this instrument suggests that this be used as a "growth chart of development", and not as a test. It is a screening procedure a pediatrician can use to assess whether an individual child is in the normal range for developmental milestones. Denver II documents the age at which children accomplish several common tasks in gross motor, fine motor-adaptive, language, and personal-social development. In addition, Denver II provides a checklist for noting specific behaviors such as attention span, interest in surroundings, fearfulness, and ability to respond to instructions. A screening manual has been developed to provide details on the proper administration of the test. A technical manual gives details on normative values and standardization techniques. Interested readers should refer to these two manuals for details.

### Table 12 C-7: Diagnostic criteria for Attention- Deficit/Hyperactivity Disorder (DSM IV-Text Revision, 2000)

**Attention- Deficit/Hyperactivity Disorder (ADHD) is characterized by "a persistent pattern of inattention and/or hyperactivity-impulsivity that is more frequently displayed and more severe than is typically observed in individuals at a comparable level of development"**

A. Either (1) or (2):

(1) six (or more) of the following symptoms of inattention have persisted for at least 6 months to a degree that is maladaptive and inconsistent with develop mental level: *Inattention*

   a. often fails to give close attention to details or makes careless mistakes in schoolwork, work, or other activities

   b. often has difficulty sustaining attention in tasks or play activities

   c. often does not seem to listen when spoken to directly

   d. often does not follow through on instructions and fails to finish schoolwork, chores, or duties in the workplace (not due to oppositional behavior or failure to understand instructions)

   e. often has difficulty organizing tasks and activities

   f. often avoids, dislikes, or is reluctant to engage in tasks that require sustained mental effort (such as schoolwork or homework)

   g. often loses things necessary for tasks or activities (e.g., toys, school assignments, pencils, books, or tools)

   h. is often easily distracted by extraneous stimuli

   i. is often forgetful in daily activities

(2) six (or more) of the following symptoms of hyperactivity-impulsivity have persisted for at least 6 months to a degree that is maladaptive and inconsistent with developmental level: *Hyperactivity*

   a. often fidgets with hands or feet or squirms in seat

   b. often leaves seat in classroom or in other situations in which remaining seated is expected

   c. often runs about or climbs excessively in situations in which it is inappropriate (in adolescents or adults, may be limited to subjective feelings of restlessness)

   d. often has difficulty playing or engaging in leisure activities quietly

If more detailed evaluation is indicated based on the screening, it is best to refer the child to a specialist in behavioral and developmental pediatrics, a neurodevelopmental disabilities specialist who can evaluate and manage the problem, or to a pediatric psychologist for detailed testing.

A sample of the specialized assessment tools are given in **Table 12C-2**.

## SCREENING FOR PSYCHIATRIC PROBLEMS

Some of the details of interviewing have been outlined earlier. Questions listed in **Tables 12C-3** and **12C-4** should help start a discussion with the parent and the child. During history taking, obtain information on the following topics: the reason why the child was brought to see the physician; details on general health, previous consultations, and treatments; any medications the child is taking; daily history of activities; details of performance in school; recreational interests; peer relationships; family

---

    e.  is often "on the go" or often acts as if "driven by a motor"

    f.  often talks excessively, *impulsivity*

    g.  often blurts out answers before questions have been completed

    h.  often has difficulty awaiting turn

    i.  often interrupts or intrudes on others (e.g., butts into conversations or games)

B.  Some hyperactive-impulsive or inattentive symptoms that caused impairment were present before age 7 years.

C.  Some impairment from the symptoms is present in two or more settings (e.g., at school [or work] and at home).

D.  There must be clear evidence of clinically significant impairment in social, academic, or occupational functioning.

E.  The symptoms do not occur exclusively during the course of a Pervasive Developmental Disorder, Schizophrenia, or other Psychotic Disorder and are not better accounted for by another mental disorder (e.g., Mood Disorder, Anxiety Disorder, Dissociative Disorder, or a Personality Disorder).

Based on the above mentioned criteria, three different subtypes may be diagnosed:

*Attention-Deficit/Hyperactivity Disorder, Combined Type: if both Criteria A1 and A2 are met for the past 6 months*

*Attention-Deficit/Hyperactivity Disorder, Predominantly Inattentive Type: if Criterion A1 is met but Criterion A2 is not met for the past 6 months*

*Attention-Deficit/Hyperactivity Disorder, Predominantly Hyperactive-Impulsive Type: if Criterion A2 is met but Criterion A1 is not met for the past 6 months*

For individuals (especially adolescents and adults) who currently have symptoms that no longer meet full criteria, "In Partial Remission" should be specified.

---

relationships; and the child's fears and anxieties. It is also important to know what the ethnic and cultural background of the family is, how intact the family is, whether there are other members of the family with mental illness, and what support structures (for emotional, physical, financial, and spiritual) are available for the family.

Other aspects of history that will help in referral and management are how the behavior affects function at home, at school, and with peers; the burden of suffering experienced by the child and the family members; additional risk factors; and strength and protective factors.

Some questionnaires that can expedite screening for psychological/psychiatric problems and initiate an interview include the Achenbach Child Behavior Checklist, and Conners Teacher and Parent report forms. If the pediatrician suspects depression or anxiety disorders, it is essential to interview the child directly. The child also may be asked to complete a Child Depression Inventory (seven to 16 years) or Revised Children's Manifest Anxiety Scale (six to 18 years) as appropriate. In addition to recognizing the presence of a psychiatric disorder, the physician has to rate the severity. Traditional classification of severity as recommended by the DSM-IV is given in **Table 12C-6**.

Mental health assessment includes a mental status examination as observed by the parent and the physician and based on an indepth interview. Write down observations in simple terms and without interpretation. The pediatrician can observe and document the mental status under the following headings: physical appearance, motor behavior, speech, social interactions, affect, and use of language and thinking process. An indepth interview requires the expertise of a mental health professional, who can collect data on feeling states, symbolic representation, fantasies, self-concept, moral judgment, and levels of adaptation.

## Specific Disorders

### Attention Deficit/Hyperactivity Disorder (ADHD)

ADHD is one of the most common developmental disorders in school-age children. The characteristic features are easy distractibility and difficulty in sustaining attention, impulsive behavior, and motor restlessness. There are three subtypes, one with predominantly inattention, one with predominantly hyperactivity and poor impulse control, and one mixed variety. Most of the children are referred because of hyperactivity in the younger age groups and for problems in the school, academic achievement, poor peer relationships, and self-esteem. Children with ADHD also should be evaluated for comorbid conditions such as conduct and anxiety disorders.

**Table 12C-7** gives an outline of the DSM-IV diagnostic criteria for ADHD. A diagnosis of this condition should be made based on the history, clinical interview, physical examination, observation in more than one setting, behavior rating scale (e.g., Conner scale), and neuropsychological testing (e.g., IQ, Educational Achievement Test). It is also important to note that the European diagnostic criteria for hyperkinetic disorder (HKD), as defined by the International Classification of Diseases (10th edition; ICD-10), is slightly different from the DSM-IV criteria. Although both sets take into account developmentally inappropriate levels of inattention, hyperactivity, and impulsivity and both require observations in more than one setting, the European criteria for HKD criteria are more restrictive. It requires atleast 6 of 8 inattentive symptoms, atleast 3 of 5 hyperactive symptoms and atleast 1 of 4 impulsive symptoms.

## *Depression*

Depression is under-recognized in childhood and adolescence. Children with a family history of depression, chronic medical conditions, physical disability, and cosmetic problems are particularly prone to depression. Feeling depressed after a major crisis in the family or after the diagnosis of a serious illness is not unusual (reactive response). This section deals with serious depression interfering with normal function.

Major depression is defined as "persistent depressed or irritable mood present for most of the day, every day for two weeks or more with a significant effect on functioning."

Answers to some of the items in the pre-visit questionnaire (Pediatric Symptom Checklist, CBCL, Adolescent Questionnaire) may give clues and these should be followed through with deeper questioning and a personal interview. The core symptoms of depression are similar in children and adults, except for variations in the expression depending on the developmental stage of the child. For example, failure to thrive may be the manifestation in infancy, academic failure in school age children, and risk-taking behavior or attempted suicide in the adolescent age group. Somatic complaints such as headache, abdominal pain, and fatigue may predominate in some children.

The pediatrician should be able to suspect the problem based on the history and clinical interview. One of the self-reported rating scales (CDI) may be very helpful. In addition, the pediatrician should be able to assess the severity and refer to a mental health professional for further management.

# BIBLIOGRAPHY

Behrman RE, Kleigman RM, Jenson HB, editors. Textbook of Pediatrics. 18th ed. Philadelphia: WB Saunders; 2007.

Cassidy LJ, Jellinek MS. Approaches to the recognition and management of childhood psychiatric disorders in pediatric primary care. Pediatr Clin N Am. 1998;45(5):1037-52.

Council on children with Disabilities; Section on Developmental Behavioral Pediatrics; Bright Futures Steering Committee; Medical Home Initiatives for Children with Special Needs Project Advisory Committee. Identifying infants and young children with developmental disorders in the medical home: an algorithm for developmental surveillance and screening. Pediatrics. 2006;118(1): 405-20.

Dixon SD, Stein MT. Encounters with Children: Pediatric Behavior and Development. 4th ed. Philadelphia: Mosby; 2006.

Frankenberg WK, Dodds J, Archer P. Denver II Screening Manual Denver, CO. Denver, CO: Denver Developmental Materials Inc; 1990.

Frankenberg WK, Dodds J, Archer P. Denver II Technical Manual. Denver CO: Denver Developmental Materials Inc; 1990.

Frankenberg WK, Dodds J, Archer P, Shapiro H, Bresnick B. The Denver II: a major revision and restandardization of the Denver Developmental Screening Test. Pediatrics. 1992;89(1): 91-7.

Hack S, Jellinek MS. Historical clues to the diagnosis of the dysfunctional child and other psychiatric disorders in children. Pediatr Clin N Am. 1998;45(1):25-48.

Hoekelman RA, Friedman SB, Nelson NM, Seidel HM, Weitzman ML, editors. Primary Pediatric Care. 3rd ed. St. Louis: Mosby; 1997.

Knobloch H, Pasamanick B. Gesell and Amatruda's Developmental Diagnosis; the Evaluation and Management of Normal and Abnormal Neuropsychologic Development in Infancy and Early Childhood. 3rd ed. Hagerstown (Md): Harper & Row; 1974.

Levine MD, Carey WB, Crocker AC, Gross RT, editors. Developmental Behavioral Pediatrics. 1st ed. Philadelphia: WB Saunders; 1983.

Perrin EC. Behavioral screening. In: The Fundamentals of Behavioral and Developmental Pediatrics. Parker S, Zuckerman B, editors. Boston: Little, Brown Co; 1995. pp. 22-9.

Reiff MI, Tippins S. ADHD: A Complete and Authoritative Guide. Elk Grove Village (Il): American Academy of Pediatrics; 2004.

Simmons JE. Psychiatric Examination of Children. 1st ed. Philadelphia: Lea & Febiger; 1969.

Wiener JM, Dulcan MK. Textbook of Child and Adolescent Psychiatry. 3rd ed. Washington DC: American Psychiatry Publishing; 2004.

# D. PHYSICAL AND SEXUAL ABUSE

A lack of suitable history to explain physical findings of trauma always makes one suspicious of possible physical abuse. In this section, sexual abuse is included together with physical abuse. Both single episode and repetitive abuses are included as well.

A thorough history obtained in a nonthreatening and nonaccusative manner is the first step. This should be well-documented. Describe the attitude, mental status, and the mannerism of the informant objectively and without judgments and opinions. Photographic documentation is essential, particularly in sexual abuse. A good diagram describing the characteristics of the lesions also may be acceptable. State laws have to be adhered to in documenting and reporting.

Document the details of exact circumstances of the injury and sequence of events such as when the symptoms or signs were noted, any preceding event such as bathing, and evolution of symptoms. It is important to obtain history about the caretakers present at the time of the injury and the presence or absence of any witnesses. History of parental or family dysfunction, such as drug abuse and alcoholism, and of spousal violence may be relevant. Parental attitudes to child rearing and availability of support system are also of importance.

It is prudent to suspect abuse as the cause of the injury under the following conditions: 1) there is no explanation or it is vague, 2) an important detail of the history is changed dramatically, 3) the explanation is inconsistent with the pattern and severity of the injury, 4) the explanation is inconsistent with the developmental and physical capabilities of the child, and 5) different witnesses provide different explanations.

The examination has to be conducted in a nonthreatening manner with special attention to the child's alertness and demeanor with careful assessment of the central nervous system, musculoskeletal system including the cervical spine, the skin, and the genitalia.

Clues to physical and sexual abuse on physical examination may be grouped under the following systems:

- Skin
- Skeletal
- Blunt abdominal injury
- Head injury
- Sexual abuse and genital organs

# INTERNET RESOURCES TO LEARN CLINICAL SKILLS

*(All accessed January 30, 2010)*

http://www.etu.sgul.ac.uk/cso (St George's University of London)
http://www.martindalecenter.com/MedicalClinical_Exams.html
http://opeta.medinfo.ufl.edu/pediatric (University of Florida)
http://www.dermnet.com
http://phil.cdc.gov/phil
http://www.entusa.com (ENT site)
http://meded.ucsd.edu/clinicalmed/ (University of California at San Diego)
http://www.sgim.org/index.cfm?pageId=588
http://www.arc.org.uk/arthinfo/medpubs/6535/6535.asp (pediatric GALS)
http://www.e-meducation.org
www.skillscascade.com (Calgary-Cambridge Guide)

# INDEX